GROUP
HYPNOTHERAPY
AND
HYPNODRAMA

GROUP HYPNOTHERAPY AND HYPNODRAMA

Ira A. Greenberg, Ph.D., *editor*

Behavioral Studies Institute and
Group Hypnosis Center for Los Angeles

Carmarillo (Calif.) State Hospital

California School of Professional Psychology

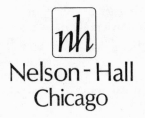

Nelson-Hall
Chicago

Library of Congress Cataloging in Publication Data

Main entry under title:

Group hypnotherapy and hypnodrama.

    Bibliography: p.
    Includes index.
    1. Hypnotism—Therapeutic use. 2. Group psycho-
therapy. 3. Psychodrama. I. Greenberg, Ira A., 1924-
RC497.G76   616.8'916'2   76-17012
ISBN 0-88229-256-0

Manufactured in the United States of America

To J. L. Moreno, M.D., (1890-1974),
an esteemed psychiatrist, psychodramatist, and sociometrist,
and a creator of hypnotic presence who gave much to mankind
and from whom many gained from his multitude of gifts.

Contents

Acknowledgments

I wish to express my appreciation to the following friends and colleagues for their critical readings of sections of this volume and for their good advice: Phillip H. Taylor, M.D., psychiatrist and nutritional therapist, Thousand Oaks, Ca.; Jacquelyn McCandless, M.D., psychiatrist, Sherman Oaks, Ca.; John Koehne, growth center operator, Elk, Ca.; Kim Blau Hufman, Ph.D., social and clinical psychologist, Camarillo, Ca., State Hospital; Mona Hodge, school teacher, Glendale, Ca.; Tom Drucker, M.A., psychologist and manager of management development, Xerox Corporation, worldwide, Westport, Conn.; Ann Dreyfuss, management consultant, San Francisco, Ca.; Gilda Martin del Campo, group facilitator and teacher, Los Angeles, and Lester R. D'Andrea, Ph.D., clinical psychologist and management consultant, Los Angeles. Also, my thanks to Linda Gordon Ramacher, M.S., Public Health researcher, UCLA, for help in correcting page proofs.

Preface: Expectations and Results

In May of 1969 I attended a four-day basic course in hypnotherapy that the American Society of Clinical Hypnosis presented in Los Angeles, and following this I began doing group hypnotherapy with patients at Camarillo State Hospital, where I had then been employed for about a year and a half. My thinking was that psychotic patients might interact better among themselves and with me while they were in the hypnotic state than they had in previous group therapy sessions. This hypothesis was not supported during my early days as a group hypnotherapist, and some six years later I am still not getting much more interaction among hypnotized schizophrenics than had been the case earlier or than I had been getting with these same patients during group sessions where they were not under hypnosis. However, during the years following my initial group hypnotherapy sessions, I no longer sought the interactions among patients. I simply found myself doing individual hypnotherapy in a group setting of from four to ten patients per session.

Another thing I had hoped for when I began my group hypnotherapy sessions was that somehow, by means of the hypnotic intervention, I would be able "to get beneath the schizophrenia," to use the words that went through my head at that time, "and get in touch with the rational part of the mind of the schizophrenic" that I presumed to be there. I saw the schizophrenia in terms of the environmental factor, and with one patient in particular, a thirty-year-old former intellectual who had been first hospitalized in 1959, I sought to use hypnosis to help him get "beneath and beyond" the psychosis, to help him regress to the period in his life when he had functioned fairly effectively and then to get at the possible traumas involved in his withdrawal. This occurred to some degree, and the patient, while in the group setting, reported some traumatic experiences that had occurred when he was fifteen and seventeen, but he was unable to experience his feelings about these events, and quickly covered them up again with strings of word-salad, his loose associations, and his lack of points of reference that had been for the previous ten years a normal part of his speech.

Nevertheless, in spite of these failures with many psychotics, I still found the group hypnotherapy sessions useful, especially with many of the non-psychotic patients who participated or with psychotic patients in fair to good states of remission. Those who had interacted to some degree in my nonhypnotic groups did about the same when called upon under hypnosis, though often their involvement was more lethargic than otherwise, which is typical of the hypnotic state. Those who had not interacted well in the waking state were about the same under hypnosis, although many would get in touch with feelings and traumas and when called upon would be able to express themselves very loudly and forcefully in terms of the emotions they were experiencing while hypnotized. But the wonderful things I had hoped for when I first began group hypnotherapy were not taking place, so then I systematically began seeking some answers to my problem.

I began a serious survey of the literature on group hypnotherapy to add to what I had previously read on the subject and in so doing managed to gather and read all of the already published material that is included in this book. I also had read the material that Dr. Irvin H. Perline of Mesa Community College's Psychology Department, Mesa, Arizona, had reported on in the journal article that is now Chapter 5 of this volume. My immediate reaction to reading the material was to regret that this valuable information was buried in various scientific and professional journals, as well as in some popular publications, and that putting this material together in book form might prove a useful contribution to the fields of hynotherapy and group psychotherapy. This I proceeded to do, and the present volume, containing as it does an additional dozen original chapters, is the result.

Part I

INTRODUCTION:
Background and Contents

1
Group Process and Hypnosis

Ira A. Greenberg

Group hypnotherapy, considered by many to be a modern psychotherapeutic modality, traces its beginnings at least as far back as classical antiquity and most certainly as far back as the eighteenth century when in 1775 the Austrian physician Franz Anton Mesmer (1733-1815) first demonstrated in Vienna his newly discovered technique. Just as the priests of Aesculapius, the Greco-Roman god of medicine, said their soothing words into the ears of patients lying in sleeplike states in the healing temples, so the modern therapist offers his positive suggestions and supportive statements to patients sitting or lying about in the group hypnotherapy room. At other times the modern group hypnotherapist might lead his hypnotized patients on a guided fantasy trip, or have them seek to uncover repressed material, or verbally interact with each other in the state of highly focused attention.

Nevertheless, group hypnotherapy, which Lewis R. Wolberg, M.D., described in his earliest important work, *Medical Hypnosis, Vol. I, Hypnoanalysis* (1948), from which Chapter 2 of this book is taken, is only in recent years beginning to gain attention in the comparatively small community of medical, dental, and psychological hypnotherapists, and the paucity of literature in the learned journals is regrettable. The group approach to hypnotherapy developed for two reasons: to enable the therapist to treat more people and to enable participants to learn from each other in their involvements during the group hypno-

therapy process. And this interaction presumably may also have occurred during the beginnings of hynosis as we know it today. Exploring
the matter, psychiatrist Jules H. Masserman, M.D., states as follows:

> Of course, Mesmer was quite sincere in his theories and felt
> himself martyred by the medical men of the day, who, along
> with Benjamin Franklin, had called him a quack. Indeed, he
> died convinced that he had discovered a universal System of
> Healing—and so he had in the sense that he had once again
> tapped a basic human yearning for encounter and relationship.
> Not "animal magnetism" (later called hypnotism) but the kind
> of communication that had been practical in the temples of
> Egypt. There, too, in a setting of diminished light, with a
> central altar upon which everybody was concentrated, the priest
> had intoned a repetitious, monotonous, rhythmic lullaby
> known to all mothers of troubled children who need reassurance
> and rest in a trusting security. Intuitively, when we are
> approached by troubled people, we still talk in this kind of
> soothing, monotonous, cadenced tone of voice. Predictably
> also, Mesmer's practice grew to such proportions that he
> couldn't give individual attention to every patient; thus, he
> began to deal with them in groups. Mesmer's patients would
> form a circle, hold hands, feel overpowered by the "magne-
> tism," fall into trances, have an intensive "corrective emotional
> experience" and leave praising the system and spreading the
> Mesmeric gospel. (1965)

Mesmer's concept of animal magnetism first appeared in part in his
doctoral dissertation, *The Planetorium Flux*, published in 1776, which
dealt with his belief of planetary influence on human bodies, and stated
that disease resulted when bodies failed to receive adequate vibrations of
this fluid. The human body was in harmony with the celestial bodies
when the fluid was appropriately and evenly distributed, and this body
became diseased when the distribution became disrupted. Following
completion of his medical studies, Mesmer developed his theory to the
point where he held that the human body was a magnet with poles at
either end connected by a "magnetic fluid," which eventually became
known as animal magnetism. Myron Teitelbaum, L.L.B., discusses
Mesmer's group hypnotherapeutic approach in his excellent book, *Hypnosis Induction Technic* [sic] as follows:

> Mesmer had considerable success in Vienna, but his critics
> forced him to leave. He took up residence in Paris, where
> patients streamed to him for cures. In order to accommodate the

patients Mesmer invented a special kind of magnet. In a large darkened room he built an oversized oak tub. In it he placed concentrically arranged bottles, ground glass and iron filings covered by water. This tub or "baquet" had many iron rods extending through the sides. A large number of patients stood or sat around the tub grasping the iron rods to absorb the magnetic fluid which they believed emanated therefrom. This was the development of the first modern method of hypnotics: the instilling within the subject the belief that approximation to a magnet would cure disease, which cure was normally preceded by convulsions. The phenomenon of the convulsions was usually suggested either directly or indirectly. The *magnetic method* was a virile one and took a long time to fall into disuse. Technics divised for its induction are legend. (1965, p. 4.)

The really modern contribution, so far as group hypnotherapy is concerned, is hypnodrama, which was invented both prior to and immediately after World War II, by the late J.L. Moreno, M.D., the psychiatrist who created psychodrama and other treatment methods, and by his student and associate James M. Enneis, M.S., a psychologist and former army lieutenant who had learned hypnotherapy in a military psychiatric setting. Just as in psychodrama, where the patient or protagonist explores a problem through action on a stage and under the guidance of a psychodrama director and uses others in the group to portray important people in his life, so in hypnodrama, the movement and emotional interaction on the stage bring forth catharsis and often immediate insight by the protagonist and by many other participants. Whether the hypnodrama employed is that in which only the protagonist is under hypnosis, as developed by Moreno and Enneis, or in which many other participants are hypnotized along with the protagonist, as was developed later, it remains a group process and belongs in a volume such as this. Hypnodrama actually belongs to two camps, namely, that of psychodrama, of which it is an offshoot, and that of group hypnotherapy, of which it can be considered one of several important divisions or categories. More than most forms of group hypnotherapy, hypnodrama calls for strong emotional bonds between and among participants, but it is not the only form of hypnotic treatment that brings this about.

As William S. Kroger, M.D., sees it, "Mass suggestion or mass hypnosis is relatively easy to establish in a group [and] the reasons for this are: There is an 'emotional contagion' that takes place with other members of the group; persons identify with what they see, [and] the inherent competitiveness is mobilized, and there is usually an intense desire to please the leader (father-figure) of the group." (1963, p. 89)

Kroger, a gynecologist, has used hypnosis to prepare large groups for prenatal training (1963, chapter 33), and found that "invariably, one third of those who are observing the volunteers being hypnotized will be hypnotized in varying degrees themselves [and] they will dehypnotize themselves when the signal is given." (1963, p. 92) Part of what may be contained in the "contagion" that Kroger speaks of may involve the sense of security that individuals get from each other when entering a new experience, especially one like hypnosis, which many people have—through motion picture films, television, and lurid magazine stories and reports—been conditioned to view with apprehension. There is safety in numbers, according to the old saying, and many individuals initially are able to experience this sense of safety in the group rather than in the individual hypnosis session. The many advantages to be found in group hypnotherapy are dealt with throughout this book, while the principal advantages of the individual hypnotherapy experience are obvious—the close attention given by and involvement with the therapist—and so need not be discussed in detail in this volume. The book, as of this time and to the best knowledge of this writer, is the only one of its kind; whereas, the books dealing with individual hypnotherapy must number in the hundreds or even in the thousands.

As to the contents of this collection, they have been organized so that if read from beginning to end the chapters will present the subjects of group hypnotherapy and hypnodrama in what is hoped to be an orderly, interesting, and enlightening manner. However, the book also may be easily read on the basis of specific areas of the reader's interests or on the basis of specific chapters in the order of the reader's choosing, since, as with any anthology, it may easily and appropriately be read or organized in many different ways. *Group Hypnotherapy and Hypnodrama* consists of seven parts or sections, with the first and last sections containing introductory and concluding material. Part I, to be more specific, consists of four brief chapters, besides this one, that deal with group hypnotherapy. The first of these presents group hypnotherapy as seen by Wolberg during the immediate post-World War II period. In this chapter he seems to have approached the matter with some sense of the importance of the prestige factor in that he saw the group establishing itself about a leader who holds himself out to be an "omniscient personage." (1948, p. 184) This is followed by two chapters describing how group hypnotherapy is practiced by William T. Reardon, M.D., with Chapter 3 being a newspaper magazine report of this psychiatrist's work, while Chapter 4 is one in which Reardon presents some of his conceptualizations along with a description of his work.

In the final chapter of Part I, "Group Hypnotherapy: a Brief

Survey," Irvin H. Perline, Ph.D., does just that, he presents a survey of the literature on group hypnotherapy up to the late 1960s. It begins with a brief review of work by the British psychiatrist Geoffrey R. Peberdy, M.D., D.P.M., of Newcastle-upon-Tyne General Hospital in northern England, who found that patients in group hypnotherapy made therapeutic gains despite an observed lack of spontaneous abreaction among group members. This is followed by a description of the work with alcoholics of R.S. Wallerstein, M.D., and by reviews of reports on the effectiveness of group hypnotherapy on weight control by F.S. Glover, M.D., by Leo Wollman, M.D., and by Herbert Mann, M.D. Perline concludes the chapter with a report on the work of J. Ilovsky, M.D., who had employed group hypnosis for the effective treatment of schizophrenics at Central Islip State Hospital in New York. Earlier in the chapter, Perline reviews works on hypnodrama by Moreno, by Enneis, and by Leonard K. Supple, M.D., all of which appear in Part IV of this book. Also in Part IV is the chapter, "Training the Unconscious by Hypnodramatic Re-Enactment of Dreams," by Rolf Krojanker, M.D., Ph.D., which is a further report on the hypnodramatic achievements of Dr. Moreno.

Part II, "Theory and Techniques: General and Specific," begins with the chapter, "The Systematic Use of Hypnosis in Individual and Group Psychotherapy," by Jack Fox, Ph.D., chief psychologist at Patton State Hospital, near San Bernadino, Calif., who presents in brief form some of the history of hypnosis, lists some of its shibboleths, and then very adequately refutes their validity. This is followed by a lengthy and exciting presentation by Florence Rhyn Serlin, Ph.D., of the Morton Prince Clinic for Hypnotherapy in New York City, who describes some of the techniques used when adding hypnosis to an otherwise psychoanalytically orthodox group therapy situation. Besides providing an excellent review of the literature, Serlin discusses such concepts as the management of resistance and of the hypnotic relationship in terms of metaphoric associations. She also offers some cases for discussion at scheduled staff meetings, along with descriptions of her office set up and of various induction techniques. The section's final chapter is entitled, "Theory and Practice of Group Hypnosis, or Collective Hypnosis, in the USSR," by N.V. Ivanov, M.D., professor at the Gorki Medical Institute in the Soviet Union. In this chapter, Ivanov examines some of the shortcomings and some of the advantages of group hypnotherapy in his country, introduces some theoretical underpinnings of this modality, and emphasizes the positive effect that collectivist society has on the group hypotherapeutic process.

Part III, "Group Hypnosis: Special Situations and Settings," consists of five chapters that include the use of group hypnosis in diverse settings and for different purposes, as well as the development of a new technique or new approach to hypnosis, namely, *hyperempiria*. In the first chapter of this section, Greenberg describes how his consulting firm, Behavioral Studies Institute, employs guided fantasies in group hypnosis for creative corporate problem solving during weekend and other type workshops with key personnel concerned with the particular problem. He also describes the teaching and personal development approach of another management consulting firm, Behavior Science Education Center, headed by Richard L. Johnson of Glendora, Calif. A short chapter, "Group Hypnotherapy in a University Counseling Center," by J.B. Hartman, Ph.D., L.L.B., explains the employment of this approach with selected students to help them overcome and/or gain from such problems as weight control, smoking withdrawl, and assertive training, plus their learning relaxation techniques, improving study habits, and functioning more effectively on written and oral examinations.

"Individual Hypnosis, Group Hypnosis, and the Improvement of Academic Achievement," by Stanley Krippner, Ph.D., follows Hartman's counseling center chapter. Krippner, president of the Association for Humanistic Psychology for 1974-1975, a research associate in the dream investigation program at Maimonides Medical Center, Brooklyn, New York, and Humanistic Psychology Institute program planning coordinator, San Francisco, provides an extensive review of the literature and then describes some of the work he had done with elementary, high school, and university students to help them reduce anxiety levels and to help them, through posthypnotic suggestion, improve their reading and study skills and to help them motivate themselves toward completing their homework assignments on time. He details some of his work in motivating students to learn and describes his work in helping them improve their language skills through methods of hypnosis. In "Principles of Gestalttherapy in Relation to Hypnotherapy," Dezso Levendula, M.D., tells how he was able to add individual hypnotherapy to the group process of Gestalt therapy to help a patient gain quick insight into a situation he was not able to work through in the group session. Finally, in the concluding chapter, "Group Hyperempiria," Don Gibbons, Ph.D., of Georgia State College at Carrollton describes the hypnotic state of hyper-alertness and presents several fantasy situations that have been useful for individuals in group hypnotherapy sessions or in group hypnosis workshops to gain important insights into some of their problems in short periods of time. Some of the chapter material is taken from Gibbons' book, *Beyond Hypnosis: Explorations in Hyperempiria* (1973).

Part IV, "Hypnodrama: the Morenean Method," contains four chapters that deal with Moreno's and Enneis' theory and clinical experiences and serves to adequately cover the field of classical hypnodrama, which is very much like psychodrama, with the exception that the one or more protagonists function while in states of hypnosis. Part V, "Hypnodrama: the Group Approach," for the most part explores a direction developed by this writer in which not only the protagonist or protagonists are in hypnosis but also the auxiliary egos (actors who help the protagonist explore his private world through the stage action), the audience, and sometimes the director. This is described in detail in "Hypnodrama and Group Hypnosis," by Greenberg, and it is followed by Leo Litwak's chapter. "Hypnodrama at the Humanistic Convention," which was extracted from a lengthy article on the 1972 Association for Humanistic Psychology convention and published in the *New York Times Magazine*. The two addenda to the Litwak Chapter are brief reports by the principal protagonist in the hypnodrama, who tells of some of her feelings during this experience, and by Greenberg, who reports on some of the things that occurred on the hypnodramatic stage after Litwak left to cover another part of the convention.

Included in this section is Krojanker's chapter, "Hypnodrama and Symbolization," which was taken from a longer work (1963) and which explains his utilization of fantasy as an adjunct to his hypnodramatic explorations. He describes one aspect of his work involving "dream correction" elsewhere in this work, which had been published originally in a journal in Ecuador, as follows: "The subject will be induced into light trance on the stage and will be asked to faithfully dream his dream again [and] the dream will be dramatized by the dreamer with the help of auxiliary egos who may be silent, or they may talk; as the psychodramatist recognizes the conflicts illustrated by the dream, he may introduce 'dream correctives' into it, which brings the dream to a more constructive ending, while the dreamer is still in trance; if necessary, the dreamer will be encouraged to continue dreaming about possible solutions to the problem for the next session, and he is awakened for the discussion period." (1963, p. 416) Krojanker further reports the beneficial effect of "having the subject relate his dream, then inducing the entire group into light trance [and] asking them to visualize their [specific] ending to the dream [and] often this is a way to collective interpretation of that dream and then evaluating the individual preferences for solving a dream conflict." (Ibid.) Krojanker's chapter is followed by two by Greenberg, "Hypnodramatics for Organizational Analysis" and "Imaginary Hypnodrama," two procedures he invented, the first being a tool or technique for management cousulting that involves the subjective appraisal of a rival group and the second being a form of individual hypnotherapy that employs some hypnodramatic techniques. The concluding chapter, "Psychodrama and Hypnosis," by Edward M. Scott, Ph.D., clinic director of the Oregon Alcohol and Drug Treatment and Training Center in Portland, brings the circle of hypnodrama to a close by describing how participants in psychodrama have on occasion gone into spontaneous states of hypnosis.

Part VI, "Therapeutics: Habit Change and Intensive Intervention," contains eight chapters that report on the employment of group hypnotherapy to treat persons with problems of weight and cigarette control, drug addiction, alcoholism, and schizophrenia, as well as to facilitate both personal and group growth and to facilitate creative problem solving of individuals in the group. The chapters include "Treatment of Obesity by Individual and Group Hypnotherapy," by Canadian psychiatrist Frederick W. Hanley, M.D., and "Group Hypnosis for Weight Reduction," by F. Scott Glover, M.D., of Houston, Texas, who reported on his work at the 1975 convention of the American Society of Clinical Hypnosis in Seattle, Washington, during which he described how he conducts a large-volume weight-reduction practice at small cost to the individuals through the multiple group approach. Other chapters in this section are "Post-Hypnotic Suggestion in Group Therapy: a Note," by William B. Singer, Ph.D., chief psychologist, Veterans Administration Hospital, Vancouver, Washington; "The Use of Extended Group Hypnotherapy Sessions in Controlling Cigarette Habituation," by Milton V. Kline, Ed.D., head of the Morton Prince Institute for Research in Hypnosis in New York City and a Fairleigh Dickinson University faculty member; "Group Therapy for Schizophrenic Alcoholics in a State-Operated Outpatient Clinic: with Hypnosis as an Integrated Adjunct," by Scott, of the Portland, Oregon, Alcohol and Drug Treatment and Training Center, and "Group Hypnotherapy Techniques with Drug Addicts," by Arnold M. Ludwig, M.D., William H. Lyle, Jr., M.D., and Jerome S. Miller, Ph.D., all of the U.S. Public Health Service Hospital, Lexington, Kentucky, with Ludwig also being chairman of the University of Kentucky Psychiatry Department. The section concludes with two chapters, also presented as papers at 1975 conventions. They are; "Behavioral Analysis of a Group Hypnosis Treatment Method," by Susan De Voge, Ph.D., assistant professor of psychology at the University of Nevada, Reno, and "Mutual Group Hypnosis for Creative Problem Solving," by Shirley Sanders, Ph.D., assistant professor of psychology at the University of North Carolina, Chapel Hill.

Part VII, "Conclusion: Appraisals and Predictions," contains the final chapter, "Group Hypnosis: Present Imperfect, Future Indicative," by Greenberg. It simply seeks to determine where we are at present, so far as the employment of this modality is concerned, and what the future might hold for both the practitioners of this and for those who seek to benefit from it. One obvious conclusion is that this book, limited as it is in scope and depth, is at this time the definitive work for both group hypnotherapy and for hypnodrama; thus, there is much that needs to be done in these two areas. The conclusion we must reach, therefore, is that this volume, despite its being, today, the final word on the subjects, remains merely a beginning. Much more must follow.

REFERENCES

1. GIBBONS, DON. *Beyond Hypnosis: Explorations in Hyperempiria.* South Orange, N.J.: Power Publishers, Inc., 1973.
2. LITWAK, LEO. " 'Rolfing,' 'Akido,' Hypnodramas, Psychokinesis and Other Things Beyond the Here and Now." *The New York Times Magazine,* December 17, 1972.
3. KROGER, WILLIAM S. *Clinical and Experimental Hypnosis.* Philadelphia and Montreal: J.B. Lippincott Company, 1963.
4. KROJANKER, ROLF. "Some New Techniques in Psychodrama and Hypnodrama." *Separata de "Archivos de Criminología, Neuro-Psiquiatría y Disciplinas Conexas."* Julio-Stbre. de 1963. Vol. XI, No. 43, pp. 410-32. *Editorial Casa de la Cultura Ecuatoriana, Quito,* 1963.
5. MASSERMAN, JULES H. "Historical-Comparative and Experimental Roots of Short-Term Therapy." Chapter in *Short-Term Psychotherapy,* edited by Lewis R. Wolberg. New York and London: Grune & Stratton, 1965.
6. TEITELBAUM, MYRON. *Hypnosis Induction Technics.* Springfield, Ill.: Charles C. Thomas, Publisher, 1965.
7. WOLBERG, LEWIS R. *Medical Hypnosis, Vol. I, The Principles of Hypnotherapy.* New York and London: Grune & Stratton, 1965.

2
Group Hypnosis*

Lewis R. Wolberg

Group hypnosis is utilized for two purposes: first, to increase susceptibility to hypnosis in prospective patients; second, as a form of psychotherapy.

Although the physician will rarely have the opportunity to prepare prospective patients for hypnosis by introducing them to a group, the technic is a useful one to know. In employing group hypnosis as a means of demonstrating the phenomena of the trance, it is always helpful to include in the group one or two good hypnotic subjects.

One of the most effective means of producing group hypnosis is to tell the group that a number of nervous symptoms are caused by an inability to relax. It is possible by simple suggestions to learn how to relax and even to enter a hypnotic-like sleep. A suggestion such as the following may be used:

"I should like to demonstrate to you how easy it is to relax. I should like to have you bring down your arms and your hands, resting them on your thighs. Place your feet firmly on the floor. Settle back in your chair, start loosening the muscles in your body, close your eyes; breathe-in deeply and regularly and relax.

"Relax your body and your mind. Relax yourself all over. Begin by relaxing the muscles of your forehead. Loosen up the muscles of your

*Lewis R. Wolberg. *Medical Hypnosis, Vol. I*, The Principles of Hypnotherapy. New York: Grune & Stratton, 1948. Reprinted with permission.

forehead. Then take the wrinkles out of your face. Shrug your shoulders. Notice how tense your back is. Shrug your shoulders and loosen your back. Let your arms feel as if they weigh a ton. Let them fall and rest on your thighs so that you have no inclination to move them. Then shift your attention to your legs. Let your legs feel heavy.

"As you sit there breathing deeply, you will feel your arms growing heavy and your legs growing heavy. Your eyes will feel tired, and your eyelids will be as heavy as lead. Your body is getting heavier and heavier. Your eyes are getting tired, very tired. They are closed and you have no desire to open them. You are going to fall asleep, deeply asleep. As you relax, it is impossible for you to help sleeping. It is impossible for you to open your eyes. They are glued together firmly. They are heavier and heavier, and they continue to stay stuck together as you feel yourself sinking into a deeper and deeper sleep. Keep breathing in deeply and go to sleep, deeply asleep. You will find now that your eyes are so firmly glued together that it is impossible to open them. The harder you try to open them, the heavier they feel. Try and you'll see that the harder you try to open them, the heavier they feel."

These suggestions should be made in a firm, confident tone of voice. As a general rule a good number of the members of the group, when challenged to open their eyes, will not be able to do so. The physician may then walk over to those who have their eyes closed and place two fingers on the eyelids, pressing them together firmly with the comment: "Continue to sleep."

After this the following statement is made: "From now on whenever I give you the suggestion to sleep, your eyes will become heavy, they will close and you will sink into a state of sleep quickly and easily. You will relax all over, and your sleep will get deeper and deeper. As you sit there with your eyes closed, I am going to give you a suggestion now that you slowly awaken. Slowly your eyes will open, and you will be awake. However, whenever I suggest that you sleep, your eyes will close rapidly, and you will go into a deep restful sleep."

Following this, the patients who have responded positively are brought to the front of the room, or seated in chairs facing the remaining members of the group. Should the physician have present one or two trained hypnotic subjects, he may proceed to induct them into a deep trance, demonstrating each step carefully. Then, the members of the group who have been selected are given the suggestion that they will relax, that their eyes will close and that they will go into a deep sleep. These suggestions are repeated until a trance has been produced. Thereafter several members may be inducted further into a trance state as deeply as they will go.

The remaining members of the group, among whom there may be patients the physician wishes especially to hypnotize, are then told that they too can easily learn to relax and sleep in the same way, and that the next time the procedure is tried, they will find it easier to sink into a state of sleep. At this point they may be enjoined to close their eyes, to relax and to go to sleep deeply. Almost invariably a certain number of the members of the group who had previously resisted falling asleep will enter a trance state. This demonstration will have a positive effect on the patient's trance susceptibility when later inducted into a trance through individual effort.

The second use of group hypnosis involves its employment for psychotherapeutic purposes. In attempting to use group hypnosis for psychotherapy, the physician must realize its limitations. It must not be confused with real group psychotherapy which is nondirective and which permits the patient to interact freely with other members of the group and with the group leader. In this interaction he expresses his customary character trends and personality patterns and gains insight into his problems and difficulties in interpersonal relationships.

The psychotherapies employed with group hypnosis are those of a directive nature, involving principles of guidance, reassurance, desensitization and persuasion. Once the trance has been produced in susceptible patients by the technics outlined above, other members of the group are urged to relax themselves, to close their eyes, and to absorb the suggestions that will be given to them. Following this suggestions are given to the group. The following persuasive suggestions from a record are exemplary:

"You have acquired faulty emotional habits that need correction. Such habits are the result of the wrong kind of thinking. You can be happy, free from worry and tension, by establishing the right habits of thinking and acting. You must tell yourself, 'I will correct those difficulties that can be remedied. I will face those that cannot be remedied. I may be unable to change the world, but I can change myself so that I will not get emotional about things. I will abolish worrying and thinking too much about myself. If anything comes up that needs solution, I will immediately review all possible courses of action and choose the one that seems to be best. Once I have made up my mind, I shall follow the plan I have evolved. I shall stop thinking and talking too much about my troubles. I shall be pleasant in my relationships with people, and shall not permit myself to be upset. I shall direct my thoughts to pleasant things, and keep in mind the kind of person I would like to be. I must think I am well, and then I will get better. If worrisome ideas keep coming up in my mind, I shall control my thoughts by picturing in my mind a time in my life when I was really happy.' ''

Group hypnosis with directive psychotherapy has definite limitations, being oriented as it is around a leader who establishes himself as an omniscient personage, whose pronouncements he expects the patient to follow. What is perpetuated here is essentially the authoritative magical figure of a parental substitute. Symptom relief is brought about as a result of a repression of conflict, and a desire on the part of the patient to comply with suggestions as a means of gaining status in the eyes of the leader. The group exists to a large extent as an appendage of the leader, and beneficial results are maintained so long as the patient is capable of maintaining an image of the former as completely powerful and protective.

Psychotherapy with group hypnosis is often effective in dependent persons whose chief motivation for therapy is to find an invincible authority on whom they can pin their faith. So long as they feel that the personage whom they endow with power will protect them, they may be capable of functioning without symptoms.

In justification of this kind of therapy, there are some individuals whose inner will to live and to develop is so diminutive that the most one can expect from them is a relief of symptoms without any real reorganization of their personality. Such persons flourish under an approach in which they are able to establish a submissive relationship to a leader. The mastery of symptoms, the institution of self discipline, the tolerance of anxiety and tension, the repression of inexpressible impulses and drives, may often result from a relationship of this type.

However, it is necessary not to over-rate the permanency of this type of therapy, inasmuch as success depends upon the ability of the patient to maintain a notion of the leader as noble, good and protective. Furthermore a clinging relationship to the leader may encourage the patient's dependency and may make it difficult for him to take up life on his own.

For these reasons attempts must always be made to encourage free interaction in the group, to get all patients who show a semblance of ego strength to enter into individual psychotherapy, or into a more dynamic form of group psychotherapy which is aimed at rehabilitating the individual in his attitudes toward life, toward people and toward himself. The emphasis should be on improving the stature of the person to a point where he is capable of dealing with his inner needs and conflicts without having to depend upon the beneficences of a protective, authoritarian figure.

3
Learning to Relax*

Joseph Shallit

The eight patients settled themselves in their chairs, closed their eyes and let their hands fall limply in their laps, as the physician told them to do.

His voice was slow, soft, soothing.

"Take a deep breath . . . let it out slowly . . . I want you to notice that heavy feeling in your legs . . . feel that surge of relaxation from the tip of your head down to your toes. . ."

The physician, Dr. William T. Reardon, moved quietly among them, watching their reactions as he continued his lulling monologue.

"With each breath, feel yourself relaxing deeper and deeper and deeper . . . that's wonderful. . ."

With one gentle suggestion after another, he led them down the velvet pathway into the shadowy world of hypnosis.

"I want you to enjoy this wonderful feeling of relaxation," the doctor's voice went on, drifting among them like a wind riffling through river reeds. "Let this feeling enter every muscle of your body. Let yourself enjoy this warm, comfortable feeling of relaxation."

Through the mechanism of his voice, the slim, white-haired doctor

*Reprinted with permission from *The Sunday Bulletin Magazine*, February 19, 1967 Copyright 1967 by The Bulletin Co.

was treating all eight patients at the same time. It was group hypnotherapy.

"You will leave this office with a new sense of calm and well-being. With your arms relaxed, you won't feel the compulsion to reach for things you know you should not have. You won't need that cigaret . . . that liquor glass . . . you won't be reaching for that midnight snack you know you shouldn't be eating. By controlling the muscles of your tongue, you can control your temper and won't be saying things you will be sorry for."

The doctor sprinkled these post-hypnotic suggestions among them, counting on each person to take the one applicable to himself and his particular problem.

"And now, whenever you feel like it, open your eyes and be wide awake . ."

This is an abbreviated account of what takes place two or three times a week in Dr. Reardon's office in downtown Wilmington. Groups of five to twenty patients are treated simultaneously for a variety of problems:

Obesity. Migraine headaches. Excessive smoking. Excessive drinking. Insomnia. Nail biting. Inability to concentrate. Uncontrollable temper.

Dr. Reardon's approach to these and similar problems is simply this: to teach the patient how to relax.

"When a person learns how to relax completely, both physically and mentally," he says, "all the irritations and pressures of life weigh less heavily. The person becomes better able to handle his problems. He faces life with more calm and more confidence, and can do his daily tasks with more efficiency and enjoyment."

The majority of patients learn the technique in six visits. Others take a longer time, depending on the severity of the problem.

The first step helps patients practice relaxation through group hypnosis under the doctor's direction. In the second and final step each learns how to relax by himself, through self-hypnosis.

In self-hypnosis, the patient puts himself into a light trance, using the same kind of relaxing suggestions the doctor has used on him. The patient does this at home or at work, any time he feels himself succumbing to tension, Dr. Reardon explains. A trance lasting two or three minutes may be enough to carry him, relaxed, through the rest of the day.

Dr. Reardon is one of a growing number of physicians who are finding hypnosis a valuable tool to add to their black bags.

Some physicians use it to put a nervous patient at ease for an examination. Others use it to supplement or replace an anesthetic during surgery or childbirth. Still others use it to aid in the treatment of ailments that have a large emotional component—such as ulcers, asthma, colitis, chronic constipation.

An increasing number of dentists are using hypnosis to deaden pain. Dr. Reardon himself recently had to have two molars extracted, and he told the dentist to forget the anesthetic—he'd use self-hypnosis. "It worked fine," he says. "I hardly felt a twinge."

Not so long ago, any doctor who used hypnosis would have kept quiet about it, to escape the odor of quackery commonly associated with this ancient and mystic technique. But following World War II, when hypnosis was used in the study and treatment of battle fatigue and other neuroses, the subject began to acquire respectability. In 1956, the American Medical Association set up a committee to study the matter, and the committee's report in 1958 approved the use of hypnosis by qualified physicians.

Today at least nine medical schools have courses in hypnosis, either for students or practicing physicians, and the science has its own publication, the American Journal of Hypnosis.

Dr. Reardon is an ear, nose and throat specialist—chief of otolaryngology at St. Francis and Wilmington General hospitals—and is a charter member of the American Society of Clinical Hypnosis.

He began looking into the possibilities of hypnosis about ten years ago, as a way to minimize the patient's discomfort and pain during examination or minor surgery.

"After taking postgraduate courses in the subject and doing independent research," he says, "I found that one could induce a hypnotic state surprisingly quickly in most patients.

"Some of them subsequently told me that this not only prevented pain but also gave them a feeling of relaxation and well-being that continued after they left the office. So then I began exploring the uses of hypnosis in conditions unrelated to my ear, nose and throat work."

At present, about half his practice involves group hypnotherapy.

The patients gathered in Dr. Reardon's office on a recent evening were typical of those seeking the benefits of this unusual form of treatment.

Ethel's problem was chronic migraine. This was her second visit. "I had a migraine attack last Sunday," she reported, "but I practiced my relaxation, and this attack wasn't nearly as bad as the ones before. I was even able to make dinner for the family. In the past, I would have had to stay in bed."

Grace was there to control the compulsive eating that prevented her from losing weight. Since her last visit, she had been on vacation and had gained five pounds.

"Didn't you do your self-hypnosis?" the doctor asked.

"I guess I didn't practice it conscientiously enough," she said.

Marie had come to the doctor with the opposite complaint: underweight, no appetite. She was also harassed by a constant, vague fearfulness, which had made her give up her secretarial job three years ago, and she hadn't worked since. This was her fifth visit. On previous visits, she had reported a new and wonderful hunger for steak. Now she had more dramatic news: "On Friday I went back to work!"

Jerry, who had been there eight times, was receiving help in mastering the nervousness that plagued him in his salesman's job. Already he had overcome a stammer that had afflicted him for twenty years.

Bill's problem was liquor. This was his first visit, and he was wary; full of questions.

"When you've put me under, will I be unconscious?" he asked.

"You'll be fully conscious," Dr. Reardon told him. "You'll be aware of everything that's going on. You'll even be able to answer questions."

"Can you put me under if I don't want you to?"

"No, that's impossible, All hypnosis is really self-hypnosis. You have to want it; you have to want to accept the doctor's suggestions. Otherwise, nothing will happen. And when you're in the hypnotic state, I can't make you do anything you wouldn't do in your waking state."

"Suppose you can't bring me out of it."

"I won't have to. As soon as you want to come out of it you will."

The man, an aircraft mechanic, thought this over with taut lips. Then abruptly he said, "Okay, doc, go ahead."

In less than a minute, he was in a trance.

The doctor gave him post-hynotic suggestions about relaxing without the aid of alcohol.

Before a patient is admitted to a hypnotherapy group, he is examined to make sure he has no physical ailment requiring treatment, and he is psychologically evaluated to make sure he is a suitable subject for hypnosis.

"At first, each hypnotherapy patient was treated separately," Dr. Reardon says, "but I and other practitioners have discovered that the patients do better when treated in a group. They seem to draw strength from one another. Before each treatment session, we have a warm-up in which each one discusses his problems and his progress, to the extent that he wants to. This gives reassurance to the ones who are pessimistic or apprehensive."

The idea of teaching patients how to perform self-hypnosis startles some people, but Dr. Reardon points out that many a person uses self-hypnosis without being aware of it.

"A woman who takes a sleeping pill every night has hypnotized herself into believing that she cannot possibly fall asleep without that little red pill," he says.

"She has to be de-hypnotized if she is ever to give up the pill and develop faith in her ability to fall asleep without it."

Dr. Reardon concedes that teaching a troubled person how to relax through self-hypnosis is not comparable to doing a thorough study of the patient's subconscious and re-patterning his personality.

"My goal is admittedly a modest one," he says. "But in many cases it's enough to answer the patient's needs."

Students who get panicky at exam time can benefit and boost their grades by learning to relax, Dr. Reardon says. He has taught his self-hypnosis method to more than 200 high school and college students.

"With relaxation," he says, "a student will ease his tensions and get rid of those stomach butterflies. He can increase his ability to concentrate, can save time in getting down to work, and can absorb material more readily."

Dr. Reardon has made several "relaxation tapes" which have been tried out in five Wilmington schools during the last year. Played on tape recorders for selected groups of students, especially under-achievers, each tape begins by telling the children to sit at ease with their eyes closed. Then, by means of suggestion but no outright hypnosis, it attempts to lead them toward a relaxed but self-confident attitude toward their schoolwork.

Dr. Reardon's file of letters from former patients includes one from a university student who reported how much better he was doing in his studies, and enclosed a belated check.

"I'm sorry to be so late," the student wrote. "I guess I've been so relaxed, I've stopped worrying about paying bills."

Dr. Reardon, with an amused shake of his head, observed, "That's carrying relaxation a bit too far."

4
A New Group Hypnotherapy*

William T. Reardon

I would like to share with you my experiences and observations from a private practice of fifteen years of group hypnotherapy. It has many things in common with some groups and differs widely from others. The results from this therapy have been very gratifying and I feel comfortable doing it. Many have been helped and to the best of my knowledge none have been harmed.

One of the greatest drawbacks to the acceptance of this therapy is that one of the ingredients used is called "hypnosis". Dr. Theodore Xenophen Barber (Director of Psychological Research at Massachusetts Medfeld State Hospital) writing in "Psychology Today" says "Since no test has been able to demonstrate the existence of the hypnotic state, there is no reason to assume that there is such a state". Barber and others have reproduced hypnotic effects by the "simple power" of suggestion.

Dr. Martin Orne of the Institute of Pennsylvania Hospital's Unit for Experimental Psychiatry says, "The nature of hypnosis is still an open question". From his experiments, he concluded that wide awake subjects could be persuaded to do everything that hypnotized subjects would do but there was a great difference in how hypnotized subjects themselves felt about what they were doing, they don't experience their

*Reprinted with permission from the *Journal of the American Society of Psychosomatic Dentistry and Medicine*, Vol. 18, No. 2 (1971).

actions the same way. Speaking of hypnoanesthesia, Dr. Orne continues, "The truth is that under hypnosis, it just doesn't hurt."

I have been privileged to be present at several group therapeutic sessions and have seen things we have in common and differences. Recently, reading "Psychic Discoveries Behind the Iron Curtain," I found a Dr. Lozanov of Bulgaria has a method very similar to the one described here. He calls his method "Suggestology". He insists it is not hypnosis and is not auto-suggestion. The state the patients enter he calls the "suggestive" state. Let me quote, "Then the psychotherapist's calm, melodious voice addresses the relaxed but fully awake patients. Relax! deeeply, deeeeply . . . there is nothing troubling you. Your entire body is fully relaxed. All your muscles are at rest. You are able to overcome all difficulties". After twenty minutes of positive suggestion while the patients relax, Lozanov concludes, "You feel completely well; you sleep well; you have a good appetite". It seems to me very much like Schultz's autogenic training and I find it difficult to separate the two.

Several processes contribute to the mutual discovery which results in the initial contact with a patient, e.g.: (a.) Professional referral; (b.) Recommendations by other patients; (c.) Self-discovery by patient via public lectures, pamphlets, radio and television discussions, newspaper articles; (d.) Discovery in my EENT Practice. Whatever the route, all patients are "screened" in a personal telephone conversation lasting from 5 to 25 minutes. Some are selected, others are rejected and some discouraged, with an approximate 50% coming for the initial and private face-to-face discussion of the problem, history taking, etc. This interview ordinarily occurs just before the new patient is to participate in a "group session". It normally provides feed-back material for permissive suggestions. Prior to this interview, most of the patients have read my 14-page pamphlet *"Modern Medical Hypnosis"* which they received via mail or waiting room.

The sessions are in a panelled room 20' x 23' with 18 contour, reclining and straight-back chairs arranged in a U shape along 3 walls. Prior to the session, patients arrive and chat or sit silently as they wish. Sometimes they re-read "Modern Medical Hypnosis," start "Psycho-Cybernetics" or other related materials which are found on the chairs.

Because the groups are "open", there is a continuous change, i.e., new patients, old patients, terminating, young, old. In this heterogeneous group the symptoms are many and varied. You find the emotionally disturbed, the problem child, the alcoholic, the obese, the smoker, insomniac, nail-biter, bed wetter, stutterer, marital problem, family problems, etc.

The so called "warm up" discussion occurs during the first 45-60 minutes depending upon the circumstances. Self-reports of progress, difficulties, successes, etc., occur at this time. The patients teach and persuade each other of the value of this treatment. I dispel the misconceptions which the "old" patients can't handle in the "new" ones by convincing demonstrations using verbal and nonverbal inductions. When I am satisfied that the group is warmed up and all questions have been answered, we proceed to the induction.

All patients are taught how to relax. "Get yourself just as comfortable as you possibly can. You may take off your shoes, loosen anything that may be disturbing you. Take a long deep breath, blow it away slowly—close your eyes. Give me your undivided attention. You are going to hear my voice on a tape recorder which will be a description of medical relaxation and a method to practice. If you follow my suggestions 'uncritically', you will enter a delightful state of relaxation you saw or experienced in the warm up". Usually, by this time, all the patients look like they are asleep and the recorder is started. The 15 minute tape has many broad spectrum, open end, suggestions. Example; "Relaxation will give you all the courage and confidence that you need to take the *t* out of the word *can't* and find out that you can do and that you will do; want it to happen, expect it to happen and it will happen".

While the tape is playing, I have a chart of the seating arrangement of the patients with notations of the specific suggestions for each patient in the group. Example:—Obesity patient—"You will be able to learn how to eat less and enjoy it more. You can learn how to place smaller portions on your spoon and fork. As you eat slowly, you allow every taste bud on the back of your tongue to enjoy every morsel of food before you swallow it. You can toss the food with your tongue forward and backward, side to side before you swallow it", etc.

In my judgment, I feel that in this relaxed state there is a very direct line of communication between the therapist and the patient. The patient has a selector and a rejector mechanism and in some way, which we do not understand, is able to take those particular suggestions for which he has a need and start to change his own behavior, attitudes and way of thinking. An important thing about this therapy is that it deals with the present. No special search is made in the memory of the past for "the traumatic" incident that could be responsible for the present behavior. One's personal problems are not special topics for discussion in the group, although many are disclosed as each chooses for himself.

I feel that the 45-60 minute warm-up is very important for developing rapport between the patient and the therapist. The patient's faith and confidence in his therapist greatly shortens the duration of the therapy.

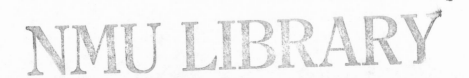

Next, the group is given a post-hypnotic suggestion to re-enter this state quickly and deeply when I place my hand on his shoulder (or his own hand) which is done to each patient. They are reminded of their homework—practice several times every day (2-3 minutes). Blink your eyes, allow them to open and be wide awake and feel refreshed all over, that's wonderful.

The question and answer discussion following the relaxed state serves a vital purpose. The patients teach each other, share experiences and clarify their own ideas about this process, thereby gaining necessary faith in its efficacy and furthering the *can do* commitment to making it useful to themselves on their own terms.

I feel that some observations are especially interesting. Everyone gets the "same" stimulus and self reports of perception differ widely. The sensations in hypnosis vary from lightness, heaviness, floating, tingling, numbness, etc. Because the sessions are unstructured as to content, the discussions may be on alcoholism, obesity, insomnia, drug abuse, bed wetting, smoking, marital problems, etc.

I believe everyone enters the group with a certain amount of apprehension. It is a new experience. The fear of the unknown is manifest in his non-verbal communications, i.e., crossed arms and legs, wringing of hands, facial expressions, body movements, etc. The patient is waiting for something to happen. Because he doesn't feel anything "dramatic" happened, I often hear, "Doctor, I don't think I was hypnotized". With this type of patient, it may take two or three sessions for him to develop awareness that he is able to do these things others are learning and reporting. I tell him I cannot hypnotize anyone but I know that if he follows my suggestions he will enter a state that Dr. Braid and others called "hypnosis". I am teaching him to relax so he can go home and practice and learn how to "do it himself". Usually when "a relaxed" patient is asked "what are you thinking about?", the answer is "nothing"—indicating mental relaxation, I believe.

Oftimes, experienced patients sit down in the therapy room, close their eyes and spontaneously relax. Patients frequently request coaching over the telephone in order to relax and better cope with a dental appointment, acute anxiety or for pain, etc.

At the close of each session appointments are made for the next visit. Usually they are once a week, but some conditions like acute anxiety, neurotic depression may require more frequent visits. Some may want a private session. Others may linger on to continue a conversation or ask questions.

In conclusion, group therapy is an efficacious method for simultaneous treatment of five to twenty-five patients while maintaining or enhancing the effectiveness of the same relaxation method as used in dyad therapy. It is short term therapy within reach of patients in the lower income bracket. Relaxation strikes at the roots of the number one mental health problem today—tension. Relaxation therapy may have a place in community medicine where we have a shortage of physicians. Qualified paramedical personnel could be used as relaxation therapists. Group therapy and treatment in groups is a fascinating field to me and I believe it merits your serious consideration.

Table I

Goals of Treatment

1. Self-Relaxation

2. Self-Awareness and their

3. Self-Application for

4. Self-Improvement via

5. Six—2 hour Weekly Sessions

1. Everyone is taught how to relax in ways similar to Jacobson's Progressive Relaxation and Schultz's Autogenic Training. Each has homework to do, practice what he experienced in the group session. It is a new tool in his own hands.

2. Patients (and therapist) learn to observe their own muscle tension resulting from anxiety, fear and worry in attempting to cope with the problems of everyday living.

3. After starting to achieve (1) and (2) patients begin to apply their new "do it yourself" tool in their own life situations.

4. This helps them change their behavior, attitude and way of thinking. They are helped to become the persons they would like to be. "You do everything better when you are relaxed whether it be physical, mental or emotional". Patients and therapist develop more awareness of their own internal states useful for self-help.

5. My groups are usually therapeutic without much "special" prompting on my part. Patients draw strength and energy from one another of the group..

Table II

A New Group Hypnotherapy

A. Procedure

1. Mutual Discovery

2. Telephone Screening

3. Direct Interview

4. Room and Warm-up

5. Induction
   Maintenance
   Suggestion
   Questions and Answers

6. Termination

REFERENCES

1.   BARBER, T.X., Questioning Hypnosis, Time Magazine, July 13, 1970
2.   ORNE, M.T., Is Hypnosis for Real? Scientists Still Cant't Agree—Evening Bulletin, August 5, 1970
3.   LOZANOV, G., Psychic Discoveries Behind the Iron Curtain, New Jersey: Prentice Hall, Inc.
4.   SCHULTZ, J.H. and Luthe, Wolfgang, Autogenic Training, New York and London: Grune and Stratton
5.   JACOBSON, E., Jacobson's Progressive Relaxation, Illinois: University of Chicago Press
6.   BRAID, J., Clinical and Experimental Hypnosis, Philadelphia and Montreal: J.B. Lippincott Co.

5
Group Hypnotherapy:
A Brief Survey*

Irvin H. Perline

This paper is an attempt to bring together under one rubric the findings from the literature of group hypnotherapy.

Much success has been reported from individual hypnotherapeutic sessions utilizing both direct and indirect suggestions (1-3). Success has been reported with such varied problems as enureses (4-6), obesity (7, 8), dentistry (9), just to mention a very few. Therapeutic hypnosis has been employed on smokers, future mothers, schizophrenics and individuals exhibiting habit disorders, along with just about every other kind of problem patient to enter the clinician's office.

There is no reason to believe that the success reported in the literature derived from individual hypnotherapeutic sessions cannot be had with group hypnotherapeutic sessions. To illustrate this point and to demonstrate what has been done with group hypnotherapy, some findings from the recent literature will be cited.

A recent study by Peberdy (10) reports on hypnotic methods in group psychotherapy. According to Peberdy, to have out-patient discussion groups is difficult, as many patients do not continue to show up, may show up erratically; many do not like to discuss their problems and

*Reprinted by permission of the author and publisher. Originally published in *The American Journal of Clinical Hypnosis* (1968), Vol. 10, No. 4, pp. 267-70. Copyright 1968 by the American Society of Clinical Hypnosis.

group composition is always a problem. In this study all patients have been suffering from morbid tension as a common theme and invariably the major suggestions have been of confidence and relaxation given with indications of post-hypnotic continuance and reinforcement. The specific symptoms of some patients were alluded to in the suggestions when these would not be incongruent with the rest of the group.

Groups composed of six patients each (10) were given time before hypnosis to discuss their feelings, fears, etc. of group hypnotherapy.[1] It was found that members often afforded each other invaluable support. The groups were composed of people in all stages of progress and in general individual hypnotic sessions were not required. Approximately sixty-five patients have been treated and detailed records of responses, reactions and results have been kept.

Peberdy noted that there was an absence of spontaneous abreaction among the group members and suggests that this may be due to a restraint dependent upon a continued awareness of the presence of other patients. However, it was found that this did not lead to any loss of therapeutic effectiveness. It was found that the communal ritual of group hypnotherapy heightens the sense of companionship and the cheerfulness of the group was always perceptible.

It was concluded that the patients' major symptom of tension was much improved in twenty-five per cent of the cases, reasonably improved in twenty-five per cent of the cases and the rest of the patients were not aided. These results achieved by Peberdy are not incongruent with the findings of R. Dorcus who researched the success rate reported by the adherents of many kinds of psychotherapy and found that approximately thirty-three percent of the cases were reported as considerably improved, thirty-three per cent slightly improved and thirty-three per cent unchanged.[2]

Wallerstein reports on a study in which group hypnotherapy was used as one of four techniques in the treatment of chronic alcoholism (11). In this study four forms of therapy, Antabuse, conditioned reflex, group hypnotherapy, and milieu therapy (control), were applied to 178 representative alcoholics in a large treatment center. The data collected over a two-and-one-half year period, plus a two year followup, revealed that Antabuse therapy was helpful to more patients than any of the other therapy modalities offered. However, the author reports that in all therapy groups sizeable numbers of patients derived significant relief from the alcoholic problem. The author concludes that choice of

[1]Peberdy reports, however, that the size of the group was due mainly to the size of the room and the ease of observation.

[2]Information obtained from Dr. S.S. Sargent, personal communication.

methods must be considered in the light of the basic psychological factors inherent in it and of the character and personality features of the patient to whom it is applied.

As Wolberg (12) points out, two factors in the effective treatment of alcoholics are: (1) the establishment of positive transference between patient and therapist and (2) support and understanding from others with similar problems. It would seem therefore that the results obtained by Wallerstein are in accordance with the expectations of current psychological theory. Certainly these two conditions were met by Wallerstein's use of group hypnotherapy.

That group hypnotherapy is an effective treatment method where spontaneity and creativity are essential is evidenced by the recent work reported on hypnodrama by J.L. Moreno and J.M. Enneis. (13) To demonstrate this point some statements and findings of these authors are cited:

> "In psychodrama the achievement of a state of spontaneous action is dependent upon stimulation of the patient by internal and external processes manipulated between the patient, director, and auxiliary egos. In hypnodrama the hypnosis acts as a psychological starter for the warming-up process in that it frees the patient from many of his inhibiting barriers, and places him in a condition of readiness to rise to a state of greater spontaneity. It is made possible for the patient to warm-up with a minimum of interference from the self." (13, p. 12)

Further, the authors note that:

> "Hypnodrama has the advantage of showing the patient's deeper personality structure early in the course of therapy. He responds verbally and kinesthetically to a situation and carries through the action on his own terms, involving the major portion of the personality. There is a minimum of defensive and evasive behavior. This enables the therapist to make a good estimate of the situation in terms of the patient's present functioning, and to base his plan of therapy more directly on the patient's needs. As the patient is treated in interaction with his social atom, the therapeutic results will be reflected in his extra-therapeutic life in a relatively short time." (p.13)

Moreno concludes in the discussion section of his book:

> "Hypnodrama has been found useful in cases where the patient is unable to express himself through other techniques, sufficiently well to gain catharsis and therapeutic success. It has

especial value in conversion hysteria and psychopathic states. It
has been found to have some success with schizoid personalities.

"When used in conjunction with psychodrama, it speeds
up the therapeutic process without loss of values attributed to
therapy given on conscious levels." (p.52)

Moreno's findings are not incongruent with those of Supple (14) who,
using hypnodrama with Moreno's techniques, found that bashfulness
and withholding were largely overcome. Supple reports that patients
seem to want to give all of their innermost and subconscious thoughts
for their own benefit and that of the group with whom they are working.
Many patients, it was found, would eagerly participate in hypnodrama
for two hours or more and reveal much deeper levels than in psychodrama. It was also noted that the patients reported favorable results from
hypnodrama.

Supple and Moreno both agree that the major principles of psychodrama apply to hypnodrama, and that the major differences that occur
between the two psychotherapeutic techniques are in the realm of
patient behavior.

While many drugs are available for over- and underweight persons,
they are often dangerous, and that group hypnotherapy is highly
effective in the treatment of weight problems is evident from the results
of the following studies to be reported. Some of these studies, it will be
found, reported significant weight loss or gain, as the case may be, in
over ninety per cent of the cases.

L. Wollman reports on the therapeutic use of hypnosis in weight
control (15). The patients taking part in this study were 525 consecutive
unselected cases consisting of 381 overweight women, 69 overweight
men, 63 underweight women and 12 underweight men. Approximately
four per cent of the patients were found to be somnambulists and only
three patients were refractory to treatment. Wollman warns against
mixing patients desiring to lose weight with those desiring to gain
weight and states that he found groups of five to be most effective.
Hypnotic suggestions were given in a directive manner to diminish or
increase by any chosen fraction the food intake of the previous week.

To relieve hunger in the obese patient a post-hypnotic suggestion
that a full meal had been eaten and enjoyed was found frequently
effective. The verbalization for the underweight group stressed heightened interest in food, greater enjoyment in eating, and pride of accomplishment as the goal is being reached.

From the results of this study it was found that there was an average
thirty pound loss over a three month period and for the same period the
underweight group gained an average of ten pounds.

Similar results were obtained by F. Glover with a much smaller group of patients. (16) According to Glover, the use of hypnosis in weight reduction is particularly effective for those who have tried other methods with little or no success. It was reported in this study that a group of twenty-seven nurses asked for aid in losing weight. The criteria set up by Glover for joining a therapeutic group to achieve these ends were (1) desire to lose weight and previous failure of attaining weight loss by other methods, (2) the individual must be at least twenty pounds overweight.

"Weighing in" preceded the group session and at this time each nurse reported her weekly calorie intake. Each nurse's loss or gain in weight was noted and posted on a chart which could be seen by any member of the group. Hypnotic suggestions were then given to the nurses in a directive manner.

After one month, two nurses having failed to lose weight were dropped from the class. Of the remaining twenty-five, none failed to lose weight. The average weight loss at the termination of therapy (four months), was thirty pounds. It was found that the greatest weight loss occurred in those most overweight. It was also noted that there was no significant difference in ability to lose weight between the older and younger nurses.

Glover concludes that group hypnotherapy is particularly adaptable for those having difficulty in losing weight.

H. Mann, in reporting on a similar study, concluded that:

> "It should be emphasized that group hypnosis in the treatment of obesity is of tremendous advantage, in that it establishes an unusual kind of interpersonal relationship and rapport, which is so well adapted to anxious, frustrated, despairing patients. It is a concise program which approaches the problem in an unusual, encouraging manner. It lends itself ideally to this type of psychotherapy, which involves guidance, reassurance and persuasion, in an atmosphere of genuine interest and enthusiasm" (17).

That group hypnotherapy may be an effective method of treatment for psychoses is indicated by a recent study of J. Ilovsky. (18) While the first group of schizophrenics treated by Ilovsky consisted of ten patients, the author states that he is beginning treatment with groups as large as 150 patients. This study reports on eighty chronic schizophrenic women whose average hospital stay was six to eight years. They were hypnotized twice weekly for six months both by the therapist and by a tape recording of the therapist's voice. Direct therapeutic suggestions were given to the patients by the therapist. The author points out that hypnosis was especially useful with paranoid schizophrenics whose "push" of hostility could be controlled and directed through hypnosis to both socially and individually satisfactory channels.

Ilovsky noted that the patients could be considered conditioned by suggestions to use their energy for working and repression instead of spending their time on expending aggression and hostility. According to the author:

> "Hypnotic suggestion introduces a complex into the unconscious mind and compels the patient to think about his problems differently. Guidance under hypnosis enables him to review his concepts and achieve a satisfactory change in his behavior and outlook."

The results of this study reveal that at the end of the year 60 percent of the patients treated were released from the hospital and that those remaining were considered more manageable. It was noted that the results with tape recordings of the therapist's voice were the same as those with direct personal hypnosis and that the rate of improvement was in direct proportion to the depth of trance achieved. Patients that failed to reach the hallucinatory stage showed no improvement but they improved rapidly as soon as they reached this depth.

It may be concluded from the many case reports cited above that group hypnotherapy was found to be an effective treatment method for such varied problems as enuresis, weight control, tension and anxiety, alcoholism and schizophrenia.

While it may be noted that most of the work being done in the field of group hypnotherapy is of a didactic and directive nature, there is no reason that future work and research will not proceed into the more non-directive areas. Certainly as more and more knowledge of hypnotherapeutics, both on an individual and group basis, is accumulated throughout future years of research and study, one may reasonably expect the expansion and acceptance of therapeutic group hypnosis into the more "traditional" areas of psychotherapy.

REFERENCES*

ESTABROOKS, G.H. *Hypnotism.* New York: E.P. Dutton & Co., Inc., 1957.

2. SCHULTZ, J.H. AND LUTHE, W. *Autogenic Training.* New York: Grune & Stratton, 1959.

*Note: "This Journal" refers to the *American Journal of Clinical Hypnosis.*

3. BRAMWELL J.J. *Hypnotism: Its history, practice and theory.* New York: Julian Press Inc., re-issue 1956.

4. MILLER, M.M. A group therapeutic approach to a case of bed-wetting and fire setting with the aid of hypnoanalysis. *Group Psychotherapy,* 1957, 10, 181-90.

5. SOLOVEY, G. AND MILECHNIN, A. Concerning the treatment of enuresis. This Journal, 1959, 2, 22-29.

6. CLAWSON, T.A. Hypnosis in medical practice. This Journal, 1964, 6, 236.

7. MANN, H. Group hypnosis in the treatment of obesity. This Journal, 1959, 1, 114-116.

8. POOLER, H.A. An instance of psychiatric complications in obesity. This Journal, 1959, 2, 90-91.

9. SOLOVEY, G. AND MILECHNIN, A. Some points regarding hypnosis in dentistry. This Journal, 1958, 1, 59.

10. PEBERDY, G.R. Hypnotic methods in group psychotherapy. *J. ment. Sci.,* 1960, 106, 1016-20.

11. WALLERSTEIN, R.S. Psychological factors in chronic alcoholism. *Amer. inter. Med.,* 1958, 48, 114-22.

12. WOLBERG, L.R. *Medical hypnosis.* New York: Grune & Stratton, 1948, Vol. 1.

13. MORENO, J.L. AND ENNEIS, J.M. *Hypnodrama and psychodrama.* New York: Beacon House, 1950.

14. SUPPLE, L.K. Hypnodrama, a synthesis of hypnosis and psychodrama: a progress report. *Gp. Psychotherap.,* 1962, 15.

15. WOLLMAN, L. Hypnosis in weight control. This Journal, 1961, 4, 177.

16. GLOVER, F.S. Use of hypnosis in weight reduction in a group of nurses. This Journal, 1961, 3, 250.

17. MANN, H. Group hypnosis in the treatment of obesity. This Journal, 1959, 1, 115-16.

18. ILOVSKY, J. Experiences with group hypnosis on schizophrenics. *J. ment. Sci.,* 1962, 108, 685-93.

Part II

THEORY AND TECHNIQUES:
General and Specific

6
The Systematic Use of Hypnosis in Individual and Group Psychotherapy*

Jack Fox

Since the days of Mesmer, who was not even aware of the psychological nature of hypnosis, its use for therapeutic purposes has undergone a variety of metamorphoses. Mesmer used it as a cure-all. Later, it was primarily used for anesthetic and analgesic purposes (Elliotson, Ward, Esdaile). During that period, the psychological nature of hypnosis was recognized by Braid. During the last half of the nineteenth century, hypnosis was extensively used for the removal of symptoms by direct suggestions. While Charcot conceptualized hypnosis as a pathological hysterical phenomenon, the Nancy School (Liebeault, Bernheim) demonstrated that hypnosis was a normal psychological state. Janet, conceptualizing psychopathology as dissociated consciousness, gave two new directions to the therapeutic use of hypnosis. He used it to recover painful dissociated memories and to re-integrate them into awareness. Morton Prince followed in his footsteps. (Boring, 1950; Brenman and Gill, 1947; Dorcus, 1945; Jenness, 1944). Breuer stumbled accidentally upon the same discovery and correctly placed the emphasis on the catharsis of the dissociated affects. Freud recognized the full significance of Breuer's discovery, pointed out that dissociation is not a passive

*Reprinted with permission from the author and publisher. Originally published in *The International Journal of Clinical and Experimental Hypnosis* (1960), Vol. 8, No. 2, 109-14.

process, but is actively brought about by the repression of unacceptable impulses and ideas, and a new, dynamic conceptualization of psychopathology was born (Freud, 1952a). Freud now used hypnosis to uncover a symptom's motivational causes and to abreact the repressed affects. Freud abandoned the use of hypnosis because there were many patients whom he could not hypnotize to the required depth (Brill, 1938; Freud, 1952b). Later, he rejected hypnosis because he felt that by its use resistances and transferences were by-passed rather than analysed (Freud, 1953a, 1953b). The further development of hypnosis as a therapeutic tool came to a relative standstill until Lindner (1944), Wolberg (1945), Brenman and Gill (1947), and others, combined psychoanalysis and hypnosis in the hypnoanalytic technique. Here, the hypnotic trance is used when free association is stopped by resistance in order to get at the resistance: to convince the patient of the reality of psychological conflicts and defense mechanisms by hypnotic implantation of artificial conflicts; to coax the patient to give up his repressed secrets by special devices, such as automatic writing and crystal gazing; to recover traumatic events; to bring about the disuse of motiveless habit patterns and to strengthen newly acquired habit patterns.

More extensive therapeutic use of hypnosis was also inhibited by the uncritical acceptance of a number of shibboleths, of which the following are the most important:

1. Only few people are capable of reaching a somnambulistic trance. It becomes ever more evident that this is largely a matter of technique and time (LeCron, 1952).

2. The hypnotized patient is a passive, somnolent "zombie," without defenses or self-assertions. This, as was clearly pointed out by Wolberg (1945), is primarily the result of the operator's attitude. When the patient is given the freedom to move, act, and talk freely and spontaneously during deep trance, he will do so, and the casual observer will never know that the subject is hypnotized. Moreover, the subject never surrenders his defenses: they manifest themselves clearly even in deep trance. They are merely dealt with in a more economical manner because material is more accessible in the trance state.

3. Direct symptom removal is only temporary: relapse is the rule, or substitute symptoms make their appearance. This shibboleth maintains itself with remarkable tenacity, in spite of much evidence to the contrary, and, thus, prevented a thorough exploration of the question as to what kind of symptoms can safely be removed by direct suggestions and what kind require an uncovering technique. One should not minimize the role which technique plays in this problem: it makes quite a difference how a suggestion is worded and whether direct or indirect suggestion is used.

4. Direct symptom removal is possible only in deep trance. Actually, suggestions are effective when repeatedly given during light trance and, if necessary, by reinforcement at periodic intervals (Van Pelt, 1956).

In hypnoanalysis, hypnosis is used as an accessory technique. The author suggests that hypnosis can be used as an integral part of, and directing agent in, the therapeutic process, which he conceives as proceeding in an orderly fashion. This conception is based on the acceptance of psychoanalytic findings that a symptom or a character attitude has a definite structure (Fenichel, 1945; Reich, 1949).

It is the function of a symptom to bind anxiety and to protect the ego from the devastating effects of too much free-floating anxiety. Each symptom, like a dream, has two legs: one rests upon a conflict during ontogenetic development, the other upon a conflict during adulthood, the latter of which may have precipitated the formation of the symptom. The symptom contains within itself the primary gain, the surreptitious expression of the unacceptable drive, and the primary defense, or the particular defense mechanism which prevents the break-through of the particular drive impulse into consciousness. Each symptom contains a number of derivatives of this original conflict. Finally, the symptom becomes integrated into the ego-structure, or ego-syntonic (Fenichel, 1945; Nunberg, 1948; Reich, 1949).

Ever since the publication of Reich's, by now classical, *Character-analysis,* it has become a more or less accepted dictum that analysis, to be successful, must proceed in a more or less orderly fashion, from the surface to the depth, or a chaotic analytic situation will develop, with more or less disastrous consequences for the patient (Fenichel, 1939; Reich, 1949). The author believes this to be also true for psychotherapy in general. Thus, it would be fruitless to confront the patient with the secondary gains which he derives from his symptoms, as long as the symptom is still ego-syntonic; or to uncover the ontogenetic leg of the symptom before its present-day leg has been uncovered; etc.

Hypnosis can be used with great advantage to give direction to this orderly process. First, it can be used to alienate the symptom by having the patient recall and/or regress to the many situations when the presence of the symptoms caused him distress and discomfort, and then to confront him with the many rationalizations by means of which the symptom became integrated into the ego-structure. After alienating the symptom, hypnosis can be used to uncover the secondary gains. This will liberate free-floating anxiety which, when followed closely, will lead to the present-day conflict. This process can be helped along by using hypnosis to locate the onset of the symptom and to unravel the precipitating events. In dealing with conflicts, present-day as well as ontogenetic, the ego-defensive aspects must be identified first. This, again, will liberate free-floating anxiety which, when followed, will lead to the identification of the drive impulses and which is facilitated by the trance state. Only when present-day drive impulses and affects are identified and abreacted may one proceed to uncover the ontogenetic leg, and this can be done by a hypnotic regression technique.

While, so far, nothing has been said about resistances and transferences, we have been dealing with them all along: an ego-defense manifests itself in therapy in the form of resistance and transference resistance. It should be noted that this technique neither by-passes nor undercuts resistances: the resistance and its underlying ego-defense is identified, uncovered, and followed in all its important ramifications. Before therapy is terminated, the hypnotic relationship itself must be analyzed, just as any other positive transference.

Hypnosis may also be used to bring about the disuse of now motiveless habit patterns and to strengthen new and more appropriate ones.

This technique appears to be particularly applicable to states of hysterical disorders and psychosomatic conditions. Also, with patients who form only very tenuous relationships, are overly defensive, given to facile rationalizations, and, thus, need the additional bond of hypnotic relationship and the encouragement to face their problems under a condition where they feel they are less responsible for their thoughts and feelings than in a state of ordinary consciousness; this group includes alcoholics, addicts, other impulse-neurotics, and psychopaths.

Psychotherapy sessions should alternate between sessions at full awareness and hypnotic sessions. One should not proceed from one stage to the next until the goal of that particular stage has been fully integrated into consciousness. One must never use the hypnotic trance to force the patient to confront something consciously which he is not ready to deal with and accept, or the patient's ego integrity will be threatened by overwhelming and unmanageable anxiety. Ego integration takes time, differs from individual to individual, and the pacing must be largely left to the patient.

In dealing with psychosomatic conditions, it is often advisable or necessary to combine the uncovering with a direct-suggestion technique, particularly, when the symptom is serious, as, for example, a peptic ulcer which may perforate the stomach wall. In such cases, direct suggestions can be used advantageously, in conjunction with medication, to control pain, relieve spasms, and to bring about a temporary state of psychological quiescence which will provide optimal conditions for healing. In using such a technique, a number of important cautions must be observed, the discussion of which is beyond the scope of this paper.

For drug addicts, alcoholics, other impulse-neurotics, and psychopaths, group psychotherapy is, in the author's opinion, the therapy of choice, for reasons which have to be elucidated elsewhere. But even group psychotherapy is difficult because these patients tend to go on "verbal jags" about their ego-syntonic symptoms, are relatively fragile and overly defensive, tend to run from therapy as soon as they begin to experience some anxiety, and often form only very tenuous interpersonal relationships. For such patients, group hypnotherapy seems particularly indicated, inasmuch as they establish a stronger therapeutic bond and develop an increasing tolerance for anxiety. Moreover, the hypnotic inquiry is most effective in cutting through the "verbal jags" and in uncovering the psychological reasons for engaging in such "dry drunks."

Before starting hypnotherapy, and particularly group hypnotherapy, a state of deep trance must be firmly established and conditioned to a signal. Before starting induction procedures, the nature of hypnosis, and especially the patients' attitudes toward hypnosis, should be thoroughly discussed, in order to dispel apprehensions, deal with resistances to the use of hypnosis, and in order to subtly reinforce the patients' belief in the possibility and efficacy of the hypnotic trance. This preparatory discussion is an essential and integral part of the induction procedures; without it, many failures may be anticipated.

The induction of the trance is most effectively accomplished in the group setting because the group contagion may be used very effectively to build the belief in the efficacy and reality of the trance. It takes approximately two to three one-hour sessions to firmly establish a somnambulistic trance. No particular method of induction need be followed; on the contrary, familiarity with a variety of methods and the therapist's flexibility to shift from one method to another one seem to be important ingredients for success. By following Mayer's (1943) principle of fractionation, involving the utilization of the patients' own experiences in building the belief in, and thus deepen, the trance state, the latter can be induced efficaciously. Some cautions must be observed. One must not challenge a patient to resist a suggestion until one is certain that he is not able to successfully resist it; otherwise, the group contagion will operate in a negative rather than in a positive direction. It is advisable to have the patients shut their eyes during the induction procedure, so that they are not able to visually observe the other patients. Suggestions should be interspersed with comments which give the patients the impression that the suggestions are effectively carried out by the other patients.

Once the somnambulistic trance is firmly established and conditioned to a signal, a few minutes should be devoted at the beginning of each hypnotic session to reinforcing the trance state, or the trance will flatten out over a period of time.

Before starting with the hypnotherapy proper, the patients should be carefully instructed, during trance, that they will be able to remain in a deep trance state with their eyes open, and that they will be able to move, act, and talk freely and spontaneously. With impulse neurotics and psychopaths, one will also find it advantageous to begin the hypnotherapeutic sessions with an experimental demonstration, by means of a post-hypnotic suggestion, of the mechanism of rationalization, in order to point up the difference between rationalization and motivational causation. Such a demonstration is very convincing and seems to enhance the therapeutic process.

With alcoholics and drug addicts it is often necessary to combine direct suggestions with the uncovering technique. The decrease and eventual disappearance of the desire for alcohol or drugs is suggested directly. Suggestion is also used to endow a harmless substitute with greater potential for gratification than the dangerous agent can provide. Such suggestions must be given repeatedly and must be reinforced throughout therapy.

Time is not available to discuss the cautions which must be observed in following such a technique. It should be clear, however, that no one should attempt it who is not thoroughly trained in psychotherapeutic techniques and who is not familiar with hypnotic techniques and phenomena.

REFERENCES

BORING, E.G. *A History of Experimental Psychology*. New York: Appleton-Century-Crofts, Inc., 1950.

BRENMAN, MARGARET, & Gill, M.M. *Hypnotherapy: A Survey of the Literature*. New York: International Universities Press, 1947.

BRILL, A.A. Introduction. In Freud, S., *The Basic Writings of Sigmund Freud*. New York: Modern Library, Random House, 1938, 3-32.

DORCUS, R.M. & Shaffer, G.W. *Textbook of Abnormal Psychology*. Baltimore: Williams and Wilkins Co., 1945.

FENICHEL, O. *Problems of psychoanalytic technique*. Albany, New York: *Psychoanalytic Quarterly*, Inc., 1939.

FENICHEL, O. *The Psychoanalytic Theory of Neurosis*. New York: W.W. Norton & Co., 1945.

FREUD, S. Early studies on the psychical mechanism of hysterical phenomena. In Freud, S. *Collected papers*, vol. V. London: Hogarth Press, 1952, 25-32. (a).

FREUD, S. Freud's psycho-analytic method. In Freud, S., *Collected papers*, vol. I. London: Hogarth Press, 1953, 264-71. (b).

JENNESS, A. Hypnotism. In Hunt, J. McV. (Ed), *Personality and the behavior disorders,* vol.I. New York: Ronald Press, 1944, 466-502.

LECRON, L. (Ed) *Experimental hypnosis; a symposium of research.* New York: MacMillan, 1952.

LINDNER, R.M. *Rebel without a cause . . . the hypnoanalysis of a criminal psychopath.* New York: Grove Press, 1944.

MAYER, L. *Die Technik der Hypnose.* Munchen/Berlin: J.F. Lehmans Verlag. 1943.

NUNBERG, H. *Practice and theory of psychoanalysis.* Nervous and Mental Disease Monographs Number 74, 1948.

REICH, W. *Character-analysis.* New York: Orgone Institute Press, 1949.

VAN PELT, S.J. *Hypnotism and the power within.* New York: Fawcett Publications, 1956.

WOLBERG, L.R. *Hypnoanalysis.* New York: Grune & Stratton, 1945.

WOLBERG, L.R. *Medical Hypnosis,* vol. I. New York: Grune & Stratton, 1948.

7
Techniques for the Use of Hypnosis in Group Therapy*

Florence Rhyn Serlin[1]

The past decades have provided strong evidence that the group process is a significant therapeutic technique (Mullan and Rosenbaum, 1962; Segrell, 1965; Silver, 1967). Similarly, hypnosis has been utilized in the treatment and management of a wide range of psychiatric and psychological disturbances (Bowers, 1960; Brown, 1965; Cedercreutz and Uusitalo, 1967; Cheek, 1966; Clawson, 1964; Crasilneck, 1968; Edwards, 1960; Fry *et al.*, 1964; Glover, 1959; Gordon, 1955; Gruenewald, 1965; Harding, 1967; Hartland, 1966; Ikemi *et al.*, 1963; Ilovsky, 1962; Jabush, in press; Mann, 1969; Mason and Black, 1963; Miller, 1957; Nuland, 1968; Sacerdote, 1962, 1965; Schneck, 1963; Schowalter, 1958; Scott, 1966; Shapiro, 1963; Smith and Burns, 1960; Solovey and Milechnin, 1958, 1959). Hypnosis also has been employed in the treatment of learning

[1]The author wishes to express her gratitude to Dr. Milton V. Kline for his unstinting advice and suggestions during the preparation of this paper. The author wishes also to express her appreciation to Dr. Nestor J. Totero for his kind permission to utilize Clinic material; and to thank Mrs. Ruth Carroll, Research Assistant, for her attentiveness to detail in the preparation of the manuscript.

disorders, speech disturbances and in rehabilitation therapy (Kroger, 1963; Salzberg, 1963; Weitzenhoffer, 1963). In addition to the heightened suggestibility of hypnosis, the emergence of transference phenomena (Kline, 1965; Totero, 1967; Watkins, 1963) is additionally significant in a group process. Since in the group setting additional difficulties lie relative to the patient's achievement of a strong transference relationship, this factor of more rapid and more intensified transference becomes particularly meaningful. The issue of resistance also becomes significant in the group setting where, for so many patients, there is such great anxiety about maintaining privacy in the threatening situation of group (Kline, 1953).

Hence, the techniques to be discussed in this paper involve particularly the problem of overcoming resistance to—not just the use of hypnosis, but the entire concept of group involvement. Pertinent to this is the fear of hypnosis generally (Alexander, 1967; Watkins, 1963); the fear of being self-revealing to a group generally (Mullan and Rosenbaum, 1962); the fear of being more revealing under hypnosis (Fox, 1960; Peberdy, 1960); and the techniques for managing the above reactions (Dorcus, 1956; Erickson, 1948; Kline, 1965).

RESISTANCE AND ITS MANAGEMENT

Common to both individual and group therapy is the patient's anxiety about the use of hypnosis. In both forms of hypnotherapy he fears loss of control; has anxiety that something might be done to him that he is unaware of while under hypnosis; and fear that the therapist may learn things about him that he may not yet be ready to reveal. In the group process however, the patient has the additional anxiety that others in the group will become aware of material about which the patient still feels an overwhelming sense of privacy and/or fear of self-revelation.

It is therefore particularly important that in the group process the patient achieve a complete sense of reassurance that whatever he experiences under hypnosis will remain a completely private experience; i.e., that his experience while under hypnosis will not come into the awareness of others in the group. To take care of this anxiety, it is frequently most helpful to emphasize prior to induction that the technique (that has been used by the writer) does not involve the patient "saying anything or doing anything" while under hypnosis . . . only that he may think about certain things that the therapist will suggest. Further, it is emphasized that it will be entirely the individual patient's own decision—after the hypnotic trance period is over—as to whether or not he will discuss any of the material that he thought of while under trance.

The anxiety that the patient generally experiences relative to other group members frequently resolves down to a conflict situation. On the one hand, the patient feels anxiety about exposing himself to other members of the group. On the other hand, the patient feels anxiety about his inability to be revealing, being convinced that unless he can be open to the other members of the group, he will receive minimal help from the non-hypnosis group therapy process. In the use of group hypnotherapy techniques, providing assurance about this area proceeds along the same typical paths as in the group therapy process. The usual assurances can be given, and these are usually substantiated by other group members.

EQUATIONS AND METAPHORIC ASSOCIATIONS OF THE HYPNOTIC RELATIONSHIP

The use of hypnosis is of particular value in the group process in relation to the elucidation of. transference phenomena. As has been frequently observed by group therapists, it is not uncommon for there to be a much greater difficulty in establishing a strong transference relationship between the individual patient and the therapist. Hypnosis has been found to be particularly meaningful in establishing strong transference relationships relatively quickly (Watkins, 1963). Hence, in a group process, where the factor of a one-to-one relationship is eliminated by the presence of one (therapist) to several (group members), it is particularly meaningful for the utilization of mechanisms that establish and intensify the strength of transference (which is a significant factor in the process of therapeutic change). In addition, however, to the factor of transference between therapist and group member, there is the significant transference relationships that occur *among* group members. This phenomenon, considered to be maximally meaningful in the group process, is frequently strengthened as a consequence of the experience of similar occurrences . . . in the case of group hypnotherapy, the similar experience being the shared occurrences of the common experience of hypnosis. Hence, the use of hypnosis in this instance may be considered an augmenting factor entirely aside from whatever gains it is assumed hypnosis achieves in the therapy procedure.

A particularly apparent incident of such co-transference being strengthened as a result of mutual experience of hypnosis occurred with a forty-one year old attorney who had sought therapy originally because of homosexual activities. He found such activity totally undesirable in his life, feeling it highly threatening to his marriage, which he wished to maintain. His particular hostilities in his homosexual experiences were usually directed toward the "Wasp" type—"White, Anglo-Saxon, Protestant." This hostility was directed in the group to a young male dancer, also involved in attempting to achieve a heterosexual existence.

The attorney had achieved some insight into the historical bases for the hostility directed against the dancer, but continued to express his feelings of such hostility nevertheless. During a group hypnotic experience, during which the therapist had suggested the members be involved with thinking about material that happened to be particularly charged for the attorney (sibling rivalry and sibling hostility), the attorney spontaneously brought himself out of the trance. It is to be noted that this was something he not infrequently did when the material was too anxiety producing for him. After the other members of the group had been awakened, and following discussion by the dancer of his own early sibling experiences, the attorney stated that "for the first time I feel sort of close to him . . . as a matter of fact, I feel more as if I want to take care of him as if he were my younger brother—or my kid, I guess, more than my brother. I feel maybe he's not so much of a *goy* . . . he could be like any one of the Jewish kids I grew up with—me in fact—going through the same bit. I think if I met him in a turkish bath, maybe I wouldn't try to hurt him so much . . . now. Maybe he *could* know what I'm feeling even if he is a white, Anglo-Saxon, Protestant . . . 'could' know, hell! he does know what I'm feeling; he was as scared as I was, I bet, when we were under. Maybe I could learn something from him, after all, because he had the guts to stay under; he didn't have to wake himself up. . . ."

Obviously, one of the primary values of the kind of phenomenon described above is that the attorney displayed a forward step in his grasping of a discrimination. Whereas initially the dancer represented a culturally-defined sibling (which may be presumed to have been symbolic of a familial sibling relationship), now, with the ability to select out the significant features of the dancer, the attorney was making inroads upon the neurotic behavior of over-generalization, and failure to discriminate. From further discussions during subsequent group meeting, it became increasingly apparent that the initial inroad to his overgeneralization relative to the dancer came as a consequence of a feeling of empathy and of a shared threat, *i.e.*, the hypnotic experience.

OVERCOMING RESISTANCE

Among the resistances most frequently encountered in the group process are those resulting from perception of the group as an invasion of privacy; viewing the group as a recapitulation of the family constellation; the experience of self-contempt as a result of a feeling of rejection by the therapist when group therapy is first suggested; the rejection of other members of the group; fear of the group's irrationalities; fear of investigation by governmental agencies as a result of the patient's revelation of particular material to members of the group who will then "betray" him; concern about group therapy being inferior; and finally, the use of the group as a refuge, so that the individual escapes the intensive interactions which he might not be able to escape in the one-to-one relationship of individual therapy (Mullan and Rosenbaum, 1962).

Some of these factors of resistance appear relatively unaffected by the use of hypnosis in the group therapy process, while others of these resistances may be particularly susceptible to breakdown by the use of hypnosis (Hilgard, 1963; Kline, 1953).

The first of these factors, resistance to the group as an invasion of privacy, may be intensified in a hypnotherapy milieu. It is for this reason that the previously discussed techniques for overcoming such feelings are particularly meaningful. The repetition of the family constellation in the group is one of the primary factors contributing to the success of the group therapy process. Hence, this area is particularly susceptible to augmentation by the use of hypnosis for examining material that initially comes up in the group process while the members are not in trance.

Relative to the area of the patient's self-concept, it is generally the consensus that change here is particularly achieved by the group process, as compared with individual therapy, as a consequence of the process of peer consensual validation. The use of hypnosis in group provides an additional mechanism for achieving a more reality-rooted adult concept, by, for example, suggesting to the patient use of such suggestions while under trance that he recall or visualize or phantasize or day-dream or dream (Kline, 1960; Schneck, 1963) instances in which he was totally successful, totally achieving, totally *pleased* with his handling of a particular situation or individual, etc. Such "ego strengthening" devices not only form a bulwark of positive experiences brought to the patient's attention, but increasingly invalidate his self-concept of total failure.

Illustrative of this phenomenon was an incident with a female patient in her middle thirties. She was a rather attractive woman, though considerably overweight. She had been married and divorced from a man several years before, whom she subsequently concluded had been a homosexual. Their relationship had been warm and loving, but with a virtual absence of sexuality. She had since been involved sporadically in relatively self destructive relationships, clinging to her lovers despite her feeling that the relationships were "masochistic." From her first group session, she expressed an emotional and sexual interest in one of the other group members, whom she knew was a homosexual. Although, on a reality basis, the two patients might be considered a compatible pair (re: age, intellectual level, cultural interests), the man expressed absolutely no interest in her except for concern as a fellow group member. She periodically expressed feelings of being totally rejected "as a woman" despite the emphasis by all of the group members that she was rejected "as a woman" because she had picked a totally unobtainable object for her interest. Go-arounds (suggested by both therapist and various group members, during various sessions) that were aimed at providing for her the information that she was *not* totally rejected as a woman, appeared to have minimal impact upon her. She would always find a way to counter the positive feelings expressed by the group members as being merely expressions designed to avoid hurting her feelings, or quite meaningless because the group member expressing such feelings was "just a kid," or "she's a woman, and knows how I must feel, but if she were a man she would feel just like every other man does," or "they're just not telling the truth! If they said what they really felt, they would say exactly what he (the homosexual patient) said to me." Pressed to repeat exactly what "he" had stated, she would invariably come up with a strong statement implying total rejection, and cling to her (erroneous) perception despite the protests of individuals or the entire group. Further, she would manipulate the homosexual patient into a position where she felt she had corroboration of his rejection of her. For example, during one session, towards the end of the period, she suddenly stated that she wished to express her feelings of deep, deep hurt. She had lost 20 pounds, and he had totally neglected to make any comment about the fact that she had achieved this goal. (It is to be noted that, in fact, the loss of the weight was quite camouflaged by her continuing to wear loose, ill-fitting clothing, and the additional fact that a 20-pound weight loss did not in actuality make a significant difference in her appearance since she was still quite overweight.) When it was pointed out by the group that the weight loss did not and could not, in reality, be expected to alter the homosexual's feelings for her on a sexual level, the patient continued to insist that his failure to make any comment corroborated her feeling that she was totally undesirable as a woman. Some time after this, while under hypnosis, it was suggested to the group that they each recall or visualize (as described in the paragraph above) an instance in which they experienced a feeling of being totally successful, totally achieving. When the group was brought out of hypnosis, she made the statement that she had visualized an episode in which one of her co-workers had expressed an interest in dating her. She had thought also of her former husband. She stated that she was realizing that many of the men with whom she had had affairs were inappropriate, but that these affairs had at least proven to her that she was desirable as a woman. If her husband could not make love to her because of his emotional problems, she was beginning to wonder, could she really blame herself for this? Further, she recognized as a possibility the fact that she chose to become interested in men who could not respond to her and that perhaps her problem was in fact her feelings rather than the objective reality that she was totally undesirable as a woman. Following the hypnotic suggestion, a significant inroad was made which had not been achieved previously despite the "consensual validation" provided by the group members, and despite rounds designed to achieve a more reality-based explanation for her experience of rejection by males in her environment.

In the area of an individual's fear of the group's irrationalities, the degree of help for the patient parallels the degree to which he can begin to see his own irrationalities as a reflection of those in others that he observes. Identification with factors in the personalities of others in the group is maximally strengthened when the patient is involved in examination under trance of those aspects of himself which he has not been particularly aware of, but which he more readily observes as being reflected in the behavior of others. One technique is to suggest to the patient in hypnosis that he reflect upon a past incident through the use of hypnotic imagery and hypnotic dream or phantasy which will reveal ways in which he is similar to other members of the group. Broadly, two kinds of material emerge from this technique. On the one hand, the patient frequently, in discussing the material visualized under hypnosis, will make such statements as: "I never realized it before, but I acted towards X (reality significant relationship) in the same way as so-and-so in the group reacts to me." With this kind of production, the patient has achieved the ability to be more comprehending of some of the reactions he has created in his own significant relationships—very frequently reactions that the patient had previously considered totally unrelated to his own actions. The second type of insight relative to this area of identification with group members is seen in the patient who achieves the realization that someone in the group has elicited reactions from him that are the same as those elicited by significant persons in his actual environment. When these reactions are irrational, and are pointed out by the group members as such, the patient frequently can generalize his clarified behavior in the group to clarified behavior in his larger environment, the outside world. A representative instance of this occurred with a male homosexual patient in his twenties who frequently had hypnotically-induced dreams of himself as a child wearing an immaculate white sweater—and thus unable to be embraced by his father, who was an automobile mechanic. If his father embraced him, his father would get grease all over the little boy's white sweater—and thus would anger the mother. Consequently, it was interpreted, the patient had the strong experience of anxiety relative to any affectional display by his father when he was a child, and to other male authority figures when he was an adult. In group sessions, he would react by withdrawing from those group members who made approving statements to him or about him. When it was suggested to the group that they be involved under hypnosis with phantasies that related to an on-going and deeply disturbing conflict situation, this male patient again had a phantasy about the white sweater. He finished telling the group about the content of the phantasy, stating that he had again experienced "that same old piece,"—and what good did having this information do him? He immediately followed this statement with: "But is that the reason that I couldn't bear my other therapist? He was a very warm man, very feeling—and it would just make me so anxious every time he tried to tell me something about myself that made me seem less of a louse. Maybe that's why I can't stand it when any of you say something decent about where I'm going these days in therapy . . . maybe it's because it sounds too much as if you like me, and might want to embrace me—and it has nothing to do with homosexual anxieties, but just anxieties about some decent guy thinking I'm a decent human being too."

That resistance which may be termed "flight into the group"—that is, resistance to intensive therapy as evidenced by avoidance of the one-to-one relationship—generally is not a factor in those persons who accept involvement in a hypnotherapy technique. This in all probability stems from the inherent concept of the use of hypnosis as being a "magical" methodology. Hence, the probability remains that the individual who seeks hypnoanalysis, whether it be in a group or individual setting, is rarely involved in attempting to escape intensive therapy. In practice, the usual defense mechanisms prevent involvements with material that is too anxiety-producing for the patient. In the use of hypnotic techniques, these defenses may take various forms such as the patient's spontaneous post hypnotic amnesia (Kline, 1966). Or the patient may move into a sleep state and not respond to the instructions of the therapist (Wolberg, 1948). A third form of resistance by the patient may simply be spontaneous awakening from the trance state (Rosen, 1953). The types of material elicited from the patient may be culled forth by such various techniques as suggesting to the patient while under trance that he have a dream about a particular area, that he experience a particular form of imagery, that he recall particular incidents that relate to areas being investigated in the group process, or that he have some thoughts that are associated with specific ideas or feelings. Revivification of past incidents or memories may also be utilized. The subject area suggested by the therapist is that which has been under discussion during the group session prior to the induction of hypnosis, or may be material which the therapist feels is being primarily avoided by the patients. Hypnosis is introduced into the group session when it is felt that the material being examined is too peripheral in effect, or when there is group resistance— *i.e.*, lethargy on the part of the entire group to involvement in particular areas or material. Following termination of hypnosis, the therapist may ask who wished to speak first. Frequently, there will be spontaneous production of the hypnotic material by one or another of the group members, however.

It is to be noted that frequently material that appears to be unrelated to the majority of patients, or related to just one of the patients, does in fact involve material that is significant for the entire group. An instance of this occurred relative to a forty-three year old male teacher who had been involved in a nine-year relationship with a woman that had terminated the previous year. It was at that time that he became involved in therapy. During the first six or so years of this relationship, the patient had refused to marry his mistress, feeling that his primary obligation was to a terminally-ill mother. The patient and his brother lived with the mother and together provided for her support and care. This care had involved a series of operations and a series of additional hospitalizations. The patient felt during that six-year period that his financial obligations to care for his parent were such that he could not form a family of his own. He rejected the significance of the fact that the woman had four children from a previous marriage, and also rejected the reality that these children would continue to be supported by the woman's first husband. In addition, he stated, he never really felt that he could depend on the woman's assurance that the financial factor was not a real obstacle, despite the woman's assurance that she fully intended to continue working after their marriage. For three years after his mother died, the patient continued the relationship with the woman, occasionally mentioning marriage—which the woman by now was rejecting. The affair terminated after nine years when the patient came to his mistress's home and found her in an intimate embrace with another man. The group readily grasped the patient's dependent relationship with his mother, his guilts relative to his mother—both before and after her death, and the patient's rejection of total responsibility for the formation of his own family of wife and children (or step-children). The other group members quite rejected any sense of identification with the patient feeling that since their mothers all happened to be alive—what basis for identification was there with the patient? Under hypnosis, a sufficient number of patients were able to get involved with their own feelings of guilt about death wishes towards the parental figure, both as child and as adult. Additionally, the group as a whole became involved with their dependency needs: their rejection of their parents as the patients had become aware (on either a conscious or unconscious level) of the switch in roles from the parent as the strong figure to be leaned upon to the parent who began increasingly to lean upon the patient (to a major or minor degree, a significant variable in this being the age of the parent and the age of the patients in the group). The significant material that resulted from this post-hypnotic discussion of relationships with the parental figure involved a community expression of ways in which each of the patients had either prematurely terminated a significant interpersonal emotional relationship, or was presently in the process of assuring the termination of such a relationship by an unconscious attack upon or refusal to fulfill the needs of persons in on-going relationships—wife, husband, lover, mistress.

Composition, Session Length, Session Environment

The composition of a hypnotherapy group, as in groups not utilizing hypnosis, may be of two types: according to symptomology, or varied composition. Groups composed according to such symptoms as alcohol addiction (Scott, 1966; Wallerstein, 1958), smoking addiction (Crasilneck, 1968), obesity (Glover, 1959; Mann, 1959) appear highly responsive to both the group process and the use of hypnosis.

It should be noted that severity of maladjustment does not appear to be a precluding factor, in that group therapy and group hypnotherapy have been utilized with relatively severely regressed schizophrenic patients (Bowers, 1960; Scott, 1966).

Certain of the character disorders do not lend themselves readily to grouping by symptom—such character disorders as homosexuality, for example, where it is found that the individuals primarily utilize the group as a social and "mate-finding" medium. On the other hand, homosexuals, whether the homosexuality be ego-syntonic or ego-alien, prove very meaningful members in a varied-composition group, along such typical lines as variability relative to sex, age, socio-cultural background, and diagnostic evaluation.

The use of hypnotherapy lends itself to the typical group therapy session length of about an hour and a half. Some work also has been done in examining group hypnotherapy in a relatively short-term marathon setting of 12 hours.

The typical group therapy setting of circular arrangements of somewhat comfortable chairs has been found adequate. Hypnosis is readily induced when the patient is in a seated position.

INDUCTION TECHNIQUES

A variety of induction techniques have been found equally effective, an induction technique most comfortable for the therapist in all probability being readily utilizable. The use of such techniques as ocular fixation, progressive relaxation, arm levitation, visual imagery—all have been utilized in group. The choice of technique for the writer had been simply that which is found to induce hypnosis in the shortest possible time. Ocular fixation has been found to be particularly successful, augmented by a deepening technique consisting of the therapist's counting from one to ten (preceded by the therapist's instruction that with each number the patient will feel himself drifting to a deeper level of sleep until at the tenth number the patient will feel as deeply relaxed, as deeply asleep as he has ever felt in the therapist's office).

With the group process, it has been found particularly effective to use a progressive relaxation technique, *beginning the induction with the eyes closed.* This eliminates the frequently encountered experience of a new patient being primarily involved with observing the other patients. It also provides an additional element of the experience of "privacy" for each patient in that there is the elimination of the negative experience of being "observed" by others in the group. It should be remembered that the condition of a group situation by itself frequently is a sufficient condition for heightened suggestibility to occur (Freud, 1922). Hence, induction will be a virtually spontaneous occurrence. The occurrence of heightened suggestibility in a group is encountered in a variety of situations. One common example is the heightened suggestibility that results in spontaneous mob action, to cite a negative instance; or the heightened suggestibility that results in mystical beliefs, stemming as far back as the ancient pagan temple and, obviously, on occasion viewed in our modern environments. Thus, it can readily be seen that the expectation of the group members who are in a group hypnosis situation would similarly result in the individual himself aiding the achievement of a group expectation . . . namely induction of hypnosis. It should be noted, a somewhat more protracted induction period is invarably required, when a new member joins a group (as is so during the first few sessions with a patient in individual hypnotherapy).

"EMERGENCY" OCCURRENCES

On occasion one of the group members may experience a particularly distressing reaction to the hypnotic experience. He may become visibly agitated, or obviously be experiencing a reaction of such intensity that the therapist may not be willing to have him continue to experience without individual attention. Under such circumstances, it is frequently advisable for the therapist to remove that patient from the group therapy room. Since there is usually at least some level of awareness on the part of the other hypnotized patients, it is advisable for the therapist to announce to the patients that they may hear the therapist leaving the room, and that there is nothing to be concerned about, that the therapist is leaving for a very brief period of time, and that the patients are to continue being involved in the thinking that they are experiencing. If the patient who is to be removed from the room has spontaneously terminated hypnosis for himself, the therapist then signals him silently to follow him, and the two leave the room. The therapist is then able to administer to him individually and ameliorate that which is occurring for the patient. If the patient to be given this individual attention is in a trance state, the therapist would add in his general statement to the group that he is going to be leaving the room with so-and-so and that he is asking so-and-so to come with him outside of the therapy room so that they may take care of something for a moment. Once outside the group room the therapist can manage the individual patient's stress reaction to the hypnotic experience. An instance of this occurred with a fifty-four year old female patient who had entered therapy primarily because of her feeling that certain physical symptoms had a psychological base. The somatic distress about which she was particularly concerned was the loss of her hair. Although there was a long history of glandular dysfunctioning, with which a loss of hair was entirely consistent, the patient was convinced that, in addition, a psychological factor of self-destructive drives was operating. During previous sessions, material had been discussed which involved the death of a playmate when the patient was three or four years of age. Although these facts had been discussed at length during the previous sessions, there had previously been no connection of this material with the patient's distress about the abundance and texture of her hair. (It should be noted that during her adolescence and youth, her hair represented her "crowning glory" as a consequence of the patient's great emotional investment in this feature of her beauty.) During a hypnotic session in which the group was instructed, while under hypnosis, to think about, or dream about, or phantasize about that which was most significant in relation to their most troubling present problem, this patient began to experience a particularly dramatic abreaction. Her entire body began to tremble, and she appeared to be shaking with sobs that she was obviously attempting to keep at as silent a level as possible out of consideration for the rest of the group. It was also apparent, nevertheless, that some of the other patients in the group were becoming aware of her reactions, and general indications of agitation appeared that had not previously been apparent when they were under hypnosis in a group situation. Therefore, out of attentiveness to both the patient's abreaction and out of concern for the other patients in the group, the therapist felt it necessary to deal with the individual patient immediately. Since it was felt that the other members of the group had not completed their thinking relative to the therapist's suggestions, it was not considered profitable to terminate the hypnotic trance for the entire group, in order to deal with the individual patient. As a consequence, the previously described technique was utilized and the patient was taken to an outer office (with the door left open between the two offices so that the therapist could maintain knowledge of occurrences in the group).

It was at that time that the patient who had been so agitated explained to the therapist that she had suddenly experienced an emotionality that she had had as a child while watching her playmate's funeral procession (which had passed in front of the patient's home). The material she had suddenly become aware of was a typical childhood reaction of feeling intense guilt at the time of the other child's death. The guilt was the typical reaction following some previous expressions of anger toward the other child when they had been playing together. This had caused the patient to believe that she had omnipotently caused her friend's death. Following the ventilation of this material, the patient and the therapist returned to the group room, the therapist concluded the trance period for the rest of the group, and there was a general discussion of the material experienced under hypnosis by the other members of the group (as well as that experienced by the particular patient under discussion). Discussion of the group's reaction to the therapist's leaving the room with the patient revealed as correct the therapist's conclusions that some of the patients had been aware while under trance of the extreme agitation of one member in the group, had themselves become agitated, and had felt reassurance from the realization that when such an instance occurred—even in a group situation—an individual was "taken care of," and that they could "count on" the therapist's attention no matter what the circumstances of therapy (*i.e.*, individual or group sessions). And, finally, they reported that due to the therapist's assurance that he would be remaining within "contact," their feeling of anxiety rapidly diminished within a few moments of the therapist's leaving the room.

An additional instance where it was felt that an individual patient should be removed from the group therapy situation while that group was in a trance state occurred when a patient, under trance, was apparently feeling great rage, and where the expression of his rage—pounding on the arms of his chair, and increasingly loud muttering—was becoming apparent to the other patients. In this instance the patient was removed from the therapy room primarily out of concern for the other members in the group. The patient was a thirty-one year old male school teacher, who had as a major problem both his denial of the experience of hostile feelings, as well as, obviously, expression of such denied affect. For example, he had spoken in the group of his mild phobic reaction to knives, and his tremendous anxiety about blood. It was generally recognized in the group that this patient had a rather severe problem relative to permitting himself the *experience* of feelings of anger because of his very great fearfulness that he would be assaultive in expressing such anger—should he become aware of such feelings. When this patient began to pound the arms of his chair and to mutter with increasing volume, some of the other patients appeared to display increasing agitation—which may have been connected with their own hypnotically induced thinking, but more probably appeared to be an anxiety reaction caused by the patient's acting-out behavior. The therapist then made the statement that one of the group members appeared to be quite upset by something he was thinking about, and that the therapist and that group member were going to leave the room. In this instance, the patient was still under hypnosis. He was taken to an outer office; the hypnosis was terminated with proper precautionary injunctions, and then the therapist and patient rejoined the group. Afterwards, discussion of this event corroborated that several members under hypnosis had been quite aware of the patient's acting-out, had begun to feel increasing anxiety about being personally attacked, and had experienced a sense of relief over the patient's leaving the room, as well as anxiety reduction with the conviction that the therapist could and would "protect" the group.

INTRODUCTION OF HYPNOSIS

The use of hypnosis has generally been found most effective in the group process under one of two circumstances: when resistance is so high in the group that only a superficial level of interaction that cannot be broken down is occurring and secondly, when the material being discussed by the group is of such moment that it would be particularly meaningful to probe into material that might be available only at unconscious levels of awareness. Hence, the group session would begin in the usual and orthodox manner of permitting group members to come to a level of interaction with each other. Whichever may be the motivation for the induction of hypnosis—resistance, or the propitiousness of the moment for examining material on a more intensive level—

the therapist suggests that this might be a good time for the use of hypnosis, and the induction is begun. The induction procedure incorporates the four points that: (a) it is "perfectly safe to go deeper and deeper into sleep," because the patient knows that he will not be asked to do anything or to say anything until after he is awake, and then he will talk about what he thought of *only* if he decides to do so; (b) he feels very comfortable about letting himself go deeper and deeper into sleep because he knows that if any of the material he is thinking about becomes upsetting to him, all he has to do is open his eyes and he will be fully awake; (c) he will not remember what he had been thinking about until he wishes to, and; (d) he feels very relaxed about letting himself go deeper and deeper to sleep because he knows that any material that is too anxiety-producing to him or too frightening or too upsetting, will not be remembered for the present.

MATERIAL ELICITED BY HYPNOSIS

The kinds of material that may be readily elicited through the use of hypnosis in the group process may be roughly fitted into two areas: first, the relation between primary and secondary material; and secondly, the balance between cognitive and affective responses. Fitting within these two categories are such areas of material as information about the patient (including historical material); attitudes toward significant other; modes that a patient utilizes in dealing with his environment; elaboration of group discussion material that had been examined during the waking state; emotion and affect; genuine feelings; cognitive mechanisms used by the patient; the patient's needs (drives); abstractions; neurotic feelings; the patient's self-image; and ego integrative and ego supportive material.

The most frequently used techniques for obtaining material in the categories listed above generally follow those techniques which are common to the mode of hypnotherapy generally (Field and Dworkin, 1967; Fromm, 1965; Kline, 1963; Meares, 1960; Wolberg, 1948). For example, it may be suggested to the patient that he will have a dream or phantasy or imagine himself sitting in a theatre watching a stage play which will be concerned with a specific theme; he will recall his earliest memory of a scene involving particular material; he is looking at a sky full of clouds and knows that a slight wind is coming up which will blow the clouds away, and that when the clouds are blown away he will see clearly revealed a scene that is at present hidden by the clouds, and which will clarify an idea or feelings; he is writing a story about a particular incident, and will now imagine how the story ends; the therapist is going to make a series of statements and the patient will immediately have a thought relating to the answer to such statements.

ELICITATION OF GROUP DISCUSSION
MATERIAL

To obtain material that may be discussed meaningfully by the group, the suggestion may be made that the patient visualize a scene that will provide him with some information or clues as to the most significant problem area for him at the present time. Alternatively, the suggestion may be made that he visualize a scene involving information that would be most helpful for him to discuss in the group at the present time. Or the patient may be involved with material relating to what he does that he is most ashamed of, whom he loves most, and least, whom he feels greatest anger towards.

Additional areas that may be examined under hypnosis are feelings of love, rage, depression, anxiety—in other words, instructions to be involved under trance with affect material. This kind of material is particularly amenable to visualization of a scene that relates to "what seems most frightening to me" or "what is most anxiety producing for me." It is frequently helpful when involved with such material that the patient be told, prior to the instructions for the scene, that he will visualize the scene but *not necessarily* re-experience the emotion that was or is attendant, in contrast, obviously, to the previously discussed technique of the affect bridge. In view of the fact that the therapist is involved with a number of patients in a group, as contrasted with individual therapy in which the therapist can readily provide total attention for his patient, it sometimes becomes a necessity to minimize levels of emotionality induced by the material introduced in trance. Since the re-experience of emotion is of major significance, if such emotionality is not experienced during the discussion period following trance, there may be reintroduction of this material during future trance states with the expectation that with "familiarity" the patient will be more readily able to cope with the level of affect which he experiences— and which the therapist can handle in a group situation.

ELICITATION OF MODES OF DEALING
WITH THE ENVIRONMENT

To obtain material in the area of modes of dealing with the environment, the patient must be involved with examination of how he interacts with significant others; how he tries to protect himself in his environment; how he deals with his aggressions.

In order to achieve change relative to such material, the patient may have suggested to him, under hypnosis, that he imagine three scenes: first, himself as he would ordinarily act in a particular situation; secondly, himself as he would most efficiently handle the same situation;

and finally, himself as he could most closely approximate the ideal in the same situation (second scene, above).

Similarly, when the patient has expressed extreme anxiety in a reality situation that should not have yielded such intensity of anxiety, hypnosis is particularly valuable for obtaining information to explain what might in effect be a "transference" situation. Watkins (1963) describes this technique, and terms this use of hypnosis for ascertaining the meaning of a symptom, the "affect bridge."

In this technique attention is focused on the affect, and the affect is intensified. A clinical example of this is the case of a patient (previously discussed) who experienced such extreme anxiety about the texture and thickness of her hair. Of significance is the fact that the patient had placed all of her feelings about her own personableness upon the single feature of lush, beautiful, thick hair. Despite group discussions that everyone's hair fell out somewhat when combed, that this was a natural process, and that her hair appeared sufficiently abundant, the patient continued to discuss feeling virtually a panic reaction during the daily ritual of combing her hair and finding strands entangled in her comb. Under hypnosis she was instructed to feel this panic, to experience an intensification of this panic, to permit the particular environment slowly to fade away, to permit recall of the precipitating event (hair entangled in her comb) to fade away and to feel only a greater and greater intensification of the panic she experienced. The patient was then instructed to let fade away the present, the room in which she spent her mornings, to forget where she was, how old she was, what year this was. (She is going back, back in time and experiencing only the extreme panic she had discussed. She is going back, back and only her extreme panic is constant. She is going back to some time when she experienced the same feelings: How old is she? Where is she?) The patient then began to talk about her feelings when she was a little girl: feelings that her daddy loved her because she was so pretty, and that if she were *not* pretty—if she soiled her dress, or if she mussed her hair, or if she got as old as her mommy was . . . would daddy still love her? Sometime later in her childhood, when the patient was in fact hospitalized for an illness, and her father rarely came to visit her (because visiting hours were in conflict with his own work hours, primarily), there had been an exacerbation of this anxiety about losing her father's love if she were ugly: in the hospital, no pretty little frocks, no pretty little hair ribbons in her hair. Quite obviously, an illness that affected the patient's "crowning glory" could be expected to provide anxiety for her and distress about her personableness; however, the degree of panic that this patient experienced relative to difficulties with her hair, must have additional meaning for her. In this instance, the additional meaning was an anxiety about loss of support, loss of protectiveness—and it may be speculated—loss of the struggle in the oedipal conflict. As Watkins points out, "When utilizing this technique any affect, lust, rage tenderness, etc. may be used as the vehicle between the present situation and the earlier experience. We select for such investigation those affects which seem to be inappropriate in the present situation, and hence, are probably transferred from early experiences. The "affect bridge" is a kind of semi-free association except that the common element that connects Experience A and the present with Experience B and the past is an affect, or feeling, not a thought or intellectual mental contact [Watkins, 1963]."

Intensifying the experience of affect, as Rosen (1960) also points out, can be of particular value with patients experiencing real or apparent medical or surgical disease, who had been organically ill for a considerable number of years. When this factor of actual organic disease occurs in a patient who experiences a little motivation for psychotherapy or defends himself by becoming convinced that his motivation for psychotherapy is a factor which, in actuality, is quite peripheral—the use of hypnosis for phantasy evocation is particularly significant. A clinical case fulfilling these characteristics is that of an attorney (n.b.: *not* the previously discussed case) who had come to psychotherapy because he felt that he was not utilizing his full potential, as evidenced by minimal earnings for someone with his capabilities, years of experience, and obligations.

This patient was sufficiently sophisticated psychologically to be able to accept the fact that there must be psychological factors involved with his disappointing yearly income, but maintained a conviction that it was his income level primarily which he wished to have ameliorated in therapy. Quite casually he discussed the fact that in his early twenties he had experienced a massive cerebral hemorrhage, which resulted in such sequelae as a considerably atrophied right arm and leg. The patient walked with a decided limp, but maintained that he was "fully adjusted" to these physical aspects. He maintained blandly that the consequences of the stroke did not in any way interfere with any aspect of his functioning; his marital relationship was excellent; he had no anxiety about his functioning or image as a "male;" his interactions with his family were fine; his interactions with his children were optimal; and he had many friends with whom he had fine relationships. Totally rejected by the patient were the group's suggestions that he had any anxiety about the possibility of a second stroke, that he viewed himself in any way inadequately, that he was at all distressed by his limp, or that he experienced any negative feelings toward his parents based on underlying anger that a "genetic weakness" had been a significant factor in his having a stroke at the rather tender age of 20 or 21. He maintained a rather bland response to the comments of the other members of the group that he *must* have some self concepts of being a "cripple." A breakthrough in this well-defended area finally occurred when the patient (along with the other members of the group) was instructed under hypnosis to visualize himself first as he was; secondly, as he would like to be, and thirdly, as he could be (*i.e.*, actual, idealized, and real selves). Of great impact upon the patient was his phantasy of his "idealized" self; the patient visualized a rather monstrous figure, half of which was miniscule in its distortion, a face pock-marked and with oozing sores, and a dismembered phallus. In discussing this material following the hypnotic period, the patient's affect was one of incredulity as well as depression: "I had no idea that's how I saw myself." Rather rapidly thereafter the patient was able to acquire a more reality-rooted concept of himself, with an ability to recognize the actuality of certain physical handicaps. Subsequently, he was able to reconstruct a self-image that included his actual capacities, as opposed to a self-image that exaggerated the incapacities that had become excessive in his repression of any conscious consideration of anatomical distortions. Hence, it might be conjectured that in this instance, hypnosis served the purpose of intensifying affect to enable movement from unawareness to awareness of repressed material which had in actuality been the real motivation for his seeking therapy . . . with his income level quite obviously being merely the material that the patient could permit into his awareness, in order to eliminate the extreme discomfort over material of which he never permitted himself to become aware.

In this area of self-image, such additional hypnotic techniques as the following may be utilized to achieve more accurate self-image or a more competently coping self.

The patient's self-image may be examined under hypnosis by having the patient first imagine the role he feels most comfortable playing, followed by seeing himself as others see him; then by seeing himself as he really is, finally, by seeing himself as he is capable of becoming. Involved in this area may be elicitation of phantasizing or dreams or scenes in which the patient sees himself in a situation that makes him feel most competent, as contrasted with situations in which the patient feels most inadequate. This may then be followed by the patient being asked to visualize a scene in which he handled everything "just perfectly," in which he displayed absolutely magnificent decision-making behavior, and followed through. It is frequently helpful to have the patient follow this by visualizing the same scene, but with the patient performing in a manner that is totally inadequate. Invariably, the patient then recognizes that he does not, in fact, function at such an inadequate level, and again a more accurate self-image results. Concomitant with such material might be the elicitation of hypnotically induced material relating to ways in which the patient feels he is "different" from what he would like to be, leading to the subsequent steps of seeing how he can eliminate such differences from his actual self. Of frequent usefulness is examination of ways in which the patient feels he shares characteristics with other group members. This kind of material obviously heightens identification with group members by intensifying feelings at an increased level for others in the group, as well as providing the obvious basis for more accurate self evaluation. Frequently, the recognition of genuine feelings follows, first, to other members of the group, and ultimately, to significant persons in the patient's "real" environment. This area is obviously of maximum significance in the facilitation of group process as well as in actual existence. Techniques include involvement under hypnosis of the patient's real feelings towards other group members; towards absent group members; towards new members.

Illustrative of this aspect of the use of hypnosis in examining all the facets of emotionality towards other group members was one patient who became extremely hostile whenever a new member joined the group. This patient was involved with attempting to minimize homosexual activity, and he readily explained that he felt angry when there were new members in the group because of his own embarrassment about revealing his homosexual activities. This seemed a readily acceptable explanation, but under hypnosis an additional motivation for his anger appeared; his feelings of inadequacy and worthlessness invariably resulted in the conviction that everyone else would be liked more than he. Hence, a new member in the group always constituted a potential threat to whatever position he achieved among the group members. In a word, very strong sibling rivalry was a more meaningful and complete explanation of this patient's rejection of new group members. Interestingly enough, this patient also would display extreme hostility to any member of the group who began discussing terminating with the group. The facile explanation that this represented a desertion of him by the terminating group member had elements of accuracy to it. In addition, however, a member leaving the group also represented for this patient the loss of an individual whose esteem he had finally earned.

Similarly, the emotions felt by members of the group about members who are absent very frequently also may reveal deeply repressed transference feelings. An instance of this occurred with a patient who was 45, married, the father of two children, and whose parents and older brothers were still meaningful in his life. Characteristic of this patient was his extremely angry expression of resentment over the absence of any group members, including an absence of a member who rarely failed to be at the meetings. The patient stated that his anger stemmed from the fact that it was "a waste of my time" every time a member was absent, because when the member did appear there would be required a recapitulation of the previous session's content. The other members of the group pointed out to him that it was rare for such a request to be made by a member when he missed a session, and that should such a request be made, the angry patient's response could always be a refusal to permit such recapitulation. Further statements were offered by other group members relative to the probability that the patient was, in fact, expressing a transferred affect, that he was experiencing feelings of rejection that in actuality belonged to significant other persons in his life. Invariably the patient would reject all such statements, insisting that his position and feelings were quite reasonable and reality-based and related to the present circumstances only. During a hypnotic session, it was suggested to the patients that they be involved with thinking of the time in their lives when they felt most "lost," most sad, most alone. During the discussion following hypnosis, this patient revealed that he had seen himself sitting alone in the therapy room—no other group members, no therapist, no secretarial force in the outer office, no other furniture except the chair in which he was sitting. Following this discussion, group hypnosis was again induced; and the "affect bridge" technique was utilized with the group. The patient recalled a time when he was a little boy and his family was moving to another city. He visualized himself standing alone in an empty room. In the discussion following the hypnotic period, the patient recalled that when he was a little boy, and, in fact, the family was moving, there was a moment when he had been left alone in the apartment while his parents were involved with directing the moving men. He recalled a moment of panic, wondering where his brothers were, although—in the present, in discussing the incident—he stated, "I must have known that it was just that everybody was being packed into the car and my brothers were already in the car, that my mother and father had just been called away by the moving men . . . in fact, I think the reason that I was still in the apartment was that I'd been in the car with my brothers and then I said that I had to go to the bathroom, and my mother took me back into the apartment so that I could go to the bathroom. We were just walking in when one of the moving men called from outside, maybe to sign the moving order or something. I don't think I was there for more than two minutes, but I think I got scared and thought they were going to forget I was still there and everybody would drive away and I didn't even know where we were moving to, and I wouldn't be able to tell anybody, and they would forget they had left me behind. . . ." The patient subsequently was readily able to associate this incident with his feelings of extreme anger over absent, as well as terminating, group members who, in effect, were "deserting" him.

ELICITATION OF MECHANISMS USED

The author's experience has been that insight into the mechanisms used by patients occurs primarily during the group discussion period (following the termination of the hypnotic period). Here, again, this is typical for the group therapy process; hence, hypnosis is utilized primarily for the elicitation of material that can subsequently be subjected to group scrutiny. As in any group process, a particularly valuable area of examination is that of the defense mechanisms.

An instance of projection, for example, was dramatically illustrated, by the attorney group member previously discussed. This is a man who very frequently characterized other members of the group as being "very vicious." He rarely displayed strong antipathy toward any of the group members, however. With the entrance of a new member, also an attorney, he very quickly verbalized strong hostility towards the second attorney. There did not appear to be any reasonable, reality-based reasons for the great hostility displayed by the first attorney; the new attorney member was also relatively unsuccessful as far as professional position was concerned—he had entered therapy because of a recognition that his earnings were markedly lower than they should be for him; the second attorney was physically incapacitated as a result of a cerebral hemorrhage during his youth; and he was a relatively pleasant as well as a relatively constricted person. The attack undertaken by the first attorney primarily took the form of sarcasm relative to the second attorney's professional capabilities. During one session, the first attorney challenged the second to a legalistic "duel"—setting up a legal situation and challenging the second attorney to circumvent the first attorney's legalistic maneuverings for this hypothetical case. Asked what there was about the second attorney that he disliked so much, the first attorney merely continued reiterating, "I don't like him, that's all. I just don't like him!" During a subsequent session, when patients were asked to imagine themselves under hypnosis as they "are," the first attorney visualized himself standing outside a public bath-house, which he was in the habit of occasionally frequenting when unable to control his drives for homosexual contact (the reader may recall that this patient was married and deeply involved in conflict about his occasional homosexual activities). During the discussion period following the hypnotic part of the session, the first attorney stated, "I guess that's why I hate his guts so much—because actually I see myself as he is—a cripple. He's crippled physically—but I'm crippled emotionally. I guess I've been putting on to him all of the feelings I have about myself. I guess I don't have to tell you what those feelings are about myself."

An illustration of another mechanism occurred when the mother of one of the patients died. During the session following the parent's death, the patient was provided extreme support by all the members of the group, except one. During that session, and the next several, the non-supportive group member's behavior consisted of covert attempts to terminate the discussion about the death of the other patient's parent by bringing in material that was unrelated, by questioning the bereaved patient about details that were quite insignificant, and by offering neither attentiveness nor solicitude. This behavior was rather rapidly picked up by the other members of the group, who began questioning the rejecting patient about his cursory level of involvement with the sadness of the bereaved patient. The reasons presented by the rejecting patient for this behavior were that he found it too upsetting to talk about the death of a parent—any parent—because of his own great affection for his mother, and his anxiety about her continued well-being. The conclusion of the group, therefore, was that the rejecting patient was involved with his own great anxieties and, therefore, that his rejection of the bereaved patient's ventilating was based on his own "hang ups," and a good bit of sympathy was extended to him. During a subsequent hypnotic period, the rejecting patient visualized himself standing by his own mother's coffin (n.b.: this patient's mother was still alive). In later discussion of this visualization, the patient made the statement that the only thing that was incomprehensible to him was that he felt no emotion as he stood and looked down at his mother's body in the coffin. It is to be noted that this was a patient very much involved with what was "right"; it was not "right" to be disloyal to one's family, and therefore it was not "right" to talk about any of his brother's cruelties to him when they were boys: it was not "right" to talk about negative aspects of his own ethnic group; it was not "right" to attack the therapist (after all, the therapist was taking on everybody else's problem, worked hard, was feeling, must be expected to make a few mistakes along the way; and so it wasn't "right" to talk about these mistakes . . . and, besides, mistakes were *not* made). And, quite obviously, it could not be "right" for this patient to be aware of, much less verbalize, negative feelings about his mother. He was able to rationalize his visualization of his mother in her coffin as being a consequence of his anxiety and fearfulness of such an occurrence. He could not rationalize the lack of affect he experienced while looking at his mother's body. In subsequent sessions, however, he became increasingly aware of the feelings that he had totally repressed, which had resulted in the full-blown reaction formation epitomized by total denial of negative, hostile, and aggressive feelings toward his mother. He was able ultimately to accept the fact that he could have negative feelings toward a parent, that such negative feelings were not the totality of feelings toward that parent, that he did not have to deny his anger toward the parent in order to maintain his feelings of love also for that parent. Ultimately, he was able to reconcile and accept the apparently conflicting emotions of great anger as well as great love . . . and that it was indeed "very right" to know and accept quite conflicting sentiments toward a parent, his wife, his children, his brothers, his peers.

ELICITATION OF NEEDS

Of major value in the use of hypnosis is the elicitation of material relative to the patient's needs or drives.

Most prominent of the needs invariably discussed in the therapy situation is the patient's need for nurturance, his needs for the fulfillment of nurturant requirements on the most elementary level. The dominance of this need was displayed during a session in which a new member joined the group. This was a twenty-eight year old woman who had entered therapy because of her pattern of choosing lovers considerably younger than herself. One of the most significant relationships had been recently terminated with the death of the young man. She had been twenty-seven; he had been seventeen, and their involvement had begun when the boy was just fifteen years old and the patient twenty-five. This material had been provided for the group during the first fifteen or so minutes of the first session that the patient attended. The statements by the other group members relative to the inappropriateness of this relationship were countered by the young woman's insistence that "he was the most grown-up man I have ever known." It was readily apparent that the patient was still in intense mourning for the boy; and she corroborated this by saying that "no other man will ever take care of me like he did . . . he wasn't a boy; he was a man; and he knew how to take care of a woman." Asked by the members of the group how the youth could possibly have "taken care of" the patient's emotional needs, the young woman retorted, "He made me feel safe with him. He made me feel that he would fight the whole world for me. He made me feel that he would love me and take care of me and be there for me until the day I died!" This feeling on the part of the patient led into hypnosis under which it was suggested to the patients that they be involved with the visualizations, phantasies, thoughts, that related to what each patient felt he "needed" in a marital partner or lover. Rather significantly, the young woman readily went into a deep trance (despite the fact that this was her first session). Following the therapist's instructions, she quickly began to sob and within a few moments was sobbing heart-rendingly. It is to be noted that obviously suitable instructions were made at this point to the group by the therapist, to the effect: "As you must be aware, one of the group members is very upset; however, nothing is going to happen to her; the therapist is still in the room; the therapist is handling the situation caringly; you will continue to be involved with the thinking that you were involved with, knowing that in a few minutes, when everyone is awake, we will be able to help the upset group member as well as you, and nothing is going to happen that cannot be handled by the therapist."

When the patients were awakened, the young woman quickly stopped crying and quite brightly said, "All I kept thinking of was 'I want a daddy; I want a daddy!'" The patient quickly added that the incongruity of this must be apparent to everyone, in view of the fact that the man she'd been so much in love with was so much younger than she, and everyone had always told her that she was involved with him in a "mothering" relationship—so obviously her yearning for a strong parental figure was totally unrelated to her proclivity for choosing lovers so much younger than herself. Questioning by the group obtained the historical material from the patient that her father had been executed in Poland for political reasons when she was an infant, that her mother had subsequently married a number of times, with one of the step-fathers having served as a significant father surrogate for the patient. The patient had always felt strongly competitive with the mother, describing her as exceedingly beautiful and charming. The typical dynamics of the patient having felt the need for a protective father figure was apparent to the patient and other group members as well. But remaining was the question of how this need tied in with the patient's choice of a mate . . . whose extreme youth precluded his serving as a strong, giving figure who could fulfill nurturant needs for her. The answer to this seeming puzzle became apparent with the patient's examination of her own feelings of worthlessness resulting from feelings of "desertion" and "rejection" by the series of "fathers"—beginning with her natural father's death. Such feelings of worthlessness resulted in fearfulness of being unable to hold onto a suitable father figure; the patient's maladaptive adjustment to this was always to select figures whom she felt she *could* hold on to, in this instance a youth, followed by a series of youths. This patient's need for both nurturance and a sense of security relative to the figure she chose resulted in distortions of perception to the degree that she convinced herself that her needs were being fulfilled despite the obvious fact that this was an impossibility. The patient further protected herself from accepting the reality of this impossibility by rationalizing: "I kept thinking while we were going together that all I had to do was wait for him to be a little older just in years, so that the world would let him take care of me the way that he was able to take care of me. And the ones who came after him—well something always happened, and the affair always ended, and I never really had to look at how *in*capable they were. . . except sexually."

The significant occurrence that led to this insight for the patient was her involvement under hypnosis in a regression experience. Regression is quite commonly a first step in any therapeutic interaction (Kline, 1963). Such regression invariably consists of and includes repetitious re-enactments of infantile relationships. Such re-enactments in the individual's external environment frequently cause trouble. Such re-enactments within the therapy room are primary aims of therapy, so that the individual can achieve insight into his modes of behavior, the immature level of such modes, and understanding of these re-enactments as the cause of difficulties in adult interpersonal relationships. The cliché about a square nut encountering a square bolt is a cliché which rarely results in adaptive adult relationships. But for the individual to acquire recognition that his behavior is that of blind attempts to resolve infantile relationships, the therapy room must serve as a place where he can display this behavior, have it pointed out to him, and become increasingly aware that this behavior exists. The obvious second step is the forgoing of such regressive behavior, and reconstruction of the ego on adult levels. The case just cited presents the patient's attempt to achieve relationships on a level that is consistent with childhood and totally inconsistent with the achievement of a complete and meaningful adult relationship. For the patient to have sought a "father figure" in a man chronologically and emotionally mature, it might be argued, would have been adaptive. For the patient to have sought a "father figure" in the very immature men with whom she felt confident she could cope . . . was quite apparently maladaptive in that a fulfilling "father figure" could hardly have been provided by her young lovers.

The need for nurturance frequently is displayed even more dramatically with the acquisition of symptoms. This was illustrated with a patient who had as her presenting complaint kleptomania. This symptom was not so overwhelming as to result in her being involved in serious legal difficulties. She had, however, become concerned enough about the symptom so that she had spoken to her parents about it and begged them for help. She had been about sixteen when the symptom was first manifested. She described her parents thus: "My father was a drunk, and my mother wanted to keep him that way, because then he always needed her to take care of him whenever he was off on a binge. Everybody begged her to have him hospitalized, and she never would do it—she wanted him to need her." During hypnosis the patient had visualized herself pilfering in a department store. Discussion of the material following the trance led the patient to the insight that her mother, being so involved with the care of her father, "didn't have time for me. But the first time that I told her I needed some therapy—help of *some* kind, because for months I had been stealing from department stores and I'd almost gotten caught that day—she sure had time to pay attention to me!" The patient's initial conclusion was simply that the stealing had been an attention-getting device. Subsequent examination of this material led the patient to the realization that, more than an attention-getting device, the objects she stole "gave me something—I don't know if it gave me something I wasn't entitled to, or if it was just that then I could go to sleep at night with—at least—some new lipstick under my pillow instead of a goodnight kiss, because my mother was so busy with my father's hangover."

It is, incidentally, almost a universal that a person—patient or not—has pilfered at some time during his life. This forms the basis for guilt feelings in a relative number of patients. This area of discussion readily leads into a discussion of the means used to substitute and to compensate for feelings of emotional deprivation, first in the early family constellation, and later in subsequent relationships. For example, the patient just discussed had—at the age of 30—become quite involved again with thinking about her previous experience of pilfering . . . at just about the time that she began to be exceedingly concerned about her husband's continued rejection of her sexually.

Concomitantly, material may be elicited involving hypnotically-induced scenes relating to feelings of being totally "cared for," totally supported. The therapist may suggest examination of: whom does the patient most want to take care of him; what feelings as a child did the patient have of being rejected, or least loved—"Recall a scene when you first felt least loved by your mother or father." Next might be an instruction to the patient to imagine a scene depicting parental figures first as they are, and then as the patient would like his parents to be or to have been. The instruction may then be to visualize a scene depicting how a "good" mother gives to a child, as contrasted with how a "bad" mother fails a child. This obviously can then be followed by scenes the patient recalls from his own childhood in which his parents fulfilled each of the above categories.

The connection between the childhood expectations regarding the parental figure and the expectation of nurturance from the marital partner became apparent for the patient last discussed as a consequence of the examination of the pilfering behavior seen as attempts by her to substitute for that nurturance which she had not received as a child from her mother . . . and again failed to receive when an adult, from her husband. In her youth, pilferage actually occurred; as an adult, ideation relative to pilferage was involved. The maladaptiveness of this substitute for behavior that would fulfill her nurturant needs ultimately became apparent to the patient.

Other basic drives may be examined similarly. Fowler (1965) has presented the position that there is a single, basic drive of the organism, and that that drive is the exploratory drive—*i.e.*, the drive for change, for variability, for that which is "new" in the environment. At the present time, this may still be considered merely a hypothetical position; but, nevertheless, this possibility provides much to examine in the therapeutic process. The patient's self-defeating and self-destructive attempts to reach goals which in actuality the patient must recognize as being meaningless become readily apparent under hypnosis. Such maladaptive functioning is readily recognized in behavior such as the individual's infidelities that threaten his marriage, when in actuality he wishes to maintain his marriage, or in the patient who engages in behavior which will probably result in the loss of a position at a time when he, in actuality, cannot afford to lose that position (as contrasted, for example, with the more efficient behavior of making the decision to leave a position, taking steps to secure a new position that is more advantageous, and then resigning from the first position). Can such behavior be ascribed to a basic drive for exploration, *i.e.* change of any kind? This remains a moot question at the present time. However, manifestations of such a drive (should it in fact exist) are frequently observed in the therapy situation. An obvious therapeutic goal is to have the patient achieve gratification of such a drive in a constructive manner rather than in a self-defeating and self-destructive mode of achieving change. More familiar theoretically-expounded drives such as the drive for sexual gratification can also be examined—in an adaptive, efficient mode, as contrasted with totally self-destructive attempts to achieve gratification. (An example of the latter is the obvious one of the homosexual who seeks his contacts in public places, thus making himself readily liable to detection, arrest, and prosecution.)

Elicitation of Abstractions

Of major value for the patient is his achievement of the differentiation between his subjective reality (sensations) and objective reality (awareness). The patient may be instructed to imagine a particular theme (involving material that had been the subject of group discussion prior to induction of hypnosis) with the patient first imagining that scene as he felt it had happened, followed by the patient imagining the scene in alternate ways. The aim is recognition by the patient of other, alternate explanations to that which he initially conceived. In sequence, then, would follow examination under hypnosis of the patient's feelings of rejection by significant others and—most significant—how the patient has rejected others . . . despite his conscious feelings that this has not occurred (which is *quite* prevalent!). This area is of particular significance, in view of its relationship with the entire scope of reality-testing material, since so often the patient views himself as having been rejected (sometimes with and sometimes without reality)—but so seldom is aware that *he also frequently has rejected other persons*—with such rejection invariably being viewed as insignificant because the other was really only using him, didn't really care about him, was totally worthless.

Elicitation of Neurotic Feelings

Since one of the greatest difficulties is having the patient achieve an accurate assessment of when his feelings are valid and when not, hypnosis is of particular value in bringing to awareness such feelings as those of persecution, being unloved, injustice collecting—as well as that huge area involving unconscious feelings of sexual taboo. It has been found by the author, incidentally, that the area of "injustice-collecting" provides particularly fertile soil for the group process, and appears to be readily amenable to more reality-rooted evaluation of such persecutory convictions on the part of the patient.

An instance of a patient who was particularly involved with injustice-collecting was a married woman in her fifties who was contemplating an affair with another man. She had never been unfaithful to her husband throughout their decades of marriage, although she had left him during the first years of their marriage because she had felt neglected as a result of his attentiveness to his work. The husband had been impotent for a number of years, and the wife continued to say she would have been able to accept this "if he had at least shown some affection to me." She was torn between leaving her husband and the financial security that she had with him and her yearning to "live, at least once, before I get too old." Outstanding in this patient's productions in the group was her insistence that the failure of her marriage—failure as far as providing gratifications for her—was totally her husband's fault. Session after session, she insisted that there was nothing for which she could blame herself. This particular patient managed to achieve an almost hysterical frenzy among the other group members by her consistent denial of any failure on her part through all her years of marriage. *Everything* was her husband's fault. The illogic of such a statement, her inability to accede that there was *anything* that she could have changed in relation to her behavior towards her husband, could not be swayed. Confronted with the accusation of the group that she was a nag, the patient vehemently denied this. Confronted by the group's accusation that her husband's permissiveness (relative to decision-making about which friends to see, when to see them, how to decorate their home, where to take vacations, what to serve for dinner) was in actuality a characteristic that provided for a husband relatively easy to live with, the patient answered that this was not so at all, that she was tired of making all the decisions, tired of his lack of interest, tired of his "leaving everything up to me." In a word, whatever feature the group attempted to have the patient see as advantageous, she could see only as an imposition upon her, a denial of her, a rejection of her. Under hypnosis, the group was asked to see a scene detailing a problem area with a significant person in their actual lives. The patient visualized a scene in which her husband came home from work, and they had a quarrel over his refusal to help her make plans for that weekend. The patients were next asked to visualize a scene in which each patient experienced the feelings, as well as being in the role of, the *other* person in the scene they had just envisioned. (It is to be noted that there were very explicit instructions in order to enable the patient to actually place himself in this role-playing position under hypnosis.) Following the trance period, the patient being discussed said, "When I was supposed to feel as if I were my husband, I felt tired. I felt myself sinking into a chair, feeling so tired. I kept thinking of the phone bill we got that morning from the telephone company, and I kept thinking of how high the bill was because of all the collect calls from my son. And then I started thinking about the fact that I was going to have to send a check out to cover the boy's tuition for next year. Then I started thinking about how I had kept wanting him to accept a scholarship he had gotten, but how much he had wanted to go to this expensive Ivy League school. And I kept thinking that it was getting harder and harder for me to drag through the hours until I could get home, and just rest, and I was thinking that even when I got home all I could do was worry. And I kept thinking that all I would like to do from Friday until Monday was just collapse in that chair and have someone serve me breakfast, and serve me lunch, and serve me dinner so that I wouldn't have to move a muscle until Monday morning when I had to start making money again. And I kept thinking I didn't want to go out Saturday night, but that, of course, I had to; that it wasn't fair to just rest, to make money. And I kept thinking that I really couldn't get up enough energy about whether or not I would enjoy going out with this one or that one, just that if I could get up enough evergy even to go out on Saturday night that it would be rather phenomenal. And I kept thinking I really didn't know which looked prettier, the end table on this side of the couch or the end table on that side of the couch; that it looked pretty both ways, and why did I have to try to make a decision about whether the furniture should be this way or that way when it really looked just fine whatever way it was. And I kept thinking that I really didn't care if I had lamb chops for dinner or a casserole for dinner; that if I had a casserole tonight we'd have lamb chops tomorrow and both tasted good enough. But most of all I just kept thinking how tired I was, how tired I was." It is of interest that during the discussion following this material the patient maintained her position that her husband was still to blame: "He has a lot of talent; he should have been able to make money easier. He shouldn't have to work so hard just earning enough money for the usual things in life— supporting a home, supporting a wife, putting a son through college." Behaviorally, however, it is to be noted that the frequency and length of the patient's expressions of anger toward her husband did decrease during subsequent discussions, and from her verbalizations, it did appear that the patient was increasingly able to "place herself in another's role."

ELICITATION OF EGO SUPPORT MATERIAL

And finally, particularly in those instances in which it appears highly desirable that the patient leave the session with some feelings of the probability of success from therapy and with some feelings of hopefulness relative to his own probable success in achieving some of his goals in therapy—ego-integrative or supportive scenes may be achieved for the patient under hypnosis with such instructions as: imagine the happiest time of your life; imagine a time of utter and complete joy; imagine a scene of total success in handling a situation. It is highly probable that the greatest value is from those scenes that have actually occurred in his own life—rather than from therapist manufac- tured tableaux (and it is rare indeed that one will encounter a patient who finds it impossible to recall at least a single instance of joy, of happiness, of feelings of competence, of hopefulness).

The value, therefore, of the use of hypnosis in the group therapeutic process, may be stated as achieving these objectives (Fromm, 1965): the field of perception is narrowed and outside stimuli are largely shut out. The range of interaction with external reality is diminished and the patient sharply funnels his attention on his inner-world reality. As the breadth of attention is decreased, its qualitative intensity seems to increase. As a consequence of this process, it may be readily stated that the achievement of the "inner world reality" of an individual's experience of competence, worthfulness, wholeness, may be communicated to his experience of himself in totality.

SUMMARY

This paper has reported on and discussed some indications of the contribution that the use of hypnosis can provide to the group therapy setting, with emphasis on those circumstances under which hypnosis appears to be particularly valid as an instrumental procedure and experience in the group therapy process. Specific techniques in the use of hypnosis and the elicitation of significant material during group therapy have been described and evaluated.

REFERENCES

ALEXANDER, L. Clinical experiences with hypnosis in psychiatric treatment. *International Journal of Neuropsychiatry*, 1967, 3, 118-24.

BOWERS, M.K. Theoretical considerations in the use of hypnosis in the treatment of schizophrenia. *International Journal of Clinical and Experimental Hypnosis*, 1960, 9, 39-46.

BRENMAN, M., AND GILL, M.M. *Hypnotherapy: A Survey of the Literature.* New York: International Universities Press, 1947.

BROWN, E. A. The treatment of bronchial asthma by means of hypnosis. *Journal of Asthma Research*, 1965, 3.

CEDERCREUTZ, D., AND UUSITALO, E. Hypnotic treatment of phantom sensations in 37 amputees. In LASSNER, J. (Ed.) *Hypnosis in Psychosomatic Medicine: Proceedings of the International Congress in Psychosomatic Medicine.* Berlin: Springer-Verlag, 1967.

CHEEK, D.B. Therapy of persistent pain states: Part I. Neck and shoulder pain of five years' duration. *American Journal of Clinical Hypnosis, 1966, 8.*

CLAWSON, T.A. Hypnosis in medical practice. *American Journal of Clinical Hypnosis*, 1964, 6, 236.

CRASILNECK. H.B. The use of hypnosis in controlling smoking. *Southern Medical Journal, 1968, 61.*

DAS, J.P. A theory of hypnosis. *International Journal of Clinical and Experimental Hypnosis, 1959, 2, 69-78.*

DORCUS, R.M. (Ed.) *Hypnosis and its Therapeutic Applications.* New York: McGraw-Hill, 1956.

EDWARDS, G. Hypnotic treatment of asthma: real and illusory results. *British Medical Journal, 1960, 2, 492.*

EDWARDS, G. Motivation and post-hypnotic effect. *British Journal of Psychiatry,* 1965, 111, 983-92.

ERIKSON, M.H. Hypnotic psychotherapy. *Medical Clinic of North America,* 1948, 571.

FIELD, P.B., AND DWORKIN, S.F. Strategies of hypnotic interrogation. *Journal of Psychology,* 1967, 67, 47-58.

FOWLER, H. *Curiosity and Exploratory Behavior.* New York: MacMillan, 1965.

FOX, J. The systematic use of hypnosis in individual and group psychotherapy. *International Journal of Clinical and Experimental Hypnosis, 1960, 8, 109-14.*

FREUD, S. *Group Psychology and the Analysis of the Ego.* London: International Psycho-Analytical Press, 1922.

FROMM, E. Hypnoanalysis: Theory and two case excerpts. *Psychotherapy: Theory Research and Practice,* 1965, 2, 127-33.

FRY, L. et al. Effect of hypnosis on allergic skin responses in asthma and hay-fever. *British Medical Journal,* 1964, 1, 1145.

GLOVER, F.S. Use of hypnosis in weight reduction in a group of nurses. *American Journal of Clinical Hypnosis,* 1959, 1, 115-16.

GORDON, H. Hypnotism in dermatology. *British Medical Journal,* 1955, 1214.

GRUENEWALD, D. Hypnotherapy in a case of adult nail-biting. *International Journal of Clinical and Experimental Hypnosis,* 1965, 8.

HARDING, C.H. In LASSNER, J. (Ed.) *Hypnosis in Psychosomatic Medicine: Proceedings of the International Congress in Psychosomatic Medicine.* Berlin: Springer-Verlag. 1967, p. 131.

HARTLAND, J. *Medical and Dental Hypnosis and its Clinical Applications.* Baltimore: Williams and Wilkins, 1966.

HILGARD, E.R. Ability to resist suggestions within the hypnotic state: Responsiveness to conflicting communications, *Psychological Reports,* 1963, 12, 3-13.

IKEMI, Y. et al. Hypnotic experiments on the psychosomatic aspects of gastrointestinal disorders. In Kline, M.V. (Ed.), *Clinical Correlations of Experimental Hypnosis.* Springfield, Illinois: Charles C Thomas, 1963.

ILLOVSKY, J. Experiences with group hypnosis on schizophrenics. *Journal of Mental Science,* 1962, 108, 685-93.

JABUSH, M. A case of recurrent multiple furunculosis treated with hypnotherapy. In press.

KLINE, M. V. Towards a theoretical understanding of the nature of resistance to the induction of hypnosis and depth hypnosis. *Journal of Clinical and Experimental Hypnosis,* 1953, 1, 32-41.

KLINE, M.V. Hypnosis and its clinical psychology. *Progress in Clinical Psychology,* Vol.IV, New York: Grune & Stratton, 1960.

KLINE, M.V. Hypnotic regression: a neuropsychological theory of age regression and progression. In Kline, M.V. (Ed.) *Clinical Correlations of Experimental Hypnosis.* Springfield, Illinois: Charles C Thomas, 1963. (a)

KLINE, M. V. Age regression and regressive procedures in hypnotherapy. In Kline, M.V. (Ed.), *Clinical Correlations of Experimental Hypnosis.* Springfield, Illinois: Charles C Thomas, 1963. Chap. 3. (b)

KLINE, M.V. *Hypnotherapy, Handbook of Clinical Psychology.* New York: McGraw-Hill, 1965.

KLINE, M.V. Hypnotic amnesia in psychotherapy. *International Journal of Clinical and Experimental Hypnosis,* 1966, 14, 112-20.

KROGER, W.S. *Clinical and Experimental Hypnosis in Medicine, Dentistry and Psychology.* Philadelphia: J.B. Lippincott, 1963.

MCLEAN, A.F. Hypnosis in "psychosomatic" illness. *British Journal of Medical Psychology,* 1965, 38, 211.

MANN, H. Group hypnosis in the treatment of obesity. *American Journal of Clinical Hypnosis,* 1959, 1, 114-16.

MASON, A.A. and BLACK, S. Allergic skin responses abolished under treatment and asthma and hayfever by hypnosis. In Kline, M.V. (Ed.) *Clinical Correlations of Experimental Hypnosis.* Springfield, Illinois: Charles C Thomas, 1963.

MEARES, A. *A System of Medical Hypnosis.* Philadelphia: W.B. Saunders, 1960.

MILLER, M.M. A group therapeutic approach to a case of bed-wetting and fire setting with the aid of hypnoanalysis. *Group Psychotherapy,* 1957, 10, 181-90.

MORENO, J.L. and ENNEIS, J.M. Hypnodrama and psychodrama. *Psychodrama Monographs,* 1950, No.27.

MULLAN, H. and ROSENBAUM, M. *Group Psychotherapy.* New York: MacMillan, 1962.

NULAND, W. The use of hypnotherapy in the treatment of the post-myocardial infarction invalid. *International Journal of Clinical and Experimental Hypnosis,* 1968, 16, 139-50.

PEBERDY, G.R. Hypnotic methods in group psychotherapy. *Journal of Mental Science,* 1960, 106, 1016-20.

PERLINE, I.H. Group hypnotherapy: a brief survey. *American Journal of Clinical Hypnosis*, 1968, 4, 267-70.

ROSEN, J. *Hypnotherapy in Modern Psychiatry.* New York: Julian Press, 1953.

SACERDOTE, P. The place of hypnosis in the relief of severe protracted pain. *American Journal of Clinical Hypnosis*, 1962, 4, 150.

SACERDOTE, P. Hypnotherapy in neurodermatitis: a case report. *American Journal of Clinical Hypnosis*, 1965, 7, 249. (a)

SACERDOTE, P. Additional contributions to the hypnotherapy of the advanced cancer patient. *American Journal of Clinical Hypnosis*, 1965, 7, 308. (b)

SALZBERG, H.C. The effects of hypnotic, post-hypnotic and waking suggestion on performance using tasks varied in complexity. In Kline, M.V. (Ed.) *Clinical Correlations of Experimental Hypnosis.* Springfield, Illinois: Charles C Thomas, 1963.

SCHNECK, J.M. *Hypnosis in Modern Medicine.* 3rd Edition, Springfield, Illinois: Charles C Thomas, 1963.

SCHNECK, J.M. Clinical and experimental aspects of hypnotic dreams. In Kline, M.V. (Ed.), *Clinical Correlations of Experimental Hypnosis.* Springfield, Illinois: Charles C Thomas, 1963, Chap.4.

SCHOWALTER, J.M. A case of allergy cured by hypnotic suggestion the modern way. *British Journal of Medical Hypnotism*, Winter, 1958, 59, 10.

SCOTT, E.M. Group therapy for schizophrenic alcoholics in a state-operated outpatient clinic: with hypnosis as an integrated adjunct. *International Journal of Clinical and Experimental Hypnosis*, 1966, 14, 232-42.

SEGRELL, B. Group therapy research problems. *Nordisk Psykologi*, 1965, 17, 449-54.

SHAPIRO, A. Experimental hypnosis and psychosomatic medicine. In Kline, M.V. (Ed.) *Clinical Correlations of Experimental Hypnosis*, Springfield, Illinois: Charles C Thomas, 1963, Chap.5.

SILVER, A.W. Interrelating group dynamic, therapeutic, and psychodynamic concepts. *International Journal of Group Psychotherapy*, 1967, 17, 139-50.

SMITH, J.M. and BURNS, C.C.L. The treatment of asthmatic children by hypnotic suggestion. *British Journal of Diseases of the Chest*, 1960, 54, 78.

SOLOVEY, G. and MILECHNIC, A. Some points regarding hypnosis in dentistry. *American Journal of Clinical Hypnosis*, 1958, 1,59.

SOLOVEY, G. and MILECHNIC, A. Concerning the treatment of enuresis. *American Journal of Clinical Hypnosis*, 1959, 2, 22-29.

TOTERO, N.J. *Transference and Counter-Transference in Hypnosis.* Lecture given at Fairleigh Dickinson University Dental School, New Jersey, May, 1967.

WALLERSTEIN, R.S. Psychological factors in chronic alcoholism. *American Internal Medicine,* 1958, 48, 114-22.

WATKINS, J.G. Psychodynamics of hypnotic induction and termination, In Schneck, J.M. (Ed.) *Hypnosis in Modern Medicine,* 3rd Edition. Springfield, Illinois: Charles C Thomas, 1963, Chap. II. (a)

WATKINS, J.G. Transference aspects of the hypnotic relationship. In Kline, M.V. (Ed.) *Clinical Correlations of Experimental Hypnosis.* Springfield, Illinois: Charles C Thomas, 1963. Chap. I. (b)

WEITZENHOFFER, A.M. The influence of hypnosis on the learning process: some theoretical considerations. II. Recall of meaningful material. In Kline, M.V. (Ed.) *Clinical Correlations of Experimental Hypnosis.* Springfield, Illinois: Charles C Thomas, 1963.

WOLBERG, L.R. *Hypnoanalysis.* New York: Grune and Stratton, 1948. (a)

WOLBERG, L.R. *Medical Hypnosis,* Vol. I. New York: Grune and Stratton, 1948. (b)

8
Theory and Practice of Group Hypnosis, or Collective Hypnosis, in the USSR*

N. V. Ivanov

INTRODUCTION

At the 1965 Congress of Hypnosis and Psychosomatic Medicine L. Chertok[4] pointed out that the study of hypnosis in most European countries had developed extremely slowly. This was due to a negative attitude towards hypnosis, dating from the turn of the century and the rise of rational psychotherapy and psychoanalyisis. In the USSR, by contrast, hypnosis was intensively explored and taught, especially in its application to groups. This has furnished an abundance of material which forms the basis of this paper on the theory and practice of group hypnosis. It should be stressed that only the scientific literature of Socialist countries has been drawn upon and no attempt has been made to cover the numerous investigations and reports that have appeared in the West.

The Russian equivalent of the term group hypnosis is *collective hypnosis,*† which is preferred for reasons to be explained below.

---

*Translated by the late Dr. B. Petrovskaia, Herrison Hospital, Dorchester. Chapter XXI in *Modern Perspectives in World Psychiatry*, edited by John G. Howells, MD, DPM. New York: Brunner/Mazel Publishers (1971), pp. 577-95. Reprinted with permission of the publisher.

†Translator's Note. In the translation the English terms 'group hypnosis' and 'group hypnotherapy' will be used but the original preferred term should be borne in mind.

The fact that Soviet psychotherapy has experienced no crisis in the field of hypnology can be linked with the historical tendency that was pointed out by V.I. Lenin that, 'in its main trends progressive thought in Russia is fortunately based on solid materialistic traditions'. In the teaching of hypnosis the materialistic tradition has stimulated a constant search for the physiological basis of hypnotic phenomena. Hypnosis was defined as a state capable of explanation in terms of organic phenomena and the natural sciences. This attitude ensured a lively and continuous scientific interest in hypnosis at a time when it was considered in the West to be pseudo-scientific or frankly mystical.

The first quarter of the twentieth century saw a rich accumulation of data testifying to the therapeutic value of hypnosis (V.M. Tokarsky[37],[38] and V.M. Bechterev[1],[2] and his colleagues). In the 1930s I.P. Pavlov[21] formulated his fundamental concept which regarded the hypnotic state as a 'partial sleep' in which irradiated sleep inhibition coexisted with still actively functioning foci of arousal. It is these zones of wakefulness that permit 'rapport', as they can be stimulated by suggestion. The 'word of command' is in itself an adequate stimulus of the secondary signal system; it operates in isolation from all other influences and becomes an absolute irresistibly acting stimulus. Thus it continues to operate as an active stimulus even after the subject has returned to a state of complete general wakefulness.

In 1937 K. I. Platonov[22] who shared I. P. Pavlov's views, wrote, 'we sometimes hear that psychotherapy should be experiencing a crisis, but this is not so in reality. Psychotherapy is only beginning to develop, and it should be all the more valuable and significant because of its materialistic foundations'.

This scientific materialistic attitude towards psychopathological mechanisms, based on organic and physiological laws, should ensure that psychotherapy is highly reliable and significant.[22]

It is on this basis that Soviet psychotherapists have been intensively investigating hypnosis and this has naturally encouraged a rational methodology in 'group hypnotherapy.'

Scientific investigation of group methods dates from 1904 when there appeared a report by I.V. Vjasemskii[41] who had carried out hypnosis on a group of five or six alcoholics. This was termed hypnotherapy for alcoholism. His practice was to induce a state of hypnotic trance in the whole group by hypnotizing each subject in turn. In this way he was able to make use of the phenomenon of mutual influence among the patients in order to reinforce their suggestibility.

Theory of Group Therapy and of
Group Hypnosis

Historical differences in the social order of Western countries and of the USSR resulted in certain differences in the development of scientific concept. In this respect let us consider the nature of personality and in particular what kinds of experiences are pathogenic in character and which are likely to respond to psychotherapeutic measures.

On reading Western philosophy and psychology, we can easily see that in the West harsh and traumatic agents are responsible for man's anxiety concerning his social experiences both present and future. It is no accident, for instance, that his fear for existence and social survival inflict upon him a constant psychic tension and lead him into a neurotic flight from reality. This is emphasized by the existentialists as being the primary, central factor in the essence of man. 'The reason for his anxiety lies in man's very existence in the world as it is' (M. Heidegger).[7]

Soviet sociologists consider that the cause of Western man's prevailing fear is to be found in his social conditions. In Western society man is forced to struggle for his individual position in society and from this there arise the primary factors that determine his peculiar isolation and alienation. Western man is surrounded more by competitors than co-workers. From this it follows that the actual conflicts engendering neuroses are the conflicts between his personality and the competitive environment.

This accounts for the specific problems of psychotherapy. In order to help the patient escape from his neurosis it is necessary to relieve his personality from the traumatic social pressures which cause his constant psychic tension. In Western countries this has given rise to the popularity of those methods of group psychotherapy which resolve social rather than clinical problems.

It would appear that the psychotherapeutic group should compensate at least temporarily for the subject's uncertainties of social existence. It assumes the psychological value of alleviating the patient's burdens of social responsibility and stressful mode of coping with life, inasmuch as within the group he re-examines his pressing problems and thereby appears to clarify them. Thus the primary value of the group appears to be more corrective than therapeutic. For instance, it is stated in Y.W. Klapman's[10] monograph that the group should represent to the patient 'a second society' in which he should re-experience his relationships with his environment from scratch.

Naturally there is no place for hypnosis in groups which emphasize the re-enacting of interpersonal relationships among its members. This is one of the reasons why group hypnotherapy has not been widely used in the West, in spite of the popularity of a number of other forms of group therapy.

By contrast the Soviet psychotherapists' attitude to essential personality problems is fundamentally different. Under the socialist order the more important social needs of personality are catered for by the Government. For the Soviet man there is no emphasis on his concern for and uncertainty about the future. Broad opportunities of education, full employment and social security eliminate his anxiety for existence and survival.

The actual factors which lead to the evolution of neurosis are usually purely psychogenic. These result in the break-down of co-ordination within the higher nervous system and thus lead to functional disorders. Therefore the dominant experience of the neurotic lies in his awareness of his illness. His affective overvaluation of difficulties creates excessive and unnecessary anxiety, and this in turn accentuates the severity of his illness. All this manifests itself as an actual situation and not as a symbolic manifestation of fundamental, nuclear personality tendencies. In such cases the basic task of psychotherapy consists of correcting and influencing the patient so as to give him an adequate appreciation of his illness and to mobilize the strengths of his personality and its defences to combat and overcome his illness. The execution of this plan lies strictly within a purely clinical sphere. The goal of the organized therapeutic group is not the establishment of a second society, but rather the facilitation of purely therapeutic measures which aim at changing the patient's attitude towards his illness and the elimination of his symptoms. By virtue of its specific therapeutic methods hypnosis can be used par excellence within the group situation. The patient on his part comes to accept hypnotherapeutic methods as completely and indisputably rational procedures.

Thus the preference of Soviet clinicians for group hypnotherapy is determined by their different theoretical approach to group psychotherapy.

These differences in definition also give rise to different views about the basic nature of psychodynamic mechanisms at work in group psychotherapy. In the West and in the United States the emphasis is on the dominant role of interpersonal relationships operating within the group. Their main goal is to achieve the intrapsychic equilibrium between the id, the ego and the superego by means of catharsis, i.e. analytically. Ultimately this process is psychoanalytic. It is directed towards the discovery of the basic causes of illness, namely the uncovering of the various complexes that have been forced into the subconscious.

The Western emphasis on establishing proper interpersonal relationships among members of the group imparts to the physician merely the role of observer. He participates only occasionally to modify the trend of the group discussion. Such an attitude generally precludes the introduction of hypnotherapeutic measures by the physician since he would then acquire a more active and controlling role.

Under the socialist order a predominant significance is assured by the organization of the collective with its characteristic specific goals. At all stages in his personality development the Soviet man is decisively influenced by the collective, which determines his main patterns of action and personality relationships. This illustrates the important psychological truth that any environmental influences become much more significant for the personality if they are supported by the collective.

In its psychotherapeutic application this principle determines the advantages enjoyed by the physician if his therapy is directed not at a single individual, but at a group of patients who have been brought together on account of similarities in their clinical characteristics. The physician's tasks of explaining, modifying and correcting are directed towards the group. They therefore carry more weight in a group situation than in a setting of personal contact. The content of the therapist's addresses to the group are received by the group as a serious scientific exposition, and accepted more readily by its members. Because of their collective awareness its efficacy is enhanced.

The therapeutic group promotes a conscious re-evaluation of subjective experiences involved in the illness and a pre-requisite is experienced psychiatric guidance. In other words the goal of a therapeutic group is a modification of personality attitudes, and the physician's function is guidance and direction, since only he can expertly appreciate and comprehend the psychotherapeutic problems. The organization of the group under a dominating or guiding physician greatly facilitates the use of hypnotherapeutic methods because the group does not counter but reinforces his function in the therapeutic process.

The obligatory guiding role of the therapist does not, of course, minimize the positive effect of mutual contact among the patients. They are encouraged actively to discuss the meaning of their illness as presented to them by the physician. Moreover, their close mutual contact gives each of them an opportunity to observe for himself the various degrees of improvement that takes place in others. These observations are so vital to the creation of a calm and beneficial psychotherapeutic atmosphere within the group. As has been pertinently remarked by V.A. Giliarovsky[3] a patient will always prefer to believe another patient rather than the physician.

The theoretical premises described above are used to determine the particular constitution of the therapeutic groups and their organization on the basis of common pathogenic categories of illness.

When the group has been constituted the psychotherapeutic sessions begin with an obligatory preliminary talk by the physician. During this there is a gradual explanation of the material necessary for the mobilization of personality. Then follows a general discussion of the data that have been presented and finally the physician proceeds to group hypnosis of all members simultaneously.

We may now assume that the place of group hypnotherapy had been clearly defined and finally assured within the general science of psychotherapy.

Even during the early exploratory stages of the study of hypnotism the possibility of simultaneous hypnosis of a group was suggested (A. Moll)[17] but although Liebault Wetterstrand[44] and Vogt[42] all noted the advantages of the reinforcement of suggestion within a group, the method did not become popular. A. Moll himself did not consider this method as suitable because it cut across the physician patient relationship of professional secrecy and allowed the patients to learn about each others problems.

Since Pratt[25] wrote on the organization of therapeutic groups and V.M. Bechterev[1] introduced the obligatory preliminary address and discussion by the physician, certain inherent advantages of group hypnotherapy have secured for it an assured place. For the Soviet clinician group hypnotherapy is not a method used in isolation but is one component in a system of psychotherapy. Such a course includes preliminary parallel work with each member of the group in private as well as the explanatory address to the whole group.

The Hungarian psychotherapist Volgyesi[43] shares similar views and elaborates his system of active and complex psychotherapy, asserting that this 'aspires to the combination of verbal (intellectual-logical and suggestion) and somato-therapeutic methods'. Thus he regards hypnotherapy as one element in general psychotherapy. However, these views have not yet found general complete acceptance. The French psychotherapist L. Chertok[4] believes that in some situations the positive results of group hypnosis may be partly due to the fact that the group protects its members from an unconscious fear of hypnosis. He does not claim any specific inherent features in group hypnotherapy. Another view is expressed by the German psychotherapist D. Muller-Heyemann,[19] who admits certain advantages in simultaneous hypnosis of several patients including that of economy of the physician's time, but he does not recommend mutual contact of patients and prefers them to be in separate cubicles. He also seems to deny that there is any specific value in group hypnotherapy. However, he is strongly in favour of and attributes inherent positive characteristics to the practice of autogenic training.

THE PRACTICE OF GROUP HYPNOTHERAPY

Physiological Foundation

The acceptance by Soviet psychotherapists of Pavlov's[21] fundamental concept of hypnosis as partial sleep inaugurated an intensive study of some physiological correlates of hypnotic states. Convincing data concerning the identity of physiological substrata of natural and of hypnotic sleep have been obtained. Some of these physiological correlates permit of explanations for the phenomena of suggestibility, rapport and the extent of influences during a hypnotic seance.

B.N. Birman,[3] who was Pavlov's closest student, provided the experimental demonstration of the presence in hypnosis of localized, active, wakeful zones in the cerebral cortex. These constitute the physiological correlates of rapport. He also showed that the degree of suggestibility is determined by the regularity of phase states. The paradoxal phase is of decisive importance. As a consequence of this paradoxal phase the weaker stimulus of the word appears more powerful than direct stimuli either conditioned or unconditioned.

V.E. Roshnov[27] carried out a series of investigations into the dynamics of the phase states during deepening hypnotic sleep. He has demonstrated that such phase states are present at all stages of hypnosis but that with the deepening of sleep the number of the vascular reactions increases and thus reflects the phase state. Plothysmographic experimental methods were used. The enhanced effect of word stimuli becomes more marked whilst the conditioned reflex responsiveness to direct stimuli clearly lessens. It has been shown that there is a simultaneous increase in the selectivity of rapport. Thus there are many more positive conditioned responses to the words of the physician than to those of other persons. However, even at the stage of somnambulism rapport is not completely limited to the hypnotizing physician, but may relate to other persons, and I.O. Narbutowich[20] has demonstrated experimentally that the reaction to certain extraneous direct stimuli also occur.

The essential practical clinical conclusions derived from experimental data are: (1.) The presence of phase states at all stages of hypnosis, including the lightest ones, permits and justifies the use of therapeutic suggestion at any stage of hypnosis; the depth of sleep is an important but not the sole determinant of the efficacy of suggestion.   (2.) Selectivity of rapport testifies to the fact that even in the deepest somnambulism the assimilation, acceptance and fulfilment of suggestion do not represent automatic obedience. To the contrary it points to a specific process of inner remaking and elaboration of the suggested data and the subsequent fulfilment takes place as a result of this working through.

The experimental physiological research conducted by A.G. Ivanov-Smolenskii[9] and his colleagues I.V. Strelchuk,[34] L.B. Gakkell[5] and F.P. Majorov,[15] has produced a wealth of material on the influence of the word as an adequate stimulus of the second signal system which creates new foci of excitation in the cortex. These new foci of activity are prepotent, and by the mechanism of negative induction or by disruption of the dynamic stereotype eliminate the pathodynamic zones that determine the illness. In practice it was these data that led to a realization of the need to create such new foci of cortical activity. Their clinical counterpart would be fresh experiences presented in the process of psychotherapy. They should counteract the morbid factors. The resultant positive affective significance of these new factors endows them with the force necessary to eliminate the illness.

The Hungarian psychotherapist Volgyesi[43] shares the opinion that hypnotherapy has as its goal 'the establishment and reinforcement of new conditioned reflex connections', and that 'therapeutic hypnosis represents an inter-cortical dynamic process in which the active neocortex of the physician comes to substitute itself for the passive neocortex of the patient'.

The physiological data demonstrate that one of the essential problems of hypnotherapy is to evolve such suggestions which will offer intensive, prepotent emotional experiences to the personality. The setting of group hypnotherapy carried with it some additional specific features which serve to reinforce and enhance this affective experience.

Methodology of Suggestion

The fundamental requirements for group hypnotherapy are a clear, systematic and sequential exposition and explanation during the physician's preliminary talks and during the subsequent suggestion introduced step by step in the seances.

As early as 1899 A.A. Tokarsky[37] formulated the requirement of such a structured sequential set of suggestions, which would provide a uniform planned system. This principle is still practised in Soviet hypnotherapy. The suggestion offered at the beginning of a course of therapy should be of a general nature, and 'have a sense of improvement in general' (Tokarsky).[37] The content of the suggestion should be continued and deepen in intensity during each seance and also from one seance to another. They should also introduce new material which in its turn will be continued, amplified and reinforced in the succeeding seances.

The explanations in the preliminary talk and conferences are also conducted step by step according to a planned sequence. At first they stress the importance and rationale of organizing the patients in a given group. Then follows a gradual exposition of the pathogenesis and evolution of illness. Finally, there is an explanation of those features of the therapeutic regimen which spring from the nature of the illness and from the peculiarities of a given group. Gradually the right attitude towards the illness is defined and its value stressed. Clear instructions are given and should be carried out punctiliously. The significance and value of these elucidated precepts is again discussed and emphasized. At the stage of formulating suggestions one of the most important considerations is to reflect and reinforce those already dealt with by the physician and the group. In this way a planned and structured system of suggestions is carried out in logical sequence to increase the potency of suggestion as a whole.

The address to the conscious 'ego', inherent in Soviet psychotherapy, necessitates the use of motivated suggestions. V.G. Sprimon (1887)[13] asserted that 'the methods of suggestion are various and should be suited to each given case. Very often words of command do not suffice, and it becomes necessary to discuss, rationalize, persuade or even furnish proof to the subject, since his individuality continues to operate even while he is in hypnosis as it does in reality'.

At the end of the nineteenth century and during the first quarter of the present century it was generally believed that the degree of suggestibility depended entirely on the depth of sleep. For this reason much of psychotherapeutic research concentrated upon methods of deepening the hypnotic sleep, and hence greater opportunities for employing concrete, imperative suggestions. Much has been achieved in this sphere, for example, by the interesting experiments of K.I. Platonov[14] and I.S. Sumbajev.[35] These experiments have shown that suggestions employing concrete imagery are much more completely fulfilled than those of an abstract logical character. However, the employment of such concrete imagery has its limitations, since they can be applied only to the more easily suggestible subjects.

Paralleled to this trend in research, problems of motivated

suggestion were being investigated. Several reports convincingly demonstrated the effectiveness of formulations which dwell upon the need to change symptomatology, and especially those which logically modify the affective experiences of the patient. Naturally, in group hypnotherapy situations motivated suggestions are the most suitable variants owing to their logical structure.

In this respect K.I. Platonov[22] elucidated specific physiological mechanisms. He stated that 'verbal influences should be motivated and as far as possible linked to the cause. . . . This is necessary in order to create broader and more numerous zones of stimulations in the higher levels of the brain' . . . and that, therefore, 'this method is less primitive than it is usually thought to be when it is considered as pursuing the narrow aims of symptomatic therapy'.

S.S. Libich[14] examined the conditions which increase the effectiveness of suggestions in collective hypnosis and formulated the following requirements: (1.) Suggestion should be sufficiently broadly framed that each patient can select from it that which he needs for himself. (2.) The general suggestion should touch on typical features of the disease which are to some extent common to all the members of the group. (3.) Suggestions should be expressed in concrete imagery, but should only outline—as if to hint at—the decision which should then be taken by the patient.

S.S. Libich[14] proposes to use 'unities of suggestion'. The complex content of any given suggestion should be subdivided with a series of elementary formulations, thus allowing the patients themselves to reconstruct the whole content from these units to suit their own individual needs.

When we come to discuss the psychotherapy of neuroses we shall give examples of how to contruct suggestions for a group.

Degree of Suggestibility

At the present time we may take it as proved that the efficacy of suggestions is not proportional to the depth of hypnotic sleep. Many cases have been cited in which the physician has obtained a radical disappearance of a symptom in this state, only to find that the symptom recurs very soon or is substituted by some other symptoms. Therefore, complete recovery is not necessarily achieved in the stage of somnambulism. Yet, sometimes a suggestion offered during the lightest sleep proves radically curative. From this it follows that the mechanisms which determine the effectiveness of suggestions are not identical with those that determine automatic obedience. They must represent some other specific processes which depend upon the physician/patient contact. In the course of this contact it is the personality of the patient which plays such a vital part in the selection and assimilation of suggestion, and it is the inner working through or reshaping of the suggestion which determines its acceptance.

We are aware of the importance of the phase states as the essential condition for carrying out suggestion, but to our regret we do not know what constitutes all the circumstances which determine the acceptance of suggestion by the individual. The physician often has recourse to the methods of trial and error, sometimes acquiring considerable influence over the patient, at other times temporarily losing it. Thus his work with patients represents for the physician a specific process of plastic adaptation to the patient's state at particular stages of the dynamics of his illness. In the final analysis the acceptance and fulfilment of the suggestion depends on the integration of fine nuances in the reciprocal relationships between the physician and the patient during a seance.

In individual hypnotherapy this integration varies considerably from seance to seance. This variability of pattern due to the nature of individual therapeutic sessions is very familiar to every hypnotherapist. In group hypnotherapy, however, there evidently emerges some factor which stabilizes the tendency to variability. We believe this factor to be the quiet, benevolent atmosphere within the group which is felt by and favourably influences the patient from the moment of his arrival at the therapeutic session. This atmosphere is peculiarly capable of modifying that individual anxiety tension which the sick man brings with him. In the group the patient immediately becomes to some extent distracted and then merges his sufferings with the organized work of the group in participating in the discussions of the material presented by the therapist. By the beginning of the hypnotic seance the sick man has already developed the anticipation and preparedness which is prerequisite to an adequate acceptance of suggestion.

We always emphasize the significance of uniformity in the conditions in which hypnotherapy should be conducted. It is necessary to maintain identical circumstances and settings for the seances, to ensure similar poses and postures in the patients, to employ similar methods in the induction of sleep, and so on. But in this connection we often overlook the fact that during a personal contact with the physician, whilst relating his experiences and anxieties, the patient brings with him something new each time—new factors which disturb the requirements of uniformity during hypnotherapy. Hence in individual therapy the physician does not always succeed in establishing the patient's transition from emotional excitement and complaints, to the desired optimum, beneficial calm in which the patient becomes entirely capable of accepting suggestion. In this respect the conditions within a therapeutic group usually offer certain advantages in that the very inclusion of the patient in the uniform group activity leads to his gradual and speedy acquiescence in the benevolent, calm, psychotherapeutic group atmosphere as a prelude to hypnosis.

The patient often comes convinced that only deep hypnosis can help him, but the group settling tends to overcome this restiveness. The group promotes the reinforcement of suggestibility and the readier acceptance of suggestion by the individual. The modification of this resistance is very difficult in individual hypnotherapy. In the group, however, the patients observe various intensities of sleep in each other and see for themselves the extent of improvement in those who experience only light hypnosis. These observations induce a change of attitude and deepen their suggestibility. Therefore group hypnotherapy produces additional beneficial factors which tend to reinforce acceptance of suggestion and thereby enhance the effectiveness of conducted hypnotherapy.

Suggestion and Personality in Group Hypnotherapy

The hypnotherapeutic seance is a channel for the physician's contact with the patient. A. Moll[17] has defined the relationship developing in hypnosis as an individual contact, but more precisely it should be regarded as a contact with various degrees of participation.

The physician always retains the leading role, but the patient engages in activity that is peculiar to himself. This is evident in his selection of suggested formulations or in the appearance of an antagonistic tendency towards unacceptable suggestions. The inner remaking through the processes of selection, acceptance and elaboration gives the patient an opportunity to endow the suggestion with fresh nuances which are dependent upon his individual patterns and relationships. One may quote a vivid example in which the patient reproduces his personal life experiences in a dream after the physician had offered only a general theme in the suggestion.

In individual hypnosis the physician's suggestion is too closely influenced by the immediate content of the patient's distress. His approach is therefore constructed as his suggestions must be directed towards the amelioration of his subject's complaints. In group hypnotherapy the suggestions may be more general. They are not entirely restricted to the feelings which the patient voices during a given session, and as a result there is greater scope for the patient to add fresh and individual elements to the content of the suggestion. Thus the physician can take more account of the patient's individual and varied activity.

The patient, in his turn, can fulfill not only the specific instructions that are suggested, but can also carry out formulations carried out by his own individual elaborations. Thereby the effectiveness of suggestion is enriched.

The data adduced above have been amply proved by the experiments of the Czechoslovak psychotherapist I. Strelchuk[34] who demonstrated the presence of a spontaneous moment when the patient chooses and exhibits spontaneous behaviour, whereas the suggestion itself has prompted only a general tendency. An obvious positive aspect of group hypnotherapy is seen in this release of 'capacity' exercised by the subject in carrying out suggestions.

A special feature of interpersonal contact in group hypnotherapy is the fact that the patient subconsciously feels a certain subordination in his attitude towards the physician. This attitude is seen in the majority of cases especially in the initial stages of treatment, causing some distrustfulness towards the forthcoming seances. These phenomena are most marked in individual hypnotherapy, when the patient is left face to face with the therapist.

In group hypnotherapy there soon develops a feeling of community, which in turn fosters a favourable acceptance of the hypnotic situation. This is another positive feature of the collective group method. We shall not dwell here upon another characteristic of group situations, namely that the fear of hypnosis which so often operates at the beginning of individual hypnotherapy, usually rapidly disappears in a group. This fact has been recorded by almost all group hypnotherapists.

Since the content of a forthcoming suggestion partially reflects previous discussions and suggestions, the patient approaches the hypnotic seance already partially mobilized to receive it. This facilitates the patient's inner working through of the material suggested, and permits greater efficiency. Here we observe the beneficial influence of previous psychotherapeutic measures, which have reinforced the personality and enhanced its defence mechanisms. Attention has been drawn to these facts by the English psychotherapist J. Hartland in his report to the International Congress on Hypnosis in 1965.

Shortcomings of Group Hypnotherapy

It may be questioned whether group hypnotherapy has any advantages in comparison with individual hypnotherapy. In cases where there has been a weakening of the immediate personal contact between the patient and the physician, can the latter ameliorate the patient's anxious complaints at any given session as well in a group setting as in an individual session? We may ask whether all the advantages of group method described above compensate for what is inevitably lost in a collective situation, by virtue of the greater distance between the therapist and the subject. Is the physician's personality too far removed from the experiential contact of the patient in group sessions?

These doubts would be justified if the contact between the physician and patient were restricted to hypnotherapeutic seances alone. But these doubts no longer arise if the treatment is organized in such a way that each group participant enjoys preliminary individual interviews with the therapist to support and maintain their psychotherapeutic relationship. This individual contact is enriched by material which has emerged at group sessions and which can and should be further utilized by the therapist at subsequent individual therapeutic interviews.

On the other hand the individual interviews enable the physician to elucidate the finer psychodynamic points involved. Later he should present this material and explain it positively in a form relevant to the group as a whole. This approach encourages the patient.

A serious risk which may be encountered in a group is the result of a lessening of a keen interest and the development of an attitude of commonplace matter-of-factness, which the patient rapidly senses. It lowers his affectivity and personal interest, and may even make him indifferent as to whether he attends the sessions regularly or with the necessary keen personal involvement. This may lead to the loss of the most important factor in collective hypnotherapy.

Certain other types of patients may also present substantial obstacles to the smooth and effective conduct of group hypnotherapy. Some may be characterized by a histrionic demonstrativeness, others may be inherently suspicious towards hypnotherapy, while others still may entertain a conviction that nothing can help them in their illness. They may be prevailed upon to give group hynotherapy a chance, but may then tend to wish to prove that no improvement is occurring or can occur. They continue in their obstinate attempts to prove to the therapist and to others present that the group does not suit them. They seem to regard the group situation as an attack upon, or threat to, their individual integrity and dignity. Whilst remaining with the group they may deliberately obstruct instructions and advice. For instance, during the hynotic seance these individuals may stubbornly insist on keeping their eyes open, indulge in motor restlessness or complain that they are uncomfortable.

In the majority of cases these refractory manifestations can be overcome if the physician ignores the patient's behaviour, especially in the early stages of a course, or perhaps if he casually and calmly remarks to such a patient 'Never mind . . . it will soon pass . . .'. When the physician assumes outward indifference and lightly ignores the patient, this same patient usually becomes an active and positive participant in group work at a later stage.

With less amenable retractory subjects there are greater difficulties in introducing them to, and involving them in, a group. Some may even stop attending. In such cases additional individual psychotherapeutic interviews may bring about the desired co-operation within the group.

But patients with a tendency to convulsive reactions, hysterical seizures or impulsive cries are contraindicated for selection to a group. They should be included only if preliminary individual psychotherapy has succeeded in removing the disturbing symptom.

GROUP HYPNOTHERAPY OF NEUROSIS

Within the present paper it would be impracticable to attempt detailed account of the Soviet attitude to neurosis. We shall confine ourselves to quoting the views of V.N. Mjassischev.[14] Mjassischev shared both Pavlov's views and his conclusions based on experimental findings regarding the role of personality and the structure of neurosis.

According to Mjassischev[16] 'Neuroses are psychogenic disorders resulting from unresolved conflicts between the personality and significant aspects of reality. These conflicts are intolerable and produce in the patient severely painful subjective experiences. These may be based on his failures in the struggle for existence, unsatisfied demands, unattained goals, unrewarded efforts or irreparable losses. His failure to reach a rational and productive solution results in his psychic and physiological disruption or disintegration'.

The physiological disruption results from a persistent neuronal overexcitation or overinhibition of the higher nervous system or to different degrees of their combination resulting in motor overactivity. These processes determine the presence and extent of functional disorders. In Pavlov's definition neuroses are a manifestation of a breakdown in the integrative functioning of the higher cortical activity.

In a systematically planned course of group hypnotherapy the clinician can isolate and define these disrupted manifestations and then control them by means of psychotherapeutic measures aimed towards reintegration. These measures are embodied in the physician's preliminary discussions and in the subsequent carefully structured hypnotic suggestion.

Let us now consider the actual characteristics of the basic, constituent stages of a hypnotherapeutic course and of the content of corresponding suggestions.

1. The patients are organized with a therapeutic group for the purpose

of instructing and familiarizing them with the nature of their illness. They should be convinced that they can be cured because their illness is functional and this should be proved to them in medical terms. From the start it is inculcated into neurotic patients that their illness is based on a disturbance of equilibrium by the disrupted fundamental processes of the higher nervous system, and that therefore their common aim within the group must be a re-establishment of a desired normal functioning. This method justifies the organization of the therapeutic group and dictates to the physician the necessity to use suggestion to induce a feeling of calm and quietness, a lessening of the central excitation and irritability and an enhancement of a general sense of wellbeing.

2. This is followed by discussions of the problems relating to the causation and evolution of the disease process. The physician uncovers the presence and significance of the anxiety or depressive manifestations or, for instance, of egocentric hypochondriasis and so on, and shows how the presence of these factors serves to perpetuate the illness.

At this stage it is again suggested to the patients that they must cultivate a calm, quiet and optimistically expectant attitude towards their illness, according to the precept 'However difficult it may be for me right now, I *know* that I shall get better, because I understand that my illness is functional'. The actual variants of the hypnotic formulations and suggestion are determined by the individual characteristics and attitudes of patients in a given group. The psychopathological attitudes are gradually eliminated by appropriate therapeutic means according to a careful plan.

3. We then proceed to a consideration of how to produce a reversal of neurotic processes. The patient is made to turn his attention from his characteristic egocentric emphasis on his illness and to focus it upon the recognition of the various emerging signs of recovery. At this state of the course, the suggestions are aimed at reinforcing the patient's emphasis on some specific aspects of his recovery. It is usually observed at this state that the patient's distress appears to recede, and that he joyfully states that his symptoms have become milder and less frequent. His conviction that he is on the way to recovery is thus further reinforced.

In formulating the suggestion it is useful to cite the patient's own comments and expressions as precisely as possible, without specifically referring to the persons present at the time in the group. As a result the patient clearly recognizes that the therapist has by now ameliorated his own peculiar painful experiences and a reinforcement of suggestibility is further secured.

4. Often in the preliminary talks the physician discusses with the patient his mode of life and the traumatic experiences that have caused the neurosis, and which at this stage still hinder his progress towards the re-

covery. At this state suggestion again reinforces the need for a calm and quiet subsequent wakeful state. The patient's interest is diverted from those difficulties and problems to which he had succumbed and his resistance to the traumatic memories is built up, until his awareness of his past stressful and painful experiences is finally eliminated.

5. Lastly, the stage is reached in which the patient is given active instruction in specific methods of combating his neurotic symptoms and of distracting himself from them. This necessary training is achieved by the mobilization of personality in the direction of modifying and correcting psychopathological patterns and by further enhancement of his self assurance and an encouragement of greater social participation and purposefulness. These instructions in specific means of combating his illness is an obligatory state in the course.

By means of discussions and suggestion instruction is given in systematic and intensive autosuggestion. The patient should create in his own mind a specific, individual formula of self-encouragement by autosuggestion. By means of this formula he consolidates his progress between the sessions; this is not practised during the seances.

In practice the effectiveness of such autosuggestions is secured if the following conditions are accepted. (1.) The creation by the patient of his own formula that tends to some degree to minimize the significance of morbid experiences, e.g. of an obsessive thought. (2.) An active transformation of the patient's morbid thoughts into those which create visual imagery or other affectively charged associations, and which permit the patient to exclude any awareness of morbid phenomena even if temporarily.

At these final stages the therapist has trained the patient in efficient methods of autosuggestion and emphasizes the need for them and reinforces their effectiveness from seance to seance. This is linked to a reinforcement of the personality.

The timing of introduction and application of fresh material depends upon the therapeutic development. Fresh material does not counter the preceding suggestion but rather serves to enrich the therapist's methods and in the end leads to significant positive results.

Organization of Group Hypnotherapy in the USSR

The basic form of organized group hypnotherapy is widely used in our country and is practised in neuropsychiatric dispensaries. These institutions serve not only those with clearly delimited psychological disorders but also those with a wide variety of peripheral borderline conditions. In particular they also offer effective hypnotherapeutic group treatment for chronic alcoholism.

The structure of hypnotherapeutic treatment of the alcoholic is also organized in a strict programme of clearly recognized stages: (1.) The initial stage is aimed at the elimination of the subjectively painful withdrawal symptoms. (2.) Then follows an elaboration of a negative attitude towards alcohol. (3.) Finally, there is a reinforcement of resistance to alcohol, of consolidating abstinence and of long term avoidance of—aversion to—situations in which a ready availability of alcohol may prove too tempting to the patient.

The basic hypnotherapeutic methods which we have outlined above are also practised in a number of specialized therapeutic departments for neuroses, e.g. in the Psychotherapeutic Department of one of the Moscow Neuro-psychiatric Hospitals under Professor M.S. Lebedinskii[12] and Assistant Professor G.K. Tarasov;[36] in the department for treatment of neuroses in the Bekhterev Neuro-psychiatric Institute in Leningrad under Professor V.N. Mjassischev[16] and Doctors R.A. Sachepizckii,[18] S. S. Libich[14] and A.Y. Straumit[33]; in the Department for Neurosis in Kharkow under Professor A.N. Shagam,[29] as well as in the Kharkow Psychotherapeutic Clinic under Professor I.Z. Velvovskii,[39] attached to the Chair of Psychotherapy of the Ukrainian Advanced Medical Training Institute. This latter offers group hypnotherapy in a sanatorium—spa environment. Similar therapeutic spa-sanatoria are also found in Kiev, Sljausk, in the Crimea and in Sochi in the Caucasus.

Group hypnotherapy is also practised in a number of units attached to clinics for internal diseases in general hospitals, and thus may be applied in cardio-vascular and gastro-enterological syndromes in which powerful neurogenic factors are known to operate. We may also mention their usefulness in the early stages of hypertension, paroxysmal tachicardia, stenocardia, bronchial asthma and moderate hyperthyroidism.

In tuberculosis sanatoria group hypnotherapy is employed to ameliorate anxiety associated with the primary condition and also to mitigate certain untoward effects of specific, organic methods of treatment.

Success is also obtained with organized hypnotherapy of selected patients suffering from purely neurological disorders. In such cases group hypnosis may attain a symptomatic relief of various sensory dysfunctions, such as causalgia or phantom limb syndrome. It is also used to aid the patient in his re-adaptation to the new way of life brought about by his illness.

Gynaecologists may utilize hypnotherapy for the treatment of menopausal disorder, mentrual disorders, pruritis, psychogenic hypogalactia etc.

In each of the foregoing spheres hypnotherapy adapts itself and evolves specific characteristics in courses of exploration, discussion and suggestion. But a detailed account of these latter systems is beyond the scope of the present paper and we have contented ourselves with only a brief mention of the basic variants of group hypnotherapy as practised in our country.

REFERENCES

1. BECHTEREV, V.M., 1911. *Hypnosis, suggestion and psychotherapy and their therapeutic value.* St. Petersburg.

2. BECHTEREV, V.M., 1928. *A new method of collective therapy of chronic alcoholics.* A collection of papers dedicated to the XXXth anniversary of work of Professor Brustein, C.A. Moscow, Leningrad.

3. BIRMAN, B.N., 1930. Psychotherapy as Social Reflexotherapy of Neurotic Illness, *J. Contemp. Psychoneurol.,* Nos. 4-6.

4. CHERTOK, L., 1959. *L'Hypnose. Probleme theoritique at pratique.* Paris.

5. GAKKELL, L.B., 1960. *Human neuroses.* A Manual of Neurology in several volumes, vol. 6. Moscow.

6. GILIAROVSKY, V.A., 1927. Collective Psychotherapy of Neurotics. *Moscow Med. J.,* No. 7.

7. HEIDEGGER, M., 1941. *Sein und Zeit.* Halle a.d. Saale, 5 Ausfl, p.180.

8. IVANOV, N.V., 1959. *Psychotherapy in neuro-psychiatric dispensaries.* Moscow.

9. IVANOV-SMOLENSKII, A.G., 1952. *Notes on the pathophysiology of the higher nervous activity.* 2nd ed. Moscow.

10. KLAPMAN, Y.W., 1948. *Group psychotherapy. Theory and practice.* London.

11. KRASNICH, S.A., 1954. *An experiment in the application of psychotherapy in a hospital for somatic diseases.* Gorki.

12. LEBEDINSKII, M.S., 1959. *Notes on psychotherapy.* Moscow.

13. LEONHARD, K., 1963. *Individual therapie der neurosen.* Ycha.

14. LIBICH, S.S., 1966. Special characteristics of collective psychotherapy in small groups. Collected papers *Problems of psychotherapy.* Moscow.

15. MAJOROV, F.P. 1950. Physiological characteristics of the somnambulistic phase of hypnosis. *Physiol. J. USSR,* 36, No. 6, 649.

16. MJASSISCHEV, V.N., 1960. *Personality and neuroses.* Leningrad.

17. MOLL, A., 1892. *Der Rapport in der Neurosen.* Leipzig.

18. MORENO, J.L., Ed. 1945. *Group Psychotherapy. A Symposium.* New York.

19. MULLER-HEYEMANN, 1957. *Psychotherapie.* Berlin.

20. NARBUTOVICH, I.O., 1958.   Researches into selective rapport in hypnosis. Collected papers *Problems of psychotherapy.* Moscow.
21. PAVLOV, I.P., 1951.   *Twenty years of experiments in objective studies of the higher nervous activity.* 7th ed. Moscow.
22. PLATONOV, K.I., 1935.   Towards a New Foundation in Psychotherapy. *J. Neuropath. Psychiatry Psychol. Hyg.,* No.11.
23. PLATONOV, K.I., 1937.   General Considerations of Means towards a Materialistic Foundation of Psychiatry. *Trans. Krasnodar med. Inst.*
24. PLATONOV, K.I., 1962.   *The word as a physiological and therapeutic factor.* 2nd ed. Moscow.
25. PRATT, Y.H., 1906.   The home sanatorium treatment of consumption. *Johns Hopkins Hospital Bull.,* 17.
26. ROSHNOV, V.E., 1954.   *Hypnosis in medicine.* Moscow.
27. ROSHNOV, V.E., 1958.   Problems of Physiological Characteristics of Various Depths of Hypnotic Sleep. Collected papers *Problems of psychotherapy.* Moscow.
28. SACHEPIZCKII, R.A., 1966.   Interpersonal relationships between physician and patient in the process of psychotherapy. Collected papers *Problems of psychotherapy.* Moscow.
29. SHAGAM, A.N., 1966.   Data relating to the theory of psychotherapy. Collected papers *Problems of psychotherapy.* Moscow.
30. SLAVSON, S.K., 1947.   *The practice of group therapy.* London.
31. SLAVSON, S.K., 1956.   *The fields of group psychotherapy.* New York.
32. SPRIMON, V., 1887.   Hypnotic suggestion as a means of treating neuroses. *J. med. Rev.,* 27, 102.
33. STRAUMIT, A.Y., 1966.   Problems in idiopathogenetic Psychotherapy. Collected papers *Problems of psychotherapy.* Moscow.
34. STRELCHUK, I.V., 1966.   Cited from Bassin, F.V. and Roshnov at the International Congress on Hypnosis and Psychosomatic Medicine (1943) Ref. *Korsakov. J. Neuropathol. Psychiatry,* No. 2.
35. SUMBAJEV, I.S., 1946.   *Theory and practice of psychotherapy.* Irkutsk.
36. TARASOV, G.K., 1966.   Problems of effectiveness of psychotherapy in small groups. Collected papers *Problems of psychotherapy.* Moscow.
37. TOKARSKY, V.M., 1890.   *Therapeutic application of hypnosis.* Moscow.
38. TOKARSKY, V.M., 1889.   *Problems of possible harmful influence of hypnosis.* St. Petersburg.
39. VELVOVSKII, I.Z., 1964.   Some aspects of the introduction of

psychotherapy into spas and sanatoria services to the sick. Collection of papers *One hundred years of Berjosorsky (The Birches) Mineral Waters.* Khartov.

40. VISH, I.M., 1959. *Psychotherapy of certain neuropsychiatric and somatic disorders.* Leningrad, Tambov.

41. VJASEMSKII, I.V., 1904. Alcoholism and its Treatment by Hypnotherapeutic Suggestion. *Korsakov J. Neurol. Psychiatry*, No. 1-2.

42. VOGT, O., 1894-95. Zur Kenntnis des Wesens und der Psychologischen. Bedentung der Hypnotisnms. *Zeitschrift fur Hypnotisnms.*

43. VOLGYESI, 1959. *Uber aktiv-Komplexe Psychotherapie und die Berwegung.* Schule der Kranken. Berlin.

44. WETTERSTRAND, L., 1893. *Hypnotism and its application to practical medicine.* (Translated into Russian from Swedish.)

Part III

GROUP HYPNOSIS:
Special Situations and Settings

9
Management Consulting with
Group Hypnosis

Ira A. Greenberg

There has long been a myth that successful business and other executives are people who seek safety in conformity and are easily threatened by personal risk taking, whether that of direct confrontation or the sponsorship of ideas, attitudes, and concepts that may be innovative or even controversial. Of course, instances of the executive who never sticks his neck out are many, but the exceptions to the stereotype are more than expected, and usually these exceptions are the true leaders among business and organizational managers. They have already, for the most part, benefited from such approaches as brainstorming, sensitivity training, simulations, role training, transactional analysis, and psychodrama; and by now these modalities have achieved ready acceptance as tools of the consulting industry's attempts to facilitate organizational development, team building, and problem solving among clients.

A fairly new approach toward helping organizations and the individuals who comprise them function more effectively involves the utilization of group hypnosis. Group hypnosis to help improve interpersonal relations or to aid in creative corporate problem solving has by no means come near achieving a wide acceptance in management consulting; nevertheless, those business and other leaders who have been exposed to this approach have found the methods and some of the results worth considering as a part of their training and problem-solving procedures. Not only have many individuals found the idea of being involved in group hypnosis exercises nonthreatening, but many more have sought out these experiences for personal and professional growth.

As yet, there are a comparatively few management consulting firms offering group hypnosis as pathways to problem solving or as means to intrapersonal development to improve interpersonal involvements. The work of two of these firms will be described to illustrate ways group hypnosis may be employed toward increasing corporate profits and increasing individual and group satisfactions with the organization concerned. The consulting firms to be described were selected primarily on the basis of this author's familiarity with them. They are Behavioral Studies Institute, founded in 1970 by this writer, who continues to serve as executive director, and Behavior Sciences Education Center, founded by Richard L. Johnson, who is its president. Behavioral Studies Institute, located in West Los Angeles,[1] offers both action methods drawn from psychodrama and role playing and fantasy work drawn from group hypnosis to facilitate organizational development and problem solving, while Behavior Sciences Education Center, located in Glendora, a suburb of Los Angeles, primarily employs group hypnosis techniques to help trainees improve themselves personally and thus improve their professional performance.

The group hypnosis approach of Behavioral Studies Institute (BSI) is one that focuses on the guided fantasy and reaches beyond brainstorming in seeking to help a corporation or institution solve problems that have not been solved by more conventional means. The problems could be in such areas as engineering, research, marketing, management, organizational structure, and interpersonal dynamics, to cite a few. The idea is to give individuals participating in the problem-solving workshop an opportunity to enlarge their perceptual field in regard to the problem at hand and in this restructuring to possibly find answers that either were new or had been overlooked previously. In other words, BSI seeks to help participants look at their problem from a new angle and from new orientations, and from these fresh viewpoints the obvious may emerge from the obscure.

BSI is not so much an organization as an association of professionals from diverse disciplines who are drawn together in teams of from two to five people to put on workshops for organizational or executive development and to help solve specific problems. The action

[1]Behavioral Studies Institute, Ira A. Greenberg, Ph.D., executive director, is at 10795 Wilshire Blvd. No. 6, Los Angeles, Ca. 90024, and Behavior Sciences Education Center, Richard L. Johnson, president, is at 122 W. Alosta Ave., Glendora, Ca. 91740.

and fantasy methods that are BSI's specialties seem to lend themselves well to dealing with emergency or crisis situations. The action techniques BSI employs for executive training, team building, and organizational development are those that for the most part have been developed in psychodrama or sociodrama, in which individuals or groups act out their problems under the guidance of a director and before a group of people from which individuals are chosen to play the parts of important others involved in the problem. These action techniques include role playing, role training, spontaneity training, and role-situation experiencing (in which individuals experience themselves in new roles and in new and often stressful situations). A recent development in management work involves the use of hypnodrama (psychodrama and hypnosis) for the exploration and diagnosing of organizational problems.[2]

For problem solving, BSI employs the guided fantasy approach that was developed in psychosynthesis (a psychotherapy that involves directed imagination, among other things), and BSI uses it with small groups of people who are either in states of hypnosis or in a relaxed waking state. In these states, people are enabled to loosen the cognitive controls employed in daily personal or business activities and thus be able to tap that vast resource that is referred to as the subconscious or unconscious mind. In a weekend workshop set up to deal with a specific problem—let us say one in mechanical engineering—the BSI workshop leader will deal directly with persons who have already been working on the problem, and these engineers and scientists together with some BSI associates—possibly an artist, an attorney, a psychiatrist, or even a philosopher—go through a series of specifically designed guided fantasy experiences and group discussions. Also involved in the problem-solving workshop is the client-firm's key person, for example, the project manager, who is the individual responsible for solving the particular problem that is delaying progress. This key person serves as an observer throughout the workshop, monitoring all that occurs, taking notes, making suggestions to the workshop leader, but not himself being directly involved in the fantasy experiences or in the other events of the workshop. Usually, this key individual is close enough to the participants in the firm's hierarchy that they may be expected to be able to be spontaneous in his presence; should the participants not be spontaneous at first, the warmup phase of the workshop is expected to

[2]See the chapter, "Hypnodramatics for Organizational Analysis," by Ira A. Greenberg, in Part V of this volume.

help overcome prevailing inhibitions. Of course, the workshop is invariably held in a pleasant environment—a good hotel or a comfortable country lodge—sufficiently removed from the place of business or from the daily lives of the participants so that the novelty of the weekend retreat[3] is in itself stimulating.

The actual fantasy in group hypnosis or in the relaxed waking state may involve the participants being guided to a room where solutions to the problem are stored or to a deeper level of their own awareness where they may then deal with the problem. They may also be asked to see the problem in their mind or imagination or inner mind and to explore it through their various senses or through their very being. For example, the problem may be one of placing a gear system that must redirect and increase a certain amount of power in a particularly limited setting without increasing its size. Besides studying the mechanism by *imaginary* sight, touch, sound, smell, and even taste, the participants can themselves "be" the gear, in the gestalt therapy sense, subjectively experiencing its structure, its materiality, and its functioning, and in the group discussion that follows comparing their experiences and whatever insights may have occurred during the experience or subsequent to it. Other ways of exploring this problem might involve studying it from the viewpoint of a particular profession; thus, an attorney might examine it in terms of the rules of evidence, an artist impressionistically or in other terms, a psychiatrist in terms of the psychopathology of the gear mechanism or in terms of its unconscious motivation, and a poet perhaps in terms of its soul or in terms of its existential being. Does a metal gear mechanism have a soul? Of course not. These are merely ways of helping individuals in a group setting stretch their minds and give vent to their spontaneity, and through this reaching or groping beyond one's ordinary cognitive functioning, the group or its individuals may come up either with solutions to the problem or with a way of thinking about it that may lead other members of the team to the problem's solution or solutions.

These are what might be expected in a weekend workshop organized to deal with a specific technical or business problem. By-products of such a workshop include a camaraderie that usually is carried over to the daily business life of the individuals, to the benefit of the organization in improved communication and cooperation among team members. The same by-products of course, would be obtained from

[3]Even in the city, a good workshop leader can help create the appropriate atmosphere of retreat and commitment to the workshop goals among participants.

the somewhat different workshops and courses presented by the Behavior Sciences Education Center.

The training program that Behavior Sciences Education Center (BSEC) has put together for the personal development and improved business functioning of corporate employees consists of five major parts,[4] which are presented in classes that may have as many as thirty or forty persons enrolled. The major categories in the BSEC program call for improvement in emotional responses, memory, cognitive skills, motor skills, and benefits from sleep. In the first category, retraining emotional responses, BSEC notes that all negative behavior responses, for example, tension, stress, and irritability, or negative emotional responses, such as feelings of inferiority, apprehension, and frustration are caused by a form of fear. Thus, says Richard L. Johnson, BSEC president, "subconscious feelings of fear will exert a strong influence on behavior in any situation." His example is that of the employee who fears rejection and therefore fails to submit an idea that might save his firm a considerable amount of money or bring in additional revenue. Johnson's way of dealing with this fear is through the cybernetics approach, first to achieve an improved self-image and second to condition new response patterns. He would then have the individual reprogram himself as follows: "Everyday I am becoming more confident in my ability to think things through accurately and completely; I am able to correct my mistakes when they do occur, and I am able to find answers to questions when I need them; therefore, it is safe to trust myself to do my very best on each task I set out to do." For the new response patterns, the program would be: "Each and every time I am criticised I will feel calm, relaxed and self-confident, [and] I will automatically say or do just the right thing in just the right way to correctly solve my problem." This, of course, is taught in the group setting, so that the entire class may benefit from the retraining.

In improving memory, BSEC points out that recall of recent information may be handicapped by excessive stress, lack of proper motivation, conditioned response, or self-image, while the success in improving recall of recent information requires the individual's correcting the cause of the problem and training the subconscious to allow a greater facility of recall. The cybernetics approach in relieving stress follows: "After relaxing, visualize the pressure cooker and picture releasing the steam as you give the following instructions: (a) Whatever

---

[4]The ideas and the material described and quoted or paraphrased are authored by Richard L. Johnson and/or his associates at Behavior Sciences Education Center and are coyprighted, 1971, as presented.

problems confront me, I am going to put them aside for now as though putting them on the shelf, [and] I will do just the right thing to correctly solve my problems one-by-one at the appropriate time; (b) the more of this steam I release from the cooker, the more relief I feel mentally and the easier it becomes to recall whatever ideas of information I need." To increase motivation: "It is important to me to be able to recall information at the moment I need it and to whatever extent it is needed; therefore, I direct my inner-mind to help me to find a reason that I can accept which will cause me to become interested in improving my recall." For conditioning appropriate responses, the instructions are, "Each and every time I see the face of someone whose name I have learned before, I will recall his name [and] each time I hear the name of someone I have known before I will recall the face," while for improving self-image, the instructions read: "I am becoming more confident in my ability to recall whatever information I need, as I need it [and] I am learning to respect myself highly enough to allow myself to do my very best at this or at any other skill I wish to employ." The quotations are taken from BSEC's Executive Cybernetics Seminar syllabus, but Johnson is quick to point out during his course that participants should use the instructions creatively for their own specific needs at specific times and not to slavishly follow the examples given, especially if they can create more appropriate programming for themselves.

For the improving of cognitive skills, BSEC's example for increasing perception and awareness states: "As I enter my prospect's place of business, my perception will include everything in my environment, [and] I will automatically become aware of any sight, sound, smell, or any other perception that will indicate my customer's need for my product," while the example for improving conceptualization is: "My inner-mind will cause me to consciously understand the significance of my perceptions and to retain them in my memory with ease until I am ready to use them in my presentation to show the prospect how my product would be a benefit to his company." An example of improving recall declares: "As I make my presentation to the prospect, I will sense his thoughts and feelings . . . [and] I will automatically recall all of the information I need, whether it is information I have prepared ahead of time or information I gained after arrival; my inner-mind will cause me to present my information in the most effective way possible to help my prospect decide to purchase my new product now." For the student who needs help in studying or test taking, the programming is as follows: "Each time I sit down to read my textbook, I will feel calm, relaxed and self-confident, [and] as I read my book I will be able to understand it as easily as though I were reading a fiction story; therefore,

I will be able to read rapidly and retain all I read with ease. Unless it is important to me to do otherwise, nothing I see or hear around me will be permitted to disturb me or distract me in any way. I will become so interested in what I am reading that I will read more rapidly than before. Time will seem to go by so swiftly that I will have finished my assigned reading almost before I realize the study time has begun. When I sit down at my desk to take my test, I will become calm, relaxed and self-confident, [and] as I read each question, I will automatically recall everything I have ever heard, read, or thought that will help me to answer that question correctly. I will be able to express the answer in precisely the way my professor wants to see it expressed."

One of the examples for programming to improve motor skills is that of bowling, with setting an objective as the initial approach, but other examples include developing copying skills, using computing skills, using selective memory, using recall, and dealing with specific problems. These same approaches may readily be employed in improving other motor skills, such as flying an airplane, operating a lathe, or handling a motion picture camera. The example given for setting an objective for a reasonable improvement over former bowling scores, states: "When I arrive at the bowling alley I will feel calm, relaxed and self-confident, [and] my inner-mind will automatically adjust my thoughts, feelings and motion in whatever way necessary for me to achieve an average score of 185 or more in the total games played this evening. While still relaxed, visualize the above instructions having been successful and causing you to bowl with correct form; picture the entire sequence from picking up the ball to seeing a strike produced; practice visualizing each step in detail with as much seriousness as one should feel toward a dress rehearsal." To employ copying skills, BSEC's example states: "I direct my inner-mind to observe this professional as I watch him on T.V. and to copy any detail from his performance that would help me to improve my skill; it is not important to me to be consciously aware of what I am copying; however, I will automatically apply these corrections in my own performance each time I bowl." For computing skills: "I direct my inner-mind to study carefully every detail about his performance as this next person takes his turn at bowling; I will automatically compute the difference between his actual performance and what he should have done to get a strike; I will automatically use the corrected procedure when I bowl so that I will be able to produce a strike."

For selective memory, still using the bowling example, instructions are: "Inner-mind, we have tried many different ideas and techniques for improving my score; some have been effective, others may have been ineffective or even counter-effective; I want you to review everything we have been doing and discard any ideas or techniques other than those that were helpful; from this point on, you will automatically select only those elements of my performance that are successful, [and] I will continue practicing my successes and will rapidly discard my failures." The example for the use of recall is: "Inner-mind, I know you still remember all of the details about my last strike; I want you to recall everything about that strike that I need to cause me to repeat it, [and] I will recall how I felt, how I stood, how I threw the ball, and I will repeat the entire process over and over until I am able to repeat the strike with ease every time I try." Finally, in dealing with specific problems: "I have read how I should be holding my wrist and I have been shown by others how my wrist-action controls the ball; [thus] inner-mind, I want you to cause me to make proper use of this knowledge by automatically applying it correctly as I throw the ball each time I bowl."

For many individuals improving the benefits gained from sleep can bring about a total change for the better in their personal and business lives, and BSEC presents a step-by-step programming procedure as follows: "(a) I direct my inner-mind to cause me to go deeply asleep immediately after entering sleep. I will remain deeply asleep all night long, awakening only at my regular time tomorrow morning, unless otherwise specified. (b) While I am deeply asleep my inner-mind will take whatever steps may be necessary to heal my thoughts, feelings, attitudes or any other thing necessary to improve my health and welfare. I will continue to remain so deeply asleep throughout the night that no unpleasant thought or feeling of any kind will be permitted to disturb my conscious mind in any way. Each and every night it will become easier and easier to follow the pattern in these instructions. (c) No matter what time of evening I may go to sleep, I will automatically adjust my sleep habits so that I will be able to awaken each morning at the appointed time feeling completely rested and refreshed. (d) The final dream that I will have tomorrow morning before awakening will be a dream in which I will feel and act very confidently, securely and spiritually strongly. When I awake in the morning I will continue to feel confident, secure and spiritually strong and those feelings will remain with me all day long, regardless of what may happen."

The programming that Johnson teaches the groups he works with and the directed fantasy experiences for creative problem-solving that Greenberg guides his workshop participants through both utilize either the hypnotic state or the relaxed waking state, and these states are brought about through quite ordinary group induction methods. Both Johnson and Greenberg first have the group members make themselves comfortable and then employ a combination of counting and the presentation of visual imagery to help group members become more and more relaxed as a means of entering the hypnotic state, or, if they wish, remaining in the waking but very relaxed state. Throughout the inductions, Johnson and Greenberg, as well as their respective associates, include positive, growth-inducing statements that are open-minded enough so that group members may utilize these statements for their own particular needs or desires. The appropriate positive suggestions are a useful part of the induction process and tend to provide an added bonus to those participating in the induction. Needless to say, the positive suggestions are aimed toward feelings of general well-being and achievement of success and do not involve anything like symptom-removal or therapeutic exploration, since such is not the purpose of these group hypnosis and other experiences.

The purpose is the employment of group hypnosis for organizational and executive development, for employee well being, and for creative problem solving as a means of helping business and other organizations to improve their methods and to achieve their goals, and an acceptance of these methods is increasing as business and other leaders become more aware of them and of what can be accomplished by them.

BIBLIOGRAPHY

1. BARBER, THEODORE X. *Hypnosis: A Scientific Approach.* New York: Van Nostrand Reinhold. 1969.

2. CHEEK, DAVID B., AND LECRON, LESLIE M. *Clinical Hynotherapy.* New York and London: Grune & Stratton. 1968.

3. COOPER, LINN F., AND ERICKSON, MILTON H. *Time Distortion in Hypnosis.* Baltimore: The Williams & Wilkins Company. 1959.

4. FROMM, ERIKA, AND SHOR, RONALD E. (Eds.) *Hypnosis: Research Developments and Perspectives.* Chicago and New York: Aldine-Atherton. 1972.

5. GIBBONS, DON. *Beyond Hypnosis: Explorations in Hyperempiria.* South Orange, N. J.: Power Publishers, Inc. 1972.

6. GILL, MERTON M., AND BRENMAN, MARGARET. *Hypnosis and Related States.* New York: International Universities Press, Inc. 1961.

7. GREENBERG, IRA A. *Psychodrama and Audience Attitude Change.* Beverly Hills, Ca.: Behavioral Studies Press. 1968.

8. ———. (Ed.) *Psychodrama: Theory and Therapy.* New York: Behavioral Publications, Inc. 1974.

9. HALEY, JAY. (Ed.) *Advanced Techniques of Hypnosis and Therapy: Selected Papers of Milton H. Erickson, M.D.* New York and London: Grune & Stratton. 1967.

10. HARTLAND, JOHN. *Medical and Dental Hypnosis.* London: Bailliers, Tindall & Cassell. 1966.

11. HILGARD, ERNEST R. *Hypnotic Susceptibility.* New York: Harcourt, Brace and World, Inc. 1965.

12. JOHNSON, RICHARD. An announcement of services. Glendale, Ca. 1971.

13. KLINE, MILTON V. (Ed.) *Clinical Correlations of Experimental Hypnosis.* Springfield, Ill.: Charles C. Thomas, Publishers. 1963.

14. _____. (Ed.) *Psychodynamics and Hypnosis.* Springfield, Ill.: Charles C. Thomas, Publishers. 1967.

15. KROGER, WILLIAMS S. *Clinical and Experimental Hypnosis:* Philadelphia and Montreal: J. B. Lippincott and Company. 1963.

16. LECRON, LESLIE M. (Ed.) *Experimental Hypnosis.* New York: The Macmillan Company. 1958.

17. MEARES, AINSLIE. *Hypnography.* Springfield, Ill.: Charles C. Thomas, Publishers. 1957.

18. _____. *Shapes of Sanity.* Springfield, Ill.: Charles C. Thomas, Publishers. 1960.

19. WOLBERG, LEWIS R. *Hypnoanalysis.* (2d ed.) New York and London: Grune & Stratton. 1964.

10
Group Hypnotherapy in a University Counseling Center*

B. J. Hartman

Hypnosis can be of significant and lasting value in student counseling. Mellenbruch (1964) included the following areas for discussion in his paper on hypnosis in student counseling: (a) study problems, (b) class attitude changes, (c) personal adjustment problems, (d) mental blocking, and (e) emotional upheavals. Summo and Rouke (1965) report using hypnosis for a number of student problems in college counseling. They include students striving beyond their capacity, parental pressure to achieve beyond their ability, overinvolvement in extra-curricular activities, reading speed and comprehension problems, and students with feelings of guilt because of neglect of study or those who have chronic feelings of inadequacy. Krippner (1963) has found hypnosis to be useful with study habit problems, test-taking behavior, and motivation problems.

In addition to the above uses of hypnosis in college counseling, the author has developed a number of specialized group hypnotherapy clinics which he is conducting on a once a week basis in the counseling center at Southern Illinois University. An announcement of the clinics is placed in the school paper at the beginning of each term. Screening interviews are held with each prospective client to determine his suitability for the particular clinic to which he is seeking entrance. Each clinic is limited to five individuals.

At present the following five clinics are in operation: weight control, smoking withdrawal, scientific relaxation, concentration and examination behavior, and assertive training.

WEIGHT CONTROL CLINIC

Before being accepted for this clinic the client must take the A-D Scale (a combination of the Taylor Manifest Anxiety Scale and the Depression Scale of the Minnesota Multiphasic Personality Inventory). If he scores high on anxiety and/or depression, he is not accepted into the group, but individual psychotherapy is recommended. Also, individuals must have had a physical examination and permission from their physician prior to being accepted for the clinic. The clinic includes eight sessions of one hour duration on a once a week basis. During the first session the misconceptions of hypnosis are discussed, and each client completes a form relating to eating habits and historical data pertinent to his overweight problem. A lecture period follows and the session is concluded with a group hypnotic induction using the progressive relaxation technique. All lecture material for this clinic is taken from the book *Mind Over Platter* (Lindner, 1965). A diet diary form is handed out at the second session, and the clients are told to list everything that they eat each day, the time of day and the number of calories. They are told to follow their physician's instructions concerning calorie intake. The remainder of the second session is devoted to group induction of hypnosis, lecture (all lectures are conducted with the clients in hypnosis), and a discussion with each client about his eating habits and overweight problem with appropriate suggestions for correcting poor eating habits.

The third session includes collecting the diet diary reports and giving a report of the number of pounds lost by the group during the previous week, group induction, lecture, ideomotor questioning with each client to determine subconscious motivation and underlying causes of the overweight problem. An ideomotor questionnaire for obesity cases consisting of 35 questions was constructed by the author for use in the clinic. The interested reader may obtain detailed information on ideomotor questioning by reading the articles by Cheek (1960) and LeBaron (1964). The third session is concluded with group training in self-hypnosis, lecture, and a description of *Dr. Lindner's "Point System" Weight Control Program* (Lindner and Lindner, 1966). Each client is given a copy of the book and told to begin using the point system rather than calories. The fourth session includes diet diary reports, group induction, lecture, continuation of ideomotor questioning and group training in self-hypnosis.

The fifth through the eighth sessions consist of diet diary reports, reports on group weight loss, and the discussion of each client's problems connected with overweight and overeating. Free ventilation is encouraged during this part of the session before hypnosis is induced. Then group hypnosis is induced and appropriate suggestions are given. The sessions end with the clients going into self-hypnosis and arousing themselves.

SMOKING WITHDRAWAL CLINIC

Individuals must have permission from their physician prior to acceptance into the clinic. The clinic is held for five weekly sessions and sixth and seventh sessions are held bi-weekly. The first session consists of lecture material from *How To Stop Smoking Through Self Hypnosis* (LeCron, 1964), a summary of the Surgeon General's Report, the misconceptions of hypnosis, group trance induction, instructions for keeping a notebook that should contain the following information: each time they smoke, the time of day, and what type of activity they were engaged in at the time. They are also given an assignment to write an autobiography of their smoking habit entitled "Why I Smoke."

The second session consists of completing a questionnaire designed to determine whether the client is a light, medium, or heavy smoker and whether his smoking is an habituation or an addiction. This is followed by group trance induction, instructions to the clients (the instructions follow the 21 day program as outlined by von Dedenroth, 1964), ideomotor questioning to determine subconscious motivation and underlying causes of smoking, and conditioning for self-hypnosis. The third session consists of group induction, lecture, suggestions to help stop smoking, further instructions (as per von Dedenroth's program), a discussion of notebooks and autobiographies with each client, and conditioning for self-hypnosis. The fourth session consists of self-hypnotic induction, a lecture entitled "Your Program For Q Day" (quit day), suggestions to help stop smoking, and a discussion of notebooks with each client.

The fifth session begins with immediate induction of the trance state and the fact that good habits have already replaced bad habits is stressed and re-stressed. This is followed by a lecture entitled "Your Program After Q Day" and suggestions to help stop smoking. The sixth and seventh sessions are meant to be reinforcement sessions. A report on each client's progress is made. Each client's problems, if any, are discussed openly. Free ventilation is encouraged during this part of the session before hypnosis is induced. Then hypnosis is induced and appropriate suggestions are given. The session ends with each client going into self-hypnosis and arousing himself.

SCIENTIFIC RELAXATION CLINIC

This is an on-going clinic meeting once a week for one hour. It consists of the differential and progressive relaxation techniques of Wolpe (Wolpe and Lazarus, 1966) and autogenic training (Schultz, 1959). The first twenty minutes is devoted to differential and progressive relaxation of the arms, facial area, neck, shoulders, upper back, chest, stomach, lower back, hips, thighs and calves, followed by complete body relaxation. The remaining thirty to forty minutes is devoted to autogenic training.

CONCENTRATION AND EXAMINATION BEHAVIOR CLINIC

This clinic consists of four sessions. The first session includes a discussion of the misconceptions about hypnosis, progressive relaxation induction technique, ego-strengthening routine (Hartland, 1965), suggestions for improving concentration and study habits and for overcoming examination panic, and conditioning for self-hypnosis.

The second, third, and fourth sessions consist of progressive relaxation induction, ego-strengthening routine, and the first, second, and third scripts for deep concentration (Lieberman et al., 1968), one for each session.

ASSERTIVE TRAINING CLINIC

This is an on-going clinic and entrance is either by referral from another staff member in the counseling center or by self-referral. In deciding whether or not assertive training is indicated, prospective group members are given the *Assertive Interaction Questionnaire* (Wolpe and Lazarus, 1966), the *Willoughby Schedule* (Wolpe, 1958) and a historical data questionnaire. The client to whom assertive training applies has unadaptive anxiety-response habits in interpersonal relationships, and the evocation of anxiety inhibits the expression of appropriate feelings and the performance of adaptive acts.

The procedure usually commences with a description of ineffectual forms of behavior in general and their emotional repercussions. Reading Salter's *Conditioned Reflex Therapy* (1961) may be assigned for its pertinent case history material. While being trained in assertive behavior, clients are told to keep careful notes of all their significant interpersonal encounters and to discuss them in detail with the therapist. It is necessary to know the circumstances of the encounter, the client's feelings at the time, the manner in which he reacted, how he felt immediately after the encounter, and his own subsequent appraisal of the situation. Upon the identification of debilitating inhibitions, the therapist firmly stresses assertive as opposed to aggressive reactions where applicable.

A form of role playing known as behavior rehearsal is used by behavior therapists in assertive training. The author has replaced behavior rehearsal with hypnodrama. Hypnodrama is a synthesis of psychodrama and hypnosis and was developed by J.L. Moreno (Moreno and Enneis, 1950).

Assertive training is a teaching situation in which the client is taught to respond in an appropriate manner in those situations which call for some type of assertive response, whether it be voicing justifiable criticism or expressing affectionate feelings. The closer that the teaching situation comes to approximating the real life situation, the greater the transfer should be from the practice session of being assertive to assertive behavior *in vivo*. This has certainly been the case with those individuals the author has observed in hypnodramatic assertive training. This approach has elicited a wealth of subconscious material which would not have been elicited with behavior rehearsal.

In conclusion, group hypnotherapy in the form of specialized clinics has been described whereby clients in a university counseling center are seen for specific problems. Many clients are referred to one of the clinics by their counselor for the particular problem area dealt with in the clinic while the counselor continues to see the client on a regular basis and continues to be responsible for the client's overall therapeutic program. Although no formal followup has been carried out at this time, indications from counselor and client reports are that the majority of clients have improved a great deal. Steady progress has been noted for all clients who have regularly attended the clinics. Research data is being collected for all clinic clients and will be published when a sufficient number have completed each clinic program.

References

CHEEK, D. Removal of subconscious resistance to hypnosis using ideomotor questioning techniques. *American Journal of Clinical Hypnosis*, 1960, 3, 103-107.

HARTLAND, J. The value of "ego-strengthening" procedures prior to direct symptom-removal under hypnosis. *American Journal of Clinical Hypnosis*, 1965, 8, 89-93.

KRIPPNER, S. Hypnosis and reading improvement among university students. *American Journal of Clinical Hypnosis*, 1963, 5, 187-193.

LEBARON, G. Ideomotor communication in confusional states and schizophrenia. *American Journal of Clinical Hypnosis*, 1964, 7, 42-54.

LECRON, L. *How to stop smoking through self hypnosis*. West Nyack, N.Y.: Parker, 1964.

LIEBERMAN, L., FISHER, J., THOMAS, R., and KING, W. Use of tape recorded suggestions as an aid to probationary students. *American Journal of Clinical Hypnosis*, 1968, 11, 35-41.

LINDNER, P. *Mind over platter*. Hollywood, Calif.: Wilshire, 1966.

LINDNER, P. and LINDNER, D. *Dr. Lindner's "Point System" Weight Control Program*. Hollywood, Calif.: Wilshire, 1966.

MELLENBRUCH, P. Hypnosis in student counseling. *American Journal of Clinical Hypnosis*, 1964, 7, 60-63.

MORENO, J. and ENNEIS, J. *Hypnodrama and psychodrama*. Beacon, N.Y.: Beacon House, 1950.

SALTER, A. *Conditioned reflex therapy*. New York: Capricorn, 1961.

SCHULTZ, J. *Autogenic training*. New York: Grune and Stratton, 1959.

SUMMO, A. and ROURKE, F. The use of hypnosis in a college counseling service. *American Journal of Clinical Hypnosis*, 1965, 8, 114-116.

VON DEDENROTH, T. The use of hypnosis with "Tobaccomaniacs." *American Journal of Clinical Hypnosis*, 1964, 6, 326-331.

VON DEDENROTH, T. Further help for the "tobaccomaniac." *American Journal of Clinical Hypnosis*, 1964, 6, 332-336.

WOLPE, J. *Psychotherapy by reciprocal inhibition*. Stanford, Calif.: Stanford University Press, 1958.

WOLPE, J. and LAZARUS, A. *Behavior therapy techniques*. Oxford: Pergamon Press, 1966.

11
Individual Hypnosis, Group Hypnosis, and the Improvement of Academic Achievement

Stanley Krippner

Group hypnosis, and the principles derived from it, have long been educational tools. Classroom teachers attempt to relax their pupils before they begin a difficult assignment or an examination. High school athletic coaches motivate their teams by delivering "pep talks." College professors capture their students' attention with colorful language and visual aids. All are using techniques of hypnosis.

Hypnosis is generally defined as a procedure which induces a state of consciousness characterized by heightened responsiveness to direct suggestion. Because suggestion is a frequent concomitant of the teaching process, it is possible that many educators have, without knowing it, used some form of hypnosis.

The utility of hypnosis, diversely employed as an educational tool, has been experimentally studied by several researchers. Scharf & Zamansky (1961), for example, used hypnosis to reduce the time required to identify words exposed on a tachistoscope. In this experiment, the word recognition thresholds of 24 college students were lowered, through hypnotic suggestion, by an average of 10 percent.

Kliman & Goldberg (1962) measured the effects of hypnosis on the reading abilities of 10 college students. In the experiment, 20 five-letter words were flashed on a screen at low levels of illumination. The candlepower required to recognize each flashing word was recorded. Subjects evidenced greatest recognition improvement while under hypnosis.

In a study by Mutke (1967), the hypnosis group reportedly was able to increase its reading speed significantly in one-fourth the time required by the control group, whose members had not been hypnotized.

Krippner (1966) reported a study involving 49 school children who were enrolled in a five-week reading clinic, in which they attended five two-hour remedial reading sessions a week. At the request of the parents, hypnosis was used with nine children to decrease tension, increase motivation, foster interest in reading, and maintain attention and concentration. It was also used to facilitate revisualizations[1] and reauditorization[2] of graphic spoken symbols, thus improving spelling accuracy. The degree of reading improvement for each child was measured by administering two different forms of the California Reading Test (Tiegs & Clark, 1957). One form was administered on the first day of the clinic and the other form on the last day. Median improvement for the total group over the five-week period was five months' reading advancement. Of those receiving hypnosis as part of the treatment program, eight children were above the median at the close of the clinic, and one fell below the median. Of the group that was not hypnotized, 16 children were above the median, and 24 fell at or below it. The children who received hypnotic treatment performed significantly better than those who did not.

Lamothe (1960) worked with 21 high school students and suggested that under hypnosis they would develop an increased capacity for remembering, paying attention, and understanding material. Statistically significant results were obtained for only three of the subjects on pretest-posttest examinations of academic achievement.

Eisele & Higgins (1962), Erickson (1961), Lodato (1968), McCord & Sherrill (1961), Sears (1962), and Summo & Rouke (1965), have also reported favourable results with hypnosis in calming anxiety, improving study habits, and increasing concentration.

Ambrose (1961) has used hypnosis with children exhibiting learning difficulties. (Betts (1957), Lichter (1968), Woody & Herr (1966), and Ziegenfuss (1962) have suggested a wider use of hypnosis with poorly motivated students, the brain-damaged, and the speech-handicapped. Estabrooks & Gross (1961) have recommended its employment with the mentally retarded, while concluding that "the real future of hypnosis as an aid to the human mind lies, however, in the education and guidance of normal youngsters, who can benefit from its employ all the way from elementary school through college."

On the other hand, Egan & Egan (1968) found no difference between

---

[1]The ability to "re-see" a word in the mind's eye.
[2]The ability to "re-hear" a word mentally.

a control group of college students and an experimental group which had been given two hypnotic sessions and had been taught self-hypnosis. Edmonston & Marks (1967) did not find hypnotic induction useful in a kinesthetic learning task, while Edmonston & Stanek (1966) found that it had no special value in a verbal learning task.

Barber (1965) has made a valid criticism of most of these experimental studies of learning and hypnosis. He contends:

> The investigation confounded two independent variables: (a) the "hypnotic trance state"; and (b) suggestions intended to elicit a high level of performance. Since suggestions for improved performance were not given under waking conditions, no conclusions are possible concerning the effects of "hypnotic trance," or the effects of suggestions for high performance, or the interaction of hypnosis with suggestions. The possibility was not considered that Ss might have performed as proficiently under a waking condition as under the "trance" condition, if suggestions for enhanced learning and recall had been given under both conditions.

He concluded that hypnosis by itself does not enhance learning or recall. He did note, however, that task-motivating suggestions may be effective at times with hypnotic subjects, as they are with non-hypnotic subjects.

Other research reviews have been presented by Fowler (1961), Glasner (1953), and Uhr (1958). In his review article, Uhr (1958) found "little if any conclusive experimental evidence treating this question" but noted that "what evidence there is . . . indicated quite definite and possibly striking improvement in learning . . . while under a well-managed trance."

GENERAL PROCEDURES

The author has worked individually and in groups with elementary and secondary school pupils at the Kent State University Child Study Center, and with college students at Northwestern University. He emphasized the use of hypnosis as an aid to the improvement of study habits, increase of concentration, reduction of examination anxiety, increase of motivation, and improvement of specific language skills.

Of those individuals able to enter "deep hypnosis," some have recalled in detail material read or heard several years previously. This type of ability is also reflected in hypnotized students purportedly able to read several pages of difficult material and recall them word-for-word the following day while writing an examination.

Because these phenomena are atypical of general hypnotic

behavior, students should not be instructed to develop a photographic memory, to read faster, or to make "perfect" examination scores. It is wiser to set more easily attainable goals which can be obtained with most individuals capable of being hypnotized.

TECHNIQUE

The students are asked to fix their attention upon a specific stimulus, such as the hypnotist's voice or a colored spot attached to the ceiling of the room. The hypnotist makes several comments to encourage relaxation and concentration on the part of the students. Hypnotic induction then proceeds according to one of the methods described by Pattie (1956).

If the students are able to perform a simple post-hypnotic suggestion, it is assumed that they can be given another suggestion that might improve their reading and studying behavior. Sometimes, only one session is needed to help a student. Sometimes, two or more sessions are needed to enable a student to alter his or her behavior. At times, a student will not react to a post-hypnotic suggestion, even after several sessions. In such a case, no further hypnotic work should be attempted; instead, other techniques should be stressed (e.g., behavioral modification, perceptual-motor training, academic skill development, megavitamin treatment, supportive counseling).

PROBLEMS IN STUDY SKILLS AND WORK HABITS

The Brown-Holtzman Survey of Study Habits and Attitudes (1956) is valuable for use with high school and college students, as it pinpoints specific problems for the educational therapist. Also effective is the practice of having students record their greatest impediments to academic efficiency.

Rapaport (1968) has defined a post-hypnotic suggestion as "a subject's execution in the waking state of a command given by the hypnotizer during the trance state." Among the post-hypnotic suggestions used by the author to improve study habits have been the following: (1.) When you are studying this evening, you will find that your concentration is so intense that you will be interested in nothing but your mathematics assignment. (2.) At 8:00P.M. you will be absorbed in completing your history term paper. For the following three hours, you will want to do nothing else. Barring emergencies, nothing will interrupt you. If your friends enter the room, you will, with as much tact as necessary, send them away. (3.) As you begin to study chemistry, your mind will quickly grasp the information at hand. Each important fact will make a profound impression upon you. You will be able to recall the information easily when future events demand it.

Academic problems often arise from a lack of organization of the work into a useful, logical, sequence. Hypnosis may facilitate a student's ability to carry through an assignment or to study effectively. Examples of suggestions which the author has given in such situations, both to individuals and groups, are the following: (1.) Before you start to study this evening, form an outline of the work you wish to accomplish so that you may, by following your outline, study very efficiently. You will accomplish a great deal as you follow this outline. (2.) When you start working on your paper, you will organize your references and other material according to an outline of the general formation of your paper. As you plan your paper, you will become very eager to make your plan a reality and put the ideas into writing.

Jeanne was a college student who had very poor study skills and work habits. She fell into the lowest 15 percent of students her age on the Brown-Holtzman Survey of Study Habits and Attitudes. We took each of the Brown-Holtzman areas where she had a problem and worked on it individually. After a new study skill was introduced and developed, it was reinforced by hypnotic suggestion. Each of Jeanne's poor attitudes toward study was discussed, and she verbally formulated a new, positive attitude. While she was in a hypnotic trance, her own words were used and she was told that she would *feel* the new attitude, as well as *think* about it. After 12 weekly sessions, Jeanne's study skills had improved so greatly that hypnosis was terminated; on re-administration of the Brown-Holtzman, she scored in the upper 25th percentile. She eventually entered graduate school and reported that her work habits were continuing at a high level.

CONCENTRATION AND ATTENTION PROBLEMS

Lack of concentration or a short attention span may present a serious block to a student's academic achievement. An example of a student suffering from these problems was Robert. After studying for a few minutes, he would feel the need to open the window, get a drink of water, or visit the candy-vending machine. He would turn on the radio or record player, or remember urgent telephone calls which had to be made. Robert claimed that it had become impossible for him to concentrate on his studies for more that 10 minutes before his thoughts would wander to other matters.

Robert was hypnotized several times in a few weeks. One by one, the bad habits were replaced with other patterns of behavior. He was told that he would ignore the room temperature while he was studying; his own sensations of thirst and hunger; the appeal of the radio, record player, and telephone. He was further told that his attention span would increase. So successful were the suggestions that, by the end of three weeks, Robert was spending several consecutive hours on his studies each night without interruption.

Lee had difficulty paying attention to classroom lectures and concentrating on the material presented. It was noticed that Lee wore a large ring; he was told that, whenever his mind wandered, he merely had to rub the front of the ring to re-focus his attention on the lecturer. This suggestion worked very well, and within a few weeks the new habit was so firmly established that the ring-rubbing technique no longer had to be utilized.

Poor concentration, a lack of attention, inability to do well on examinations, and other poor study habits often handicap children who have become reading disability cases. If serious emotional disturbances lie behind these problems, educational hypnosis must be part of a more comprehensive psychotherapeutic program. If not, hypnotic procedures may be effective when the approach is merely one of counseling in specific areas.

ELIMINATION OF ANXIETY

Test anxiety is a frequent study affliction. Many individuals claim to be well prepared when they enter the examination, only to forget essential data, make minor errors, and let nervous reactions lower their score once they begin the test. Hypnotic suggestions can be given to increase accuracy, reduce nervous tension, and improve recall.

Students desiring to improve their test-taking behavior are warned that several sessions are required. Students should not report for hypnosis with the hope that it will help them on an examination the following day. Instead, suggestions are presented and developed over a period of several days or weeks. Hypnotic suggestions are made regarding the interest students will find in the subject matter. They are told to think of their long-range goals and to realize how important their academic records will be in the attainment of these goals.

As might be suspected, those students without vocational goals or with little concern for the future have the most difficulty in benefitting from this type of hypnotic suggestion. Hypnosis, after all, does not implant new ideas in the mind; it merely reenforces those that have been there all along. Therefore, it is ineffective if there is nothing to reenforce.

Hypnotic suggestions can also be made concerning the ability to concentrate on crucial items. The students are told that no outside stimuli will distract them. They will be paying such close attention to the test that nothing else will interest them unless an emergency arises.

The hypnotist tries to keep the students from developing nervous symptoms and feelings of undue anxiety. A modicum of anxiety often helps to sharpen reactions during a test; too much hampers effectiveness.

Therefore, the students are told that their self-confidence will be very high as a result of their thorough preparation for the examination. Because their self-confidence will be very high, there will be no reason for them to develop fear reactions toward the test situation. They are told that they will approach the examination with an alert, but not over-anxious, attitude; they will be attentive, but not tense, while answering the examination questions.

At times, suggestions are also given to enable the students to sleep soundly the night before the test. They are discouraged from spending the night studying and are instructed to begin preparing for the examination well in advance.

Harry was a "B" student in the field of engineering; his IQ was 138 on the Wechsler Adult Intelligence Scale (WAIS). He felt that "examination panic" prevented him from doing well in a test situation. He also claimed to make careless errors which lowered grades.

During one academic quarter, Harry was put into a hypnotic trance before several of his examinations. He was given suggestions to decrease anxiety and fears, as well as suggestions to improve recall and memory. He was told that he could easily revisualize material which appeared in texts and reauditorize material from classroom lectures. For comparative purposes, he took alternate examinations without having previously entered a hypnotic trance.

On the latter examinations, Harry made a "B" average during the quarter. On those he took following hypnosis, he received without exception, grades of "A." He was later taught self-hypnosis, which enabled him to achieve the same results without the aid of a hypnotist.

Carl claimed that he needed a high grade in a Spanish examination to pass the course. He was so anxiety-ridden over the test that he had been unable to concentrate on the subject matter and had had difficulty getting to sleep. Hypnotic sessions began one week before the scheduled test.

The night before the examination, Carl was put into a light hypnotic trance and informed that he would spend the next several hours studying. He was told that he would study so intently that he would not worry about the test itself, talk to his roommate, or leave his desk—except to answer the telephone or go to the bathroom. Furthermore, he was told that at midnight he would become very tired, have a pleasant night's sleep, and awake at 7:30 A.M. He was told that he would feel in excellent condition in the morning and do well on his Spanish examination.

So well did the suggestions take effect that Carl refused to speak to anyone who entered his room that evening. He left his desk only once; on his way to the bathroom he was heard to mumble, "I must get back to that Spanish book." He later reported that he had adequately covered the material by 11:45. However, he was unable to close his book and reviewed the material again until 12:00. At this point he felt drowsy and went to bed. After a sound night's sleep, he awoke refreshed; took the Spanish examination; and received a "B," the highest grade he had ever received in that subject.

MOTIVATION AND INTEREST

Another area in which hypnosis can make a valuable contribution to the learning process is that of motivation. The difference between an excellent student and a poor student is often as much a matter of interest as it is of intelligence.

An interview with a student will often reveal what has impelled him to attend college. He may state his vocational ambitions, academic intentions, and life-long goals. Under hypnosis, these comments can be strengthened and reenforced so that the subject commits himself to these statements, feels strongly about them, and acts upon them.

Motivational problems seemed to afflict Rosie. Although her high school record was excellent and her IQ on the WAIS was 123, she found college difficult. She claimed that she would do well academically only if she liked a professor, enjoyed a course, and was "in the right mood" for studying. Rosie proved to be adept at self-hypnosis (LeCron, 1964; Sprinkle, McInelly, & Newman, 1966). Eventually, she was able to put herself into a light trance and tell herself that she would take a keen interest in an assignment. By this method, she was able to follow her assignments through to completion; as a result, her academic record showed a marked improvement.

Walter felt little motivation toward learning. He knew that a college education was necessary for the attainment of his vocational objectives but could not develop an interest in his course work, even in business, his major field. Walter's exact words regarding his long-range goals were repeated to him under hypnosis. Eventually, he was permitted to state these goals himself while in the hypnotic trance. Finally, he discussed his goals with the hypnotist while in hypnosis. The positive statements about career objectives were reenforced in this manner and gradually began to bring about a change in his academic performance. It can be seen in this case and the other cases that the student is encouraged to take as active a part in the procedure as possible. Success in carrying out hypnotic suggestions depends more on the student than on the hypnotist.

Problems in motivation and persistence also affected Guy, who characteristically fell asleep during class and while doing his homework. He had an IQ of 127 on an individually administered intelligence test (Wechsler, 1955) but refused to take any personality tests or submit to a psychiatric interview. On several occasions, hypnotic trances were induced, but Guy fell asleep while in a trance and no suggestions could effectively be introduced. In other words, he went from an "hypnotic sleep," in which the individual is very conscious of what is occurring, to an actual sleep, in which he is not aware of what the hypnotist is attempting. During the few sessions in which Guy remained awake, he did not go into a deep enough trance for post-hypnotic suggestions to be effective. Some months later, Guy's college career was terminated when he was found to be the producer of counterfeit drivers' licenses and falsified student identification cards.

The case of Guy demonstrates that deep-seated problems cannot be treated effectively by hypnotic suggestion unless they are preceded by personality change. In most cases, extensive psychotherapy would be required to bring about these changes. Although Guy's consciously stated attitudes regarding college were positive, his unconscious motives were too strong to be easily countermanded. Hypnosis, as we have previously asserted, can be seen as an efficient reenforcer of drives already present; however, it cannot reenforce a drive which is either non-existent or in conflict with some stronger one.[3]

DEFICIENT LANGUAGE SKILLS

Revisualization and reauditorization are necessary abilities if accurate spelling is to develop. Myklebust (1956) has stated that the proficient speller unconsciously revisualizes and reauditorizes words simultaneously. The Radaker technique (1963), which involves revisualization practice, was used with many clients exhibiting spelling problems. It was combined with reauditorization practice and educational hypnosis for those clients seen by Krippner (1966). The following language was used with a hypnotized client having difficulty spelling the word "car."

---

[3]In this connection, it might be asked what special qualifications a professional person must have in order to utilize hypnosis successfully in an educational setting. This is a crucial point because it is likely that the lack of trained personnel, rather than the lack of student interest, is the major factor inhibiting development in this field. A sound knowledge of educational psychology as well as a solid background in hypnosis are necessary. The hypnotist must understand the psychological and psysiological concomitants of reading improvement and study habits. Membership in either the American Society of Clinical Hypnosis or the Society for Clinical and Experimental Hypnosis is recommended.

Try to imagine a big, white moving picture screen. Nod your head when you have imagined the movie screen in your mind's eye. (Pause.) In just a moment you will be able to imagine some big, black letters appearing on the white screen. The letters will be very clear and they will stay on the screen until the right word appears. Imagine that the letter "C" is appearing on the left-hand side of the screen. To help you imagine this, I am going to trace a "C" on your forehead. (At this point the writer traced a "C" on the left side of the client's forehead.) Nod your head when the letter "C" appears on the screen. (Pause.) Very good. Next, imagine that the letter "A" is appearing in the middle of the screen. To help you imagine this, I am going to trace an "A" on your forehead. Nod your head when the letter "A" appears. (Pause.) Very good. Next, imagine that the letter "R" is appearing on the right side of the screen. To help you imagine this, I am going to trace an "R" on your forehead. Nod your head as soon as the letter "R" appears. (Pause.) Very good. "C-A-R" spells "car." Can you see all three of the letters on the movie screen? Nod your head if you can. (Pause.) Very good. Now hold these letters in your mind's eye and concentrate on them. Make the letters a dark, dark black and make the movie screen a bright, bright white. Concentrating on the letters will help you to remember how to spell "car" when you open your eyes. Now imagine that you can hear someone saying "car." Think of what it would sound like if someone said "car." Listen for this word in the back of your mind and you will hear it. Nod your head when you have heard it. (Pause.) Fine. Now keep looking at the movie screen and see how dark and black you can make the letters. At the same time, listen for the word "car" in the back of your mind. See if you can see and hear the word at the same time. If you can, nod your head. (Pause.) Very good. From now on, it will be easier for you to spell the word "car." Even without thinking too much about it, you will automatically see the word "car" in your mind's eye and hear the word "car" in the back of your mind. You will soon be able to do this for other words as well. Seeing and hearing words with your eyes closed is good practice for remembering how to spell words with your eyes open. For example, you are going to open your eyes in a few minutes and you will be able to take a pencil and paper and spell the word "car."

Some poor spellers have problems discriminating between two letters because of those letters' directionality. For example, they confuse "b" and "d," "p" and "q" "n" and "u," etc. These problems are often associated with lack of proper space orientation of body parts. A child who cannot tell his left hand from his right hand frequently confuses the letters "b" and "d," as well as such words as "saw" and "was." The author has helped in such cases to foster proper orientation through balancing, coordination, and lateral dominance activities. At times, he has also employed hypnosis (Krippner, 1966).

> Raise your right arm. Hold it high in the air. Your hand is so firm and so strong that you could hold it there for an hour. Remember that this is your *right* arm. I am going to take your right hand and trace the word "right" on it. "R-I-G-H-T" spells "right." This is your *right* hand and your *right* arm.

Once the client could discriminate between the right and left sides of his body, he would generally make better discriminations between such letters as "p" and "q." Letter knowledge was reenforced under hypnosis by having the client revisualize the letters, tracing the letters on his forehead, and having him trace the letters in the air while in the hypnotic trance.

CONCLUSION

The use of hypnosis with individuals and groups in educational settings deserves additional study and further application. At this point, no controlled research is available demonstrating the superiority of educational hypnosis over other task-oriented procedures. However, clinical reports indicate the possible utility of hypnosis in ameliorating students' study problems, improving concentration, reducing test anxiety, increasing motivation, and facilitating the learning of specific language skills. Hypnosis is not a panacea and must be used in combination with other methods and techniques. It does merit greater consideration by a society committed to the maximum development of the talents and skills of its citizens.

REFERENCES

AMBROSE, G. *Hypnotherapy with children.* (2d ed.) London: Staples Press, 1961.

BARBER, T.X. The effects of "hypnosis" on learning and recall: A methodological critique. *Journal of Clinical Psychology*, 1965, 21, 19-25.

BETTS, E.A. Using clinical services in the reading program. *Education*, 1957, 78, 27-32.

BROWN, W.F., & Holtzman, R.H. *Brown-Holtzman survey of study habits and attitudes.* New York: Psychological Corporation, 1956.

EDMONSTON, W.E., & Stanek, F.J. The effects of hypnosis and motivational instructions on kinesthetic learning. *American Journal of Clinical Hypnosis,* 1967, 9, 252-55.

EDMONSTON, W.E., & STANEK, F.J. The effects of hypnosis and meaningfulness of material on verbal learning. *American Journal of Clinical Hypnosis,* 1966, 8, 257-60.

EGAN, R.M., & EGAN, W.P. The effect of hypnosis on academic performance. *American Journal of Clinical Hypnosis,* 1968, 11, 30-34.

EISELE, G., & HIGGINS, J.J. Hypnosis in education and moral problems. *American Journal of Clinical Hypnosis,* 1962, 4, 259-63.

ERICKSON, M.H. Historical note on the hand levitation and other ideometer techniques. *American Journal of Clinical Hypnosis,* 1961, 3, 196-99.

ESTABROOKS, G.H., & GROSS, N.E. *The future of the human mind.* New York: E.P. Dutton, 1961.

FOWLER, W.L. Hypnosis and learning. *Journal of Clinical and Experimental Hypnosis,* 1961, 9, 223-32.

GLASNER, S. Research problems in the educational and psychological applications of hypnosis. *Journal of Clinical and Experimental Hypnosis,* 1953, 1, 42-48.

KLIMAN, G., & GOLDBERG, E.L. Improved visual recognition during hypnosis. *Archives of General Psychiatry,* 1962, 7, 155-62.

KRIPPNER, S. The use of hypnosis with elementary and secondary school children in a summer reading clinic. *American Journal of Clinical Hypnosis,* 1966, 8, 261-66.

LAMOTHE, G.V. La hypnosis en la enseñanza. *Acta Hypnosis Latino América,* 1960, 1, 15-30.

LECRON, L.M. *Self-hypnotism.* Englewood Cliffs, N.J.: Prentice-Hall, 1964.

LICHTER, S. The potential use of hypnosis in schools. *The American Way of Living,* 1968, 1, 1.

LODATO, F.J. Hypnosis: An adjunct to test performance. *American Journal of Clinical Hypnosis,* 1968, 11, 129-30.

MCCORD, H., & SHERRILL, C.I. A note on increased ability to do calculus post-hypnotically. *American Journal of Clinical Hypnosis,* 1961, 11, 129-30.

MUTKE, P.H.C. Increased reading comprehension through hypnosis. *American Journal of Clinical Hypnosis,* 1967, 9, 262-66.

MYKLEBUST, H.R. Language disorders in children. *Exceptional Children,* 1956, 23, 163-66.

PATTIE, F.A. Methods of induction, susceptibility, and criteria of hypnosis. In R.M. Dorcus (Ed.), *Hypnosis and its therapeutic applications.* New York: McGraw-Hill, 1956.

RADAKER, L.D. The effect of visual imagery upon spelling performance. *Journal of Educational Research*, 1963, 56, 370-72.

RAPAPORT, D. *Emotions and memory.* (2d ed.) New York: International Universities Press, 1968.

SCHARF, B., & ZAMANSKY, H.S. Reduction of word-recognition threshold under hypnosis. *Perceptual and Motor Skills*, 1963, 17, 499-510.

SEARS, A.B. Hypnosis and recall. *Journal of Clinical and Experimental Hypnosis*, 1962, 4, 165-71.

SPRINKLE, R.L., McINELLY, W.A., & NEWMAN, B.R. *A student guide to self-hypnosis.* Laramie: University of Wyoming, 1966.

SUMMO, A.J., & ROUKE, F.J. The use of hypnosis in a college counseling service. *American Journal of Clinical Hypnosis*, 1965, 8, 114-16.

TIEGS, E.W., & CLARK, W.W. *California reading test.* Subtest of California achievement tests. Monterey: California Test Bureau, 1957.

UHR, L. Learning under hypnosis: What do we know? What should we know? *Journal of Clinical and Experimental Hypnosis*, 1958, 6, 121-35.

WECHSLER, D. *Wechsler adult intelligence scale.* New York: Psychological Corp., 1955.

WOODY, R.H., & HERR, E.L. Psychologists and hypnosis. Part II. Use in educational settings. *American Journal of Clinical Hypnosis*, 1966, 8, 254-56.

ZIEGENFUSS, W.B. Hypnosis: A tool of education. *Education*, 1962, 82, 505-7.

12
Principles of Gestalttherapy in Relation to Hypnotherapy*

Dezso Levendula

Although Gestalttherapy derives from Gestalt Psychology, it also includes much of Freudian psychology, and also some para-Freudian developments.

Academic Gestalt Psychology claims that we become aware of an object not by summing up its parts, but rather by perceiving it as a total. A most important tenet of Gestalt Psychology is that one part of the total is usually in sharper focus than the rest of the perceptual field. This focal point of awareness is called the "Gestalt," a German word meaning "figure" or "configuration." The perceptual field surrounding the Gestalt is called "the background." Gestalt and background are perceived simultaneously as a unit. The need of the moment determines which part of this unit holds our interest, thus becoming a Gestalt, while the rest of the perceptual field recedes in attention and becomes the background (1).

Kurt Goldstein enlarged upon Gestalt Psychology when he developed the organismic concept which includes, beside the awareness of externalities, the inner happenings, thoughts, ideas, and emotions. Accordingly, awareness of the inside world also obeys the Gestalt principle.

The literature of Gestalttherapy is rather scant. The main contribu-

*Reprinted with permission of the author and publisher. Originally published in the *American Journal of Clinical Hypnosis* (1963), Vol. 6, No. 1, pp. 22-26. Copyright 1963 by the American Society of Clinical Hypnosis.

tion is a book, *Gestalttherapy*, written by Perls, Hefferline, and Goodman (2). Gestalttherapy is eminently suitable for group therapy, but it can be applied in individual therapy. The group sessions are active, intense, and informal. Ideally, the therapist is friendly, fair, but not afraid to express his opinion. He does not advise the patient and does not become a crutch, but is supportive by his acceptance and respect. The group leader keeps the session controllable but not controlled. All these desired qualifications of the Gestalt group leader could be equally well applied to any group therapeutic endeavor.

The sessions are directed toward experiencing, feeling, and expressing, and not to interpretation nor to intellectualization. The patients develop the theme spontaneously. The focus of the Gestalt therapist is upon using what is immediately available, namely the structure or the actual situation in the therapeutic hour. A basic difference from psychoanalytic therapy is that the Gestalt therapist does not consider the actuality of the experience only as a "clue" to the unconscious, but rather accepts it as a reality.

Another significant difference is the striving towards sharp Gestalt formation as a foundation of awareness. The patient is urged to experience and express his actual feelings as they occur "right here and now" as a response within the therapeutic situation. Talking "about" how he once felt "there and then," Perls terms "only broadcasting."

The therapist does not use free association to unblock the repressed, and he does not circumvent the resistances. On the contrary, he concentrates his therapeutic efforts on the resistances and blocks. He does not urge the patient not to resist; on the contrary he encourages him to form a sharp Gestalt of the feelings which accompany the resistances. For example, if the patient is sad, he is urged to elaborate on the sadness and thus to discover how he handles his feelings.

Another important tenet of Gestalttherapy is that motor behavior is the essential instrumentality of emotional expression. Aggressive drives to hit, to bite, and to kick are checked by tensing the opposing muscles. These motor controls are utilized consciously at first, but later the responses become automatic and habitual. Repression, in certain aspects, may be equated with automatic, unconscious muscle control.

The Gestalttherapist believes that muscle action during the therapeutic session becomes an important and telling sign of inner struggle. For example, when an emotionally significant situation is experienced during the session, the patient may have palpitation, he may have shortness of breath, or he may tremble through muscle action, or he may feel a tightness in his abdomen due to the contractions of the involuntary smooth muscles of the gastrointestinal tract, etc. The patient may look pale or red because the smooth muscles of the blood vessels were called upon unconsciously. The muscular manifestations are either visible to the therapist or are felt by the patient. Even if the patient does not actually know what these muscle changes represent, he can learn through self-observation that they occur only in situations with a characteristic emotional content.

The Gestalttherapist seldom asks "Why?" because he believes that the answer usually is a rationalization which comforts the patient but does not solve questions. On the other hand, the therapist will frequently ask, "What?" and "Where?" and "How do you feel it?" and "What do you do to prevent yourself from feeling it and expressing it?" because he wants to teach the patient to form a sharp Gestalt of his sensations. Gestalttherapy postulates that it is unessential to recall the conflictual episodes of the past. It is of greater significance for the patient to understand that his emotional responses toward existing life problems are faulty, habitual, and stereotyped. Current experiences in reality situations are of prime importance in effective therapy.

As the therapy progresses, the patient will gradually recognize his defense reactions, and that they are automatic. He will become aware that certain situations which are meaningless and harmless to others are menacing only to him. The patient reaches the conclusion with the help of the therapist that these situations are filled with anxiety only because they may be patterned after original repressed emotions. His anxiety is increased by the fact that he does not remember its origin. Eventually, the patient will learn not only to face the anxiety he attempted to block, but also to experience it, to express it, and finally to discharge it.

Gradually, by learning the Gestalten of his habitual responses, the patient learns to integrate the new knowledge about himself, thereby strengthening himself. The unfinished emotional phase of the situation which once menaced the child becomes a finished finality in the actuality of the "here and now" of the session, not in restriction to understandings of past feelings, even though the actual repressed ideational content of the original conflict may never become conscious.

CLINICAL EXAMPLE

In a group Gestalttherapy situation, a participating psychiatrist suggested an experiment. He asked the group members to place their right hand on the best liked person, their left hand on the next best liked person, and their foot on the most disliked member of the group. Immediately, a great discussion started. How could a person hurt someone's feelings so openly? Finally, the originator of the experiment placed his foot on a certain participant, and nearly all the group members selected this same individual as the target of their dislike. No one offered the hand of comfort. After the experiment, the victim proudly announced that the whole thing did not bother him; on the contrary, he felt quite important to be worthy of so much hate. But in a short while he became depressed, and when urged by the group leader to make the sadness a clear Gestalt, he began to cry. He gave the reason that suddenly he could not get it out of his mind that his parents were killed in a concentration camp, and that he had never allowed himself to cry about their cruel fate. He cried bitterly in the high-pitched tone of a child, protesting that even God had forsaken him by permitting his parents to die. Choked with tears, he asked for a Bible and read the twenty-third Psalm of David in order to give his parents the funeral which they had never had. A wave of sympathy arose within the group. Some conforted him, and one member of the group, who had been most intent in her dislike of him before, now sat at his feet to dry his tears. Then he uttered accusations against civilization which tolerated those barbaric crimes, and finally scolded the group members because they were quite content to enjoy life while innocent people were destroyed.

The patient, and also the group, were first sincerely convinced that the memory of the parental cruel fate had caused the overwhelming strong emotional reaction. He accused the originator of the experiment of being a rude person who exposed him to the humiliating mob reaction. Later, when asked to focus on his feelings, the true significance of the event gradually became clear to him. He realized that when he was rejected by the group, he could not bear it. It was a catastrophic experience to be unloved. It did not help to tell the group that the whole thing did not bother him, and when the denial as a defense failed, he unconsciously regressed toward childhood. Apparently, this was a more appropriate defense against the emerging anxiety. He looked first for his parents, and then realizing they were dead, he turned to God. He was amazed in retrospect at the effective choice his unconscious had made. His crying gave him a tremendous relief, and, at the same time, turned the hatred of the group, if not into love, at least into concern and sympathy. His unconscious choice in describing his parents' fate permitted him to scold the group members for being poor parent substitutes. Through this one experience with the group, he thereby learned to understand that there is an unconscious mind which protects one from overwhelming anxiety. As a result of this single therapeutic experience, he fully realized that he could never tolerate being disliked. His engaging manners then served him well to win the regard of the people around him.

This man had had severe headaches all his life, but as a result of this therapeutic encounter, he realized that to be loved at all costs was such an important thing in his life, and that he had never dared to express resentment openly against anybody. One cannot go through life without becoming angry. Therefore, he turned his aggressions against himself, which resulted in the migraine attacks. The therapeutic gain was considerable, although the specific underlying repressed childhood trauma was not recalled during the group therapy session.

The patient was then seen in individual therapy. He was hypnotized and it was suggested to him to re-experience the same emotion he had felt when in the group. He started to cry bitterly. He was asked to listen intently to his own crying until he could clearly remember when he had cried and felt the same way before. After some urging, he recalled that when he was about three years old, his parents went frequently to visit his grandparents in the evening. The parents had no mode of transportation other than walking, and they carried his baby brother in their arms. He was left at home locked in the dark house, immensely frightened, and when the parents returned hours later, they always found him crying and tearful. The patient had the vague feeling that his father urged his mother not to pay too much attention to his crying.

He achieved deep insight by experiencing in the actuality of the hypnotic session the dread of being abandoned and unloved. He understood how every situation in his life in which he was threatened by dislike became a facsimile of the childhood experience. He realized with sadness that he never truly forgave his parents for abandoning and locking him in the dark room. It was quite a shock but a revelation also to learn that this severly traumatic experience had so long influenced his life.

Let us analyze first the approach of the Gestalttherapist in the described case. He created an experimental conflict, then increased the awareness of the emotions and facilitated the acting out in the psychodrama, and guided the patient to the spontaneous realization that he could not tolerate being disliked. This specific example also demonstrated the basic tenet of the Gestalttherapy, that resistances need not be circumvented, but rather are to be faced.

Contemporary hypnotherapy shows a similarity to the techniques of Gestalttherapy. Induced experimental conflicts as in the clinical case mentioned, intensifications of emotions, the understanding of a past emotional situation, are utilized by both therapists. The Gestalttherapist would be in a more advantageous position if he would combine his approach with hypnotic techniques. For example, the Gestalttherapist teaches the increasing of awareness through experimental exercises. The hypnotherapist can achieve this much more easily by directing the patient's attention to become sharply aware of an idea or sensation or memory which thereby becomes "a bright Gestalt" while the rest of the perceptual field recedes into a background. The hypnotic state itself corresponds to the Gestalt-background principle, and the Gestalt formation becomes more or less an automatic function of it.

The hypnotherapist becomes a Gestalttherapist when he does not aim to circumvent resistances, but teaches the patient to become aware of them. It is better to let the patient face the realities from which his resistances arise and to permit him to experience the apprehension in fantasy during the hypnotic session until he becomes immunized against his difficulties. The emotionally safe and understanding environment of the therapeutic situation is easier to tolerate and to benefit from than are the underlying unknown causes.

To summarize: The Gestalttherapist does not strive to unearth the traumatic conflict. Though the therapeutic situation is only a facsimile of the original hurt, it achieves a therapeutic effect because through it, the patient is led to express and tolerate and eventually to finish—if not at the ideational, at least at an emotional level of reaction—the underlying traumatic incidents of the past. In encouraging and teaching the patient to focus upon his bodily responses during emerging emotional experiences, he is urged to become consciously aware of psychosomatic interactions. It should be emphasized that the resistances are not circumvented, but rather are focused upon and permitted to be fully experienced. The Gestalttherapist does not advocate abolishing all resistances, because it is only natural that many of them are culturally necessary as they prevent us from yielding to detrimental urges. It would be correct to state that Gestalttherapy aims to put the resistances on a conscious choice basis.

The hypnotherapist has a greater variety of techniques at his disposal than the "pure" Gestalttherapist. By an identification with the "school," the Gestalttherapist avoids studiously the exploration of the unconscious, which may be an error. As the clinical case described in this paper showed, the subject came to a greater understanding of himself and to a more profound therapeutic benefit by exploring the unconscious roots of his fears in connection with being unloved. Rigidity and unquestioning adherence to rigidly conceived schools of thought, principles, and ideas are out-moded in psychotherapy. The therapist who owes no allegiance to *any specific therapeutic dogma*, but willingly has knowledge and understanding of the majority of them is in an advantageous position to administer to his patient. Nevertheless, the combination of Gestalttherapeutic principles with hypnosis enriches both approaches.

The hypnotherapist has techniques at his disposal to reach the unconscious which are unique to hypnosis. Hypnotic revivification enables the patient not only to recall a past happening but also to re-experience the effect originally experienced. There, a memory may become an actuality within the context of the therapeutic hour fulfilling the ideal of the Gestalttherapist, who aims not just for reminiscences, but rather for the uniting of the remembrance of the event with the emotions of the "here and now."

Hypnosis is particularly effective to achieve an integration of newly gained knowledge, and on the basis of corrective emotional experiences, to evolve a new and better philosophy of existence. Studying the literature of hypnotherapy, one becomes aware that Gestalttherapy principles have been utilized by many leading hypnotherapists. Milton H. Erickson gave evidence already in his earlier publications that he did not especially aim at the removal of the resistances, but rather at utilizing them (3).

The unbiased student cannot help but notice the marked similarities between the Gestalttherapist's approach and that of the contemporary hypnotherapists. It is suggested that the purposeful synergistic combination of Gestalttherapy and hypnotherapy may lead to a forceful and effective psychotherapeutic concept.

REFERENCES

1. KOHLER, WOLFGANG, *Gestalt Psychology*. New York: Liveright Publishing Corporation, 1947.
2. PERLS, F.S., HEFFERLINE, R.F., and GOODMAN, P., *Gestalttherapy*. New York: the Julian Press, Inc., 1951.
3. ERICKSON, M.H., Special techniques of brief hypnotherapy. *J. clin. exper. Hypn.*, 1954, 2, 102-29.

13
Group Hyperempiria, the Awareness Experience

Don Gibbons

The term *hyperempiria* is taken from the Greek prefix *hyper,* which means "increased" and from the word *empiria,* which means "experience" or "awareness," and the term is used to indicate a form of hypnosis in which the subject is taught to enter a state of increased awareness or alertness from the start of the induction procedure. It is the induction that generally differentiates hyperempiria from standard hypnosis, and it is the induction that subsequently brings about a trance of increased alertness as opposed to increased drowsiness or lethargy. Although it was developed during individual inductions, hyperempiria lends itself especially well to group work, and a number of inductions that may be effectively employed with groups are included in this chapter.

To begin with, hyperempiria is an experience, and from a phenomenological point of view the essential factor in determining the effect of an experience upon a particular individual is its meaningfulness rather than its intensity or the number of times it is repeated. A single meditative insight may change one's life almost at once, while an orgiastic experience, or a series of them, may have little permanent effect unless they are also existentially meaningful. Thus, in working with individuals through hyperempiria, the operator seeks to help the subject or patient experience specifically meaningful fantasy events while in this state.

However, there are certain types of experiences which are universally meaningful in that they deal with the central concerns of human existence: time, life, death, the Deity, and the bounds of one's own identity and awareness. A group hyperempiric induction differs from group fantasy experiences in hypnosis in that the former includes specific suggestions to the effect that the subjects will experience an altered state of consciousness or a change in the perception of their own awareness. This provides a conceptual framework and an ideological rationale to facilitate the acceptance of subsequent suggestions which may be at variance with everyday experience.

Like a hypnotic induction, a group hyperempiric induction is most effective if it is administered in an appropriate setting. The subjects should be comfortably seated or lying down, and the lighting should be fairly dim if the induction is conducted indoors. Appropriate background music may be provided to enhance the effect of the imagery which is employed in the induction procedure.

The first induction utilizes imagery associated with entering a cathedral. However, imagery associated with a wide variety of other situations may be substituted to suit the needs and tastes of various groups. It is only necessary that the modified procedure contain, in addition to the appropriate facilitating imagery, specific suggestions to the effect that the subjects are entering a state of hyperempiria and a description of the changes in conscious perception which are being brought about as the induction takes its course.

After the hyperempiric induction has been completed, suggestions may be provided to facilitate group interaction as illustrated. The example given results in a "snowballing" or delayed-action effect which is able to capitalize on the enhanced responsiveness of the more suggestible members of the group as they interact with the less suggestible members over the course of time to produce an ever increasing degree of cohesiveness on the part of the group as a whole.

Further information on hyperempiric induction procedures, together with a number of techniques which are useful either in individual or in group settings after the induction has been completed, may be found in Gibbons (1973).

THE CATHEDRAL OF THE MIND: A HYPEREMPIRIC INDUCTION

Just make yourself comfortable, and close your eyes; and as you listen to my voice I am going to show you how to release your consciousness so that it may rise to a higher level than you have known previously. First of all, I would like you to picture yourself standing in front of a large wooden door, which is the door to a great cathedral. . . .

If you accept the image of the scene as I describe it, without trying to
analyze what I am saying, your imagination will be able to let you
experience the situation just as if you were really there. . . . So just let
yourself stand there a moment, gazing at the carved wooden panels of the
door as you prepare to enter. . . .

Soon the doors will open and you will go inside, as I guide you into
a higher state of awareness called hyperempiria. You will begin to
experience very pleasant feelings of increased alertness and sensitivity as
your consciousness commences to expand. . . . Just let yourself be
guided by my voice now, as the doors begin to open and your awareness
commences to increase. . . .

As the doors swing open and you enter the cathedral, you first
traverse a small area paved with stone, stopping at the font if you desire,
and then you pause before a second pair of doors which leads to the
interior. . . . You are beginning to enter a higher level of consciousness
now; for this Cathedral presents your mind with an image which is able
to portray within itself all of the vast reserves of strength and spiritual
power contained within your own being, and within the Universe as
well. . . . And as you enter, you begin to feel all of these vast resources
flowing into your own awareness. . . . As you pass through the second
pair of doors and into the dimly lit interior, you can hear gentle tones of
music floating upon the quiet air. . . . Let yourself breathe slowly and
deeply now, as you inhale the faint aroma of incense, and your consciousness drifts higher. . . . Breathe slowly and deeply, and listen to the
music and the chanting. . . . Just let the music merge completely with
your own awareness, and carry it along. . . . And soon you will feel as if
you were holding within your own consciousness an awareness of the entire Universe, and all its beauty. . . . You are entering into a higher level
of consciousness now, one in which your ability to utilize your full
capacity for experience is greatly enhanced. . . . You are experiencing
exaltation in your ability to use your consciousness so much more effectively, as your awareness continues to expand, more and more. . . .
Your perceptual abilities are becoming infinitely keener as the music
swells within you, yet you can still direct your attention as you would
normally, to anything you desire. . . . It's such a pleasant feeling as
your awareness expands more and more, multiplying itself over and
over again. . . .

You are experiencing a wonderful feeling of release and liberation
now, as all of your vast, previously untapped potentials become freed for
their fullest possible functioning; and in just a short while your entire
capacity for experience will be fully released. . . . Your perceptions of
the world around you will take on new and deeper qualities, and they

will possess a greater depth of reality than anything you have been able to experience previously.

Some distance away from you stands the High Altar, bordered by banks of softly glowing candles. As the music continues and your awareness continues to increase, you can feel yourself being drawn irresistibly towards it. . . . And as you begin to approach, the closer you get the more your awareness expands, the more beautiful the experience becomes. . . . As you feel your consciousness expanding more and more, you are feeling an ever growing sense of joy as all of your perceptual abilities are becoming turned to their highest possible pitch; and it's not fatiguing or tiring in the least.

As you approach nearer and nearer, you feel your capacity for awareness and for experience becoming infinitely greater than it could possibly be in any other state. . . . In just a few seconds now, all of your perceptual abilities will be tuned to their highest possible pitch, and you will be able to concentrate infinitely better than you can in the everyday state of consciousness. . . . Now, you are ready. All of the vast reserves within you have been freed for their fullest possible functioning. And while you remain within this state of hyperempiria, you will discern new and greater levels of reality and of meaning, and discover new dimensions of experience, greater and more profound than anything you have previously undergone. . . .

Suggestions for Facilitating Group Interaction

The suggestions which you are about to receive will increase in strength and effectiveness as long as the group continues to function. They may start out weakly at first; but their force will increase, like a snowball rolling downhill, with each moment that passes. . . .

With each moment that passes you will find yourself communicating more easily with those around you. . . . *With each moment that passes* you will become more aware of a growing sense of warmth and fellowship, good will and mutual understanding as communication continues to flow more freely. . . . And with each moment that passes you will be freer to express your own feelings of warmth and fellowship in return.

Each passing moment will find you *more* alert, *more* involved, and more responsive to the needs of others. . . . And you will respond in a manner which meets your own needs as well. . . . And as you do you will find yourself gaining new knowledge, new insights, and new experience which will be of great help in the pursuit of your own personal growth and in facilitating the growth of others.

(At the conclusion of these suggestions, the subjects may be told that at the count of five they will be able to open their eyes and move about as they would normally, while remaining in hyperempiria until the group is terminated, at which time they may be asked to close their eyes once more while suggestions to return to normal awareness are provided. In the meantime, a wide variety of commonly used group techniques may be employed with enhanced effectiveness.)

RETURN FROM THE HYPEREMPIRIC STATE

In a moment I am going to count backwards from ten to one, and by the time I get to the count of one you will be back in the usual, everyday state of consciousness in which we spend most of our waking lives. . . .

After you come down, you will be feeling absolutely wonderful. Your mind will be clear and alert, and you will be thrilled and delighted by the pleasant experiences which you have had. Your hyperempiric experiences will be of great help to you as you continue your own personal growth. But equally important will be your desire to communicate and to share these experiences with others. . . .

And now I will return you to your usual state of consciousness by counting backwards from ten to one. . . . Ten. Coming back now, coming all the way back. . . . Nine. Coming down more and more now, and feeling perfectly wonderful as you continue to come down more and more. . . . Eight. . . . Seven. . . . Six. Down and down, coming down more and more now. . . . Five. Soon you will be all the way down, feeling thrilled and delighted by the pleasant experiences you have had. . . . Four. Almost back now. Soon you will be down completely. . . . Three. Nearly back now. In just a few seconds you will have completely resumed your everyday state of consciousness, feeling wonderful. . . . Two. Almost back. One. You can open your eyes now, feeling wonderful!

"Good morning!"

SIX IMPOSSIBLE THINGS

"Now I'll give *you* something to believe. I'm just one hundred and one, five months and a day."

"I can't believe *that!*" said Alice.

"Can't you?" said the Queen in a pitying tone. "Try again: draw a long breath, and shut your eyes."

Alice laughed. "There's no use trying," she said. "One *can't* believe impossible things."

"I daresay you haven't had much practice," said the Queen.

"When I was your age, I always did it for half an hour a day. Why, sometimes I've believed as many as six impossible things before breakfast. . . ."

—Lewis Carroll,
Through the Looking Glass

In order to illustrate the variety of effects which may be produced if one has the kind of background which enables him to "believe impossible things," I would like to share with you six suggestions which I have found to be particularly effective in group settings.

A hypnotic or hyperempiric induction should be provided beforehand, of course, in order to supply the necessary veneer of plausibility which permits those who are able to do so to behave in an "Alice-in-Wonderland" fashion in the real world. And oh, yes: one thing more. Unless you happen to be the Red Queen yourself, don't try all six of these suggestions at one time—even if you *have* had breakfast!

RECOVERING THE TREASURES OF THE UNCONSCIOUS

Now I would like you to visualize yourself in ancient Egypt, standing completely alone before the cavelike entrance to a large pyramid which towers above you, its top completely lost to view in the darkness of a desert sandstorm. . . . Let yourself visualize the scene more and more clearly as you stand there, gazing at the entrance-
. . . . Hear the wind whistling in your ears, and feel the driven sand stinging your cheeks and forcing you to squint your eyes. . . . As you project yourself more clearly into the situation, the feeling of reality surrounding these images will continue to grow, until you are able to actually live the experiences as I describe them. . . . Just let yourself stand there a few seconds more, gazing at the entrance to the pyramid as you prepare to enter and the feeling of reality continues to grow stronger. . . .

Now you are ready to enter the pyramid itself, and as you do, you discover that the passageway is brightly lit by torches which are fastened to the wall at regular intervals. . . . The passage slopes suddenly downward as you continue along its length, but you continue to follow it eagerly; for this pyramid presents your mind with an image which will enable us to explore together the deepest levels of your awareness.
. . . Let yourself continue to be guided by my voice now, as you travel ever downward, plunging to greater and greater depths. . . . For you are plunging also into greater and greater depths of your own unconscious, leaving the world of everyday awareness far behind as you continue to sink down and down . . . until suddenly, at the very end of

the passage, you come upon a vast storehouse, filled with treasures of every description. . . .

You have entered into the storehouse of all the vast untapped resources within you, wherein resides all of the potential for good and for achievement which you have not yet turned to your advantage. . . . All of this treasure is rightfully yours, for it has been stolen from you through the force of circumstance—and unless you carry it back into the world outside, to enjoy and to share with others, it will eventually be sealed up inside this chamber and lost forever. . . .

Your gaze is suddenly drawn to one particular jewel which is infinitely more brilliant than all the rest, embedded in the forehead of a huge, forbidding statue in the center of the room. . . . As you continue to look at it, the jewel appears to glow with an eerie light of its own. . . . This statue, holding within its forehead this softly glowing stone, is the very embodiment of all the negative and sinister forces of failure and defeat within the personality of each one who looks at it; and it has been placed in this room as a guardian of the treasure here, making all other guardians unnecessary. . . .

In order to liberate this vast storehouse of your potential, you must first overcome the tendencies within you which are acting to prevent this, personified and embodied in the statue before you. . . . Seizing a dagger from beneath your belt, you spring upon the statue and strike the stone from its forehead in one quick blow. . . . And as it rests upon the ground, you see that the stone no longer appears to glow, but lies dark and ugly before you like a lump of coal. . . .

Stooping quickly to scoop up as much of the treasure as you can, you hurriedly retrace your steps to the entrance. . . . And as you step outside, you discover that the sandstorm has abated. . . . The way is clear before you, and you can see for miles in every direction. . . . You stride purposefully away, knowing that your return to the world of your everyday life will allow these treasures to manifest themselves in new habits, new ideas, and new directions. . . . And each time you return to the pyramid you will be able to recover more treasure from the storehouse of your potential. . . . And no matter how much treasure you may gather, this storehouse will never be empty.

Something Beautiful

As you continue to interact with those around you, you will discover something beautiful in the personality of everyone here; and you will be able to convey to that person your recognition and appreciation of this discovery.

ENHANCING SPORTS PERFORMANCE

As a result of what I am about to tell you now, you will find that any negative aspects of your performance in sports that might have troubled you will have greatly diminished in importance; and as time goes on, this process will continue of itself. With each passing day, you will find yourself adopting a much brighter outlook, in which the positive aspects of playing and winning, and the lure of success, have taken on a great deal more appeal. And in this more positive frame of mind you will come to experience wonderful new feelings of strength and energy as you find yourself looking forward eagerly to each new challenge, wanting more than ever to play and to win. . . .

Of course, you may be able to feel *some* anxiety and tension now and then; for a *little* tension can be a means of giving your performance an extra push. But if you should ever find yourself in need of an additional measure of reassurance, you will only have to close your eyes for a moment, cross your fingers and silently say to yourself the word "calm"; and this action will serve as a stimulus which will release from the depths of your mind a great wave of steadiness, confidence, and calm which will be more than adequate for all your momentary needs. . . .

As a result of the suggestions you are receiving now, any barriers or obstacles which might have kept you from performing at your very best will be eliminated. . . . You will be able to look forward to each new game secure in the knowledge of your own abilities and of the vast resources within you for further growth. . . . Nothing is holding you back any longer. . . . You are completely free now to develop all of the vast potential within you to its fullest extent. . . .

And as you proceed, the success of winning will be experienced as infinitely richer and more rewarding than it has been, while the sting of any occasional setback you may still encounter will be so considerably diminished that you will scarcely notice it. . . . You will be able to accept any occasional reversal calmly and philosophically as the small price which must be paid in order to experience the rich joys of playing and winning. . . . And because playing itself has become so enjoyable, you will be able to derive satisfaction from *any* game, regardless of the outcome. . . . All these changes will, of course, result in marked improvements in your training, your preparation, and in your actual performance. You will find that you will easily be able to get all the rest that you require, and that you will be able to do whatever else may be necessary as part of your training. You will sleep soundly and well, without wasting time and energy worrying about your past or future performance; for each time you play, you will find your timing and coordination improving. . . . Each time you play, you will see definite gains in your strategy and skill. . . . And each time you play, you will find that you are advancing closer and closer to the goal of becoming the player you want to be.

Esthetic Appreciation and Enjoyment

The next time you read a novel, see a movie, or go to a play, what I am about to tell you now will set in motion a number of changes in your sensitivity and responsiveness; and these changes will greatly enhance your appreciation and understanding of what you experience, multiplying your enjoyment many times over. . . .

You will find that all of your senses will suddenly begin to feel immeasurably keener at the outset, and that your emotional responsiveness is also vastly increased. . . . These changes will enable you to become more and more deeply involved in the experience as it unfolds, for you will be able to follow it not with just your senses alone, but with your entire being. . . .

And this enhancement of your natural abilities will help you to discover new depths of responsiveness within your own personality, and an ever-increasing capacity to experience life itself in a richer and a more profound manner.

The Celebration of Life:
An Exercise to Strengthen the
Forces of Personal Growth

I would like you to visualize yourself now as a tiny songbird which has not yet hatched out of its shell. Perhaps you might wish to curl up where you are, in order to help capture the sensation more clearly. . . . Just hold that image in your mind and continue to focus on it, and soon you will be picturing it so clearly that the feeling of reality will become clearer and stronger with each second that passes. . . . As you continue to project yourself into the situation and the image becomes clearer and clearer, you are ever more able to experience the full reality of the scene. . . . Beginning to feel just as if you were a baby bird now, encased in its shell and ready to peck its way out into the world. . . .

Let yourself experience all of the full reality of the situation now. . . . Feel how cramped you are in the shell, and let yourself experience the urge to break out growing stronger and stronger. . . . The surging life forces within you may not be denied any longer: the shell within which you have lived up to now is no longer able to contain you. . . . You must break through to the world that lies waiting outside; for the forces of growth are becoming stronger and more insistant with each passing second. . . .

You are beginning to peck away at the shell now, slowly at first and then with ever more rapid movements. . . . And the shell begins to crack and to give way before your insistent efforts. . . . Now a tiny piece of the shell has fallen away, and you catch a glimpse of the tantalizing world outside. . . . It appears to be a fascinating place of indescribable beauty; and you feel a renewed surge of strength and joy as you redouble your efforts in response to the promise of what is to come. . . .

More pieces of the shell are falling away now, and you are able to push your head completely through the opening which you have created. . . . With a great burst of strength you cause a crack to appear along the entire length of the shell, and the crack becomes larger and larger with each repeated shove. . . . Until at last your shell has broken apart, and with a great surge of triumph you stand blinking upon the threshold of a new life. . . . You are completely free of all the constraints of the past. . . . Completely free from everything that has been holding you back. . . .

You are ready to begin a new phase of your existence, and ready to unfold and use the new talents and abilities that you have been quietly unfolding in the darkness. . . . And as you experience yourself standing upon this threshold of a new life, you feel the stirrings of a song rising within you. . . . A song of joy and of victory; a song of growth and a celebration of life. . . . The song rises up within you, and as you flex your wings for the first time the notes burst forth clear and strong. . . .

This feeling of triumph and of joy will remain with you, and you will still be able to feel the forces of life and growth, experiencing them ever more clearly as your own personal development continues. . . .

And now, as you remain in an altered state of awareness for a time, the scene is fading and you are becoming aware of yourself as a person once more. . . . But the feelings of triumph and of joy will remain. . . . The scene is almost gone. . . . Now you are fully aware of yourself as a person once more. . . . But you will continue to carry the lesson of this experience with you; and each time the exercise is repeated the beneficial effects will be ever greater.

FACILITATING INTERPERSONAL EFFECTIVENESS

The experiences which you have today will provide you with much more confidence in yourself, which will be reflected in the greater ease and skill with which you are able to deal with others. . . . You will be a great deal less aware of yourself, and much more clearly aware of the thoughts and feelings of those around you. . . . You will be much more interested in what they have to say, and easily able to lose yourself in the current topic of conversation. . . .

As you derive more enjoyment out of talking to people and

developing new friendships with them, you will find it much easier to relax in social situations. You will develop a keener interest in other people and in their ideas, and a greater ability to understand and appreciate the other person's point of view. . . .

As your confidence and skills improve, you will become exquisitely more sensitive to the emotional needs of those around you, and you will find new sources of wisdom and understanding within yourself which will enable you to meet those needs. . . . There will be many more people who will be able to look upon you as a friend to whom they can turn for comfort and advice; and there will be many more people whom you will be able to look upon as a friend in return. . . .

As your confidence and skills improve, you will be able to establish a number of deep and rewarding relationships which will be a source of great personal satisfaction both for you and for other people. . . . Your life will take on a great deal more meaning and be considerably enriched because of the many new friendships which you will be able to form, which will also enrich the lives of many others. . . .

REFERENCE

GIBBONS, DON. *Beyond Hypnosis: Explorations in Hyperempiria.* South Orange, N. J.: Power Publishers, Inc., 1973.

Part IV

HYPNODRAMA:
The Morenean Method

14
Hypnodrama and Psychodrama*

J.L. Moreno

I divide psychiatry into three categories: Confessional psychiatry, Shakespearean psychiatry and Machiavellian psychiatry. An illustration of confessional psychiatry is psychoanalysis. An illustration of Shakespearean psychiatry is psychodrama; it heals and explores the truth by means of dramatic methods. I call it Shakespearean because Shakespeare, more than anyone else, has contributed, not to this form of therapy but to its content. Illustrations of Machiavellian psychiatry are electric shock therapy, insulin shock therapy and lobotomy. I call them after Machiavelli because he has advocated the cruellest methods in the government of human affairs, the means being justified by the end.

Psychodrama, among the three categories, is in a strategic position because it brings the three efforts into a synthesis. After the study of heredity, of anatomy, of physiology, of internal medicine, of histology, of neurology, after you have been psychoanalyzed and even after you have had your lobotomy you must enter the process of living itself, a world full of unknown opportunities and boundaries, or at least, full of uncertainties; a world ever changing, filled with unknown objects and people. After you have acquired all the knowledge your learnings need a finishing touch, you still have to learn how to live. This is what

*Reprinted with permission, Group Psychotherapy (April 1950) Vol. 3, No. 1, 1-10.

psychodrama and its allied methods and techniques propose to do for people: to provide them with the science and skills of living, a "life practice."

Historically the psychodrama grew out of the principle of play. Play has always been there; it is older than Man, it has accompanied the life of organisms as one of its excesses, anticipating growth and development. In our culture it was particularly Rousseau and Froebel who directed our attention towards the educational value of play. But a new vision of the principle of play was borne when in the years before the outbreak of the first World War I began to play with children in the gardens and streets of Vienna: play as a principle of cure, as a form of spontaneity, as a form of therapy and as a form of catharsis; play, not only as an epiphenomenon accompanying and supporting biological aims but as a phenomenon sui generis, *a positive factor linked with spontaneity and creativity*. Play has gradually been separated from its metaphysical, metabiological and metapsychological connections and shaped into a methodical and systematic principle. All this has brought the idea of play to a new universality, unknown heretofore; it has pushed and inspired the development of play techniques, play psychotherapy, theatre of spontaneity, therapeutic theatre, culminating in the role playing, psychodrama, sociodrama of our time.

After the Viennese "garden revolution,"[1] the opening of the first therapeutic theatre—The Spontaneity Theatre—in Vienna (1921) was the greatest triumph of the play principle. Supplemented two years later by my book *Das Stegreiftheater* it signalized the surpassing of psychoanalysis by revolutionizing the *vehicle form* and *concept* of treatment. The psychoanalytic vehicle was the couch. The antiquated couch was transformed into a multidimensional stage, giving space and freedom for spontaneity, freedom for the body and for bodily contact, freedom of movement, action and interaction. Freud's free association was replaced by psychodramatic production and audience participation, by action dynamics and dynamics of the groups and masses. With these changes in the research and therapeutic operation the framework of psychoanalytic concepts, sexuality, unconscious, transference, resistance and sublimation was replaced by a new, psychodramatic and sociodynamic set of concepts, the spontaneity, the warming up process, the tele, the interaction dynamics and the creativity. These three transformations in vehicle, form and concept, however, transcended but did not eliminate the useful part of the psychoanalytic contribution. The couch is still in the stage—

[1]J.L. Moreno: Homo Juvenis (in "Einladung zu einer Begegnung") Anzen gruber Verlag, Vienna, 1914, p. 12.

which is like a multiple of couches of many dimensions, vertical, horizontal and depth—sexuality is still in spontaneity, the unconscious is still in the warming up process, transference is still in the tele; there is one phenomenon, productivity-creativity for which psychoanalysis has given us no counterpart except a defective one, sublimation. Because of the extremely dialectic character of our century, being in a transition from one type culture to another, this change in concepts and operations is hidden, insidious and Machiavellian in itself.

Some Comments on the Dynamics of Psychodrama Therapy

The question of dynamics in psychodrama is often the cause of misunderstandings. The logic of psychoanalysis is to take advantage of the transference of the patient, to work through the resistance he has against returning the repressed to consciousness. The logic of pyschodrama is different and more complex because of the novel elements entering the situation. The transference to the therapist exists here, too—to begin with, but the relation is far more realistic, it often assumes the character of a real battle between therapist and patient. The patient feels far more threatened because the therapist wants so much more from him; not only does he want him to speak freely but to expose his whole inner drama in action and words and not only his own, but also that of people who are closest to him and whose secrets he fears to reveal. So he tries to put up a fight, as if against an attack. The therapist in turn is not the quiet, passive listener in psychoanalysis, he himself must put up a good battle in order to get the patient to produce. The transference, therefore, begins at times from *his* side and is overwhelming in character, like that of a man who is in love with a woman and takes the initiative. Therapist and patient warm up to each other, it is a battle of wits. The therapist wants something from the patient right away, but he refuses to give. This picture of an overwhelming resistance of the patient because of the therapist's need of an overwhelming transference should not mislead the reader. In most cases the resistance against being psychodramatized is small or nil. Once a patient understands the degree to which the production is of his own making he will cooperate. It is obvious that we are here using the concept of transference in a way which goes far beyond the ordinary definition and destroys its meaning. The fight between therapist and patient is in the psychodramatic situation extremely real; to an extent they have to assess each other like two battlers, facing each other in a situation of great stress and challenge. Each of them has to draw spontaneity and cunning from their resources so that whatever amount of projected transference operates from the patient towards the therapist is pushed into the background or reduced to a small element. Positive factors which are shaping the relationship and interaction in the reality of life itself take their place: spontaneity, productivity, the warming up process, tele and role processes.

But because of the dialectic character of the psychodramatic methods this first phase is rapidly eliminated and replaced by another. The therapist, after having made so much ado to get the patient started, recedes from the scene; frequently he does not take any part in it, at times he is not even present. From the patient's point of view his object of transference, the therapist, is pushed out of the situation. The retreat of the therapist gives the patient the feeling that he is the winner. Actually it is nothing but the preliminary warm up before the big bout. To the satisfaction of the patient other persons enter into the situation, persons who are nearer to him like his own mother and wife or individuations which are part and parcel of him like his delusions and hallucinations. He knows them so much better than this stranger, the therapist. The more they are in the picture the more he forgets him and the therapist wants to be forgotten, at least for the time being. The dynamics of this forgetting can be easily explained. Not only does the director-therapist leave the scene of operation, the auxiliary ego therapists step in and it is between them that his share of *tele*, transference and empathy is divided. In the course of the production it becomes clear that *transference is nothing by itself, but the pathological portion of a universal factor, tele*, operating in the shaping and balancing of all interpersonal relations. As the patient takes part in the production and warms up to the figures and figureheads of his own private world he attains tremendous satisfactions which take him far beyond anything he has ever experienced; he has invested so much of his own limited energy in the images of his perceptions of father, mother, wife, children, as well as in certain images which live a foreign existence within him, delusions and hallucinations of all sort, that he has lost a great deal of spontaneity, productivity and power for himself. They have taken his riches away and he has become poor, weak and sick. And now the psychodrama, as if by the grace of God, gives back to him all the investments he had made in the extraneous adventures of his mind. He takes his father, mother, sweethearts, delusions and hallucinations back unto himself and the energies which he has invested in them, they return by actually living through the role of his father or his employer, his friend or his enemy; by reversing the roles with them he is already learning many things about them which life does not provide him. But when he himself can be the persons he hallucinates, not only do they lose their power and magic spell over him but he gains their power for himself. His own self has an opportunity to find and reorganize itself, to put the elements together which may have been kept apart by insidious forces, to integrate them and to attain a sense of power and of relief, a "catharsis of integration" (in difference from a catharsis of abreaction). It can well be said that the psychodrama provides the patient with a new and more extensive experience of reality, a *"surplus" reality,* a gain which at least in part justifies the sacrifice he made by working through a psychodramatic production.

But this second phase in psychodrama is gradually replaced by a third. Now the audience drama takes the place of the production. The therapist vanished from the scene at the end of the first phase; now the production itself vanishes and with it the auxiliary egos, the good helper and genii who have aided him so much in gaining a new sense of power and clarity. The patient is now divided in his reactions; on one hand he is sorry that it is all gone, on the other he feels cheated and mad for having made a sacrifice whose justification he does not see completely. The patient becomes dynamically aware of the presence of the audience. In the beginning of the session he was angrily or happily aware of it. In the warming up of the production he became oblivious of its existence, but now he sees it again, one by one, strangers and friends. His feelings of shame and guilt reach their climax. However, as he was warming up to the production the audience before him was warming up too. But when he came to an end they were just beginning. The *tele*-empathy-transference complex undergoes a third re-alignment of forces; it moves from the stage to the audience, initiating among the audio-egos intensive relations. As the strangers from the group begin to rise and relate their feelings as to what they have learned from the production, he gains a new sense of catharsis, a group catharsis; *he has given love and now they are giving love back to him.* Whatever his psyche is now, it was moulded originally by the group; by means of the psychodrama it returns to the group and now the members of the audience are sharing their plights with him as he has shared his with them.

The description would not be complete if we would not discuss briefly the role which the therapist and the therapeutic egos play in the warm up of the session. As this part has numerous versions I will limit· myself here to their contribution to the treatment of mental disorders, especially in the psychoses. It is in the treatment of the psychotic personality that psychodrama has reached some of its most astonishing results.[2] The theoretical principle is that the therapist acts directly upon

[2]See "Psychodrama and the Psychopathology of Inter-Personal Relations," *Sociometry*, Volume 1, 1937; "Psychodramatic Shock Therapy," *Sociometry*, Volume 2, 1939; "Psychodramatic Treatment of Psychoses," *Sociometry*, Volume 3, 1940; "A Case of Paranoia Treated Through Psychodrama, *Sociometry*, Volume 6, 1943.

the level of the patient's spontaneity—obviously it makes little difference to the operation whether one calls the patient's spontaneity his
"unconscious"—that the patient enters actually the areas of objects and
persons, however confused and fragmented, to which his spontaneous
energy is related. He is not satisfied, like the analyst, to observe the
patient and to translate symbolic behavior into understandable, scientific language but he enters as a participant-actor, armed with as many
hypothetic insights as possible, into the spontaneous activities of the
patient, to talk to him in the spontaneous languages of signs and
gestures, words and actions which the patient has developed. This is, of
course, dangerous psychiatry. Psychodrama does not require a theatrical
setting, a frequent misunderstanding; it is done in situ—that is, wher-
ever the patient is found. According to psychodramatic theory a considerable part of the psyche is not language-ridden, it is not infiltrated by
the ordinary, significant language symbols and it assumes that these
silent parts of the psyche play a great role in the development of the
psychoses. Therefore, bodily contact with such patients, if it can be
established, touch, caress, embrace, hand shake, sharing in silent
activities, eating, walking or confused activities, are an important
preliminary to psychodramatic work itself. Bodily contact, body therapy
and body training continue to operate in the psychodramatic situation.
An elaborate system of production techniques has been developed by
means of which the therapist and his auxiliary egos push themselves
into the patient's world, populating it with figures extremely familiar to
him, with the advantage, however, that they are not delusionary but half
imaginary, half real. Like good and bad genii they shock and upset him
at times, at other times they surprise and comfort him. He finds himself,
as if trapped, in a near-real world. *He sees himself acting, he hears
himself speaking, but his actions and thoughts, his feelings and perceptions do not come from him, they come, strangely enough, from another
person, the therapist, and from other persons, the auxiliary egos, the
doubles and mirrors of his mind.*

INTRODUCTION INTO HYPNODRAMA

Hypnodrama is a synthesis of psychodrama and hypnosis. The idea
of hypnodrama came to me through an accident. In the summer of 1939
the late Dr. Solby brought a young woman for treatment. She suffered
from paranoid delusions accompanied by nightmares, every night the
devil came to visit her. She was unable to get into a psychodramatic
contact with the incident. After trying the self-directed technique and
methods of mild prompting without results I became highly directive;
this put the patient unexpectedly into a hypnotic trance. I decided to try

a psychodrama under these novel circumstances. With the aid of two male auxiliary egos she was able to portray two meetings with the devil, one as it had happened the night before, one as she expected it to happen the following night. Apparently hypnosis operated as a "starter" and spurred her spontaneity.

I tried the technique several times since; it was particularly successful a few years later with Bill, a man who blamed his deep depressions and ideas of reference to a mysterious incident in a doctor's office. It was the beginning of his inability to produce, to love, to work and to enjoy things. He ran away, leading the life of a tramp until he was found and hospitalized. Like Marie, Bill had a vivid recollection of every detail of past and present experiences, but he could not evoke the spontaneity to speak about them or dramatize them. The inability to produce gradually spread over all his physical, mental and social functions, leading to a general loss of spontaneity to what I have called a "productivity neurosis."[3]

Here follows a description of the technique, some observations and recommendations. It is assumed that the hypnotic operation has a psychodramatic nucleus which has to be mobilized and treated in order that it should attain real effect. The hypnotic operation itself is reconstructed from a psychodramatic point of view in all its aspects, a) in the role of the hypnotist himself; he becomes a psychodramatic director, assisted by a staff of auxiliary egos, b) in the acts of bringing about the hypnotic sleep; it helps the warm up if the patient improvises on the stage the genius loci—his bedroom—if he goes to bed and assumes the position of the sleeper; and c) during the hypnotic trance of the subject the verbal suggestion of the hypnotist is replaced by a psychodramatic production. The patient is treated during the trance like a subject in a psychodrama session, he is changed into a psychodramatic actor; he is the protagonist who, in cooperation with the hypnotist-director and auxiliary egos externalizes the internal structure of his mental world.

Although hypnosis is the starting point of a hypnodrama, the hypnotisand takes part in the production as the central character, he is exposed to a bombardment of psychodramatic stimuli and is suggested by the chief therapist to interact during the session with every auxiliary ego. The auxiliary egos materialize the persons, objects, images and scenes as they are projected by the patient. He often gives, upon instructions of the hypnodramatist, a soliloquized echo of every part played by an ego. Thus either he acts out or shapes the production step by step. The usual routine of hypnosis of giving simple, verbal orders to

[3]See "Creativity and Cultural Conserves," *Sociometry*, Vol. II, 1939.

the subject is transformed in the hypnodramatic experiment into a complete psychodrama.

When Freud left Breuer he dropped a forceful element, the Mesmeric-hypnotic component which he did not know how to handle rationally. It was a logical move and consistent with pyschoanalytic philosophy. The Mesmeric-hypnotic component is a dramatic, an action element which as an operation cannot be made part of psychoanalysis except post mortem, after the hypnosis is over. The two operations contradict one another, the hypnotist tries to make the patient unconscious of himself, the psychoanalyst tries to bring to consciousness unconscious experiences. The relation of hypnosis to psychoanalysis is somewhat similar to the relation of play to psychoanalysis. Play productivity and psychoanalysis do not fit together; they are opposite forms of warming up. With the advent of psychoanalysis Mesmeric hypnosis became antiquated, a form of magic, and rightly so. With the entrance of psychodrama into the arena of the medical therapies, however, a change has been taking place, as the literature of the last few years discloses. The conversion of hypnosis can proceed into two directions, a) submitting the patient to a material analysis *after* the hypnosis trance is over, which hypnotists or psychoanalysts trained in hypnosis have frequently tried to do. But the hypnotic operation, turning the patient unconscious and the psychoanalytic operation, turning the patient conscious, contradict each other. The other conversion was to combine hypnosis with dramatic methods and use analysis supplementary to the process of psychodrama as it unfolds. These two directions, hypnosis plus psychoanalysis, and hypnosis plus psychodrama are actually in the process of developing, the one under the label of hypnoanalysis, the other as I have called it, hypnodrama. But if one watches some of the hypnoanalysts (as well as the hypnotists) of today as to what they actually practice, even if they camouflage it in writings, the more explicit it becomes that psychodramatic elements are becoming an intrinsic part of their operation and that they are becoming more and more conscious of these elements. When they interpret them they may or may not use psychoanalytic concepts but what they *do* has little similarity to free association; it does have great similarity to psychodrama. The same conclusion can be made as to the dynamic factor underlying the effect of sodium pentothal; it is the warming up of the patient by the therapist and the use of auxiliary ego techniques. The effect can be attained without sodium pentothal which is a handicap to full production.

In Mesmer's sessions the group was frequently a natural part of the procedure. But the psychoanalysts pushed the group out of therapeutic existence and turned psychotherapy extremely individualistic; this has had its salutary effect and may never be entirely abandoned. However, with the advent of psychodrama the group has come back into therapy and is again moving into a place of honor. By this I do not mean only the closed group method, but particularly the "open" group method (open to all comers) used in psychodramatic sessions. The group is coming back in full swing, in a controllable way, not in the uncontrolled way in which Charcot, Freud and others found it. In addition to the group factor, other elements will be added by future therapists which neither hypnotist nor analyst have ever considered in their schemes, the process of "training and retraining" in situ. The hypnotist and analyst delimit their therapy to the consultation room and left it unrelated to the actual living of the patient in the community. But it is on the action and reality level that the patients must find themselves, that is why these areas had to be integrated into the treatment situation. By means of role training, spontaneity training and so forth, this deficiency in medical psychotherapy has been overcome. The hypnotic operation is in itself of limited value, it can gain a new momentum as a psychological starter to psychodramatic production. It can serve a similar purpose as the psychochemical starters, insulin, electric shock, alcohol, sodium amytal, pentothal, etc., and replace them in many instances.

The usefulness of a starter for the patient can be noted in two areas: a) the area of communication, b) the area of productivity. There are, for instance, psychochemical starters which may make uncommunicative patients more communicative, for instance alcohol and insulin, but they may often lower the productivity of the patient, that is their "therapeutic" productivity. Many therapists who use psychodramatic methods superficially are identifying the phenomenon of abreactivity with therapeutic productivity. A distinction should be made for theoretical and clinical reasons between abreactive and integrative catharsis. Abreactions per se are often harmful, reinforcing rather than dissolving certain symptoms; this clinical experience is one of the reasons why Freud considered catharsis resulting from abreaction as unsteady and unsatisfactory, and why he replaced it by transference analysis. The abreactions, however, can be turned into reliable therapeutic contributions. Because of their dramatic character they can gain within the psychodramatic framework a new, appropriate, homeopathic character. Here they are not isolated, uncontrollable elements, previously at best food for analytic interpretation, but elements which are turned positive and integrative, as they can be structured into the psychodramatic production in process. Therefore as soon as the psychoanalyst tackles the abreactions and the unconscious *directly*, or if he tries to "provoke" abreactions, then he turns into a psychodramatist and stimulates the patient to react psychodramatically towards him. Whatever the role is which the doctor assumes, he operates then as an analytically oriented psychodramatist would. The modern Mesmerist is in a similar situation. He becomes unknowingly and gradually a hypnodramatist.

IN CONCLUSION

It may be significant to quote here Ferenczi who is usually referred to as the author of active therapy in psychoanalysis and to place his statements side by side with quotations from my own writings. In order to indicate the contrast as clearly as possible I select some quotations from the most characteristic writings of the two authors which appeared at approximately the same time.

S. FERENCZI (1921):

> "The fundamentals of psychoanalytic technique have undergone little essential alteration since the introduction of Freud's "fundamental rule" (free association) . . . For most patients the treatment can be carried out without any special "activity" on the part of either doctor or patient, and even in those cases in which one has to proceed more actively the interference should be restricted as much as possible . . . Psychoanalysis as we employ it today is a procedure whose most prominent characteristic is *passivity*." (See *Theory and Technique of Psychoanalysis*, p. 198 and 199.)

S. FERENCZI (1925):

> " . . . One should not employ activity if we can assert with a good conscience that all available methods of the not-active (the more passive) technique have been brought into use . . . The analyst is therefore first and last inactive and independent and may only occasionally encourage the patient to do particular actions." (Op. Cit., 220 and 224.) The kind of activity Ferenczi refers to is for instance, a patient keeps her legs crossed during analysis on the couch and he, Ferenczi, forbids the patient to adopt this position because in so doing she is carrying out a larval form of onanism. (Op Cit., p. 191.)

J.L. MORENO (1919):

> "If you . . . would produce your dramas on this stage they would exert upon you, the original and permanent hero, and everyone in the audience a comical, liberating and purging

effect. In playing yourself you see yourself in your own mirror on the stage, exposed as you are to the entire audience. It is this mirror of you which provokes the deepest laughter in others and in yourself, because you see your own world of past sufferings dissolved into imaginary events. To be is suddenly not painful and sharp, but comical and amusing. All your sorrows of the past and present, outbursts of anger, your desires, your joys, your ecstasies, your victories, your triumphs have become *emptied* of sorrow, anger, desire, joy, ecstasy, victory, triumph, that is, emptied of all *raison d'être.*" (See "Die Gottheit Als Kommoediant," *Daimon,* April, 1919, Vienna. Transl. *Psychodrama,* Vol. I, p.24.)

J.L. MORENO (1923):

"The persons play themselves . . . they do not want to analyze reality, they bring it forth. They produce it, they are master; not as fictitious beings but their true existence . . . The whole of life is unfolded, with all its mutual complications . . . not one instance is extinguished from it, each moment of boredom is retained, every fit of anxiety, every moment of inner withdrawl comes back to life." Here total production of life is brought into view, not total analysis. (Das Stegreiftheater, p. 90-91.)

The ideal objective of psychoanalytic therapy is *total analysis.* It aims to give the patient more analytic insight than the routine of living activates in him spontaneously. The objective of psychodramatic therapy is the opposite; it is *total production* of life, it tries to provide the patient with more reality than the struggle with living permits him to achieve spontaneously, a *"surplus" reality.* The excess of life realization helps the patient to gain control and mastery of self and world through practice, not through analysis. Analysis occurs and is given to the patient whenever necessary but it is an adjunct to psychodrama and not the primary source of catharsis.

15
The Hypnodramatic Technique*

James M. Enneis

While hypnosis as an adjunct to therapy has been in use for some time, hypnodrama serves as a vehicle for merging older uses of hypnotherapy with newer concepts of psychodrama. The term and concept of hypnodrama have been introduced by Moreno;[1] he was also the first to experiment with the technique. Although this technique has been found useful in certain types of cases, the full scope of its applicability has not yet been determined. It is hoped that this, the first in a series of papers on the subject, will stimulate interest in its application and result in research on a broad scale, thus enabling us to make a more accurate evaluation of the technique.

It is probable that workers in the field of hypnotherapy have been using dilute hypnodrama. In abreaction and other procedures which utilize the patient's ability to place himself in situations, the therapist often consciously or unconsciously takes the role of one or more of the people involved, thus becoming an auxiliary ego. In addition, through suggestion he causes the patient to create hallucinatory auxiliary egos.

*Reprinted with permission. *Group Psychotherapy* (April 1950), Vol., 3, No. 1, 11-54.

[1] J.L. Moreno, "A Case of Paranoia Treated Through Psychodrama," *Psychodrama Monographs*, No. 15, Beacon House, 1945, p. 16; see also Glossary of Terms, Sociatry, Vol. 2, No. 3 & 4, 1949, p. 435; and "Hypnodrama and Psychodrama," immediately preceding.

The patient reveals his relationship to these persons and to the situations through verbalization and modified motor activities. Since the patient is usually mildly restrained by the therapist, his actions are inhibited. This constitutes a major block to catharsis, since the organism is not free to express itself in action. The patient is limited in his expression mainly to those feelings and emotions which fall within his vocabulary range.

In hypnodrama the patient is free to *act*, and is given auxiliary egos to help portray his drama. Under these circumstances situations become more real and are more productive in the therapy of the patient.

SOME THEORETICAL CONSIDERATIONS

The Warming-Up Process and Spontaneity States

In psychodrama the achievement of a state of spontaneous action is dependent upon stimulation of the patient by internal and external processes manipulated between the patient, director, and auxiliary egos. In hypnodrama, the hypnosis acts as a psychological starter for the warming-up process in that it frees the patient from many of his inhibitory barriers, and places him in a condition of readiness to rise to a state of greater spontaneity. It is made possible for the patient to warm up with a minimum of interference from the self.

There are two main types of spontaneity states[2]. One may be thought of as a comedy role. In this state the individual plays on many emotions without becoming deeply involved with any one emotional tone. He plays the role of the creator of the drama and at the same time is a critical observer of the action. In the other type of spontaneity state he takes one emotional tone and plays it through before going to another. In most psychodramas there are mixed types of spontaneity. The patient will play one or more single emotions through and then go into a short comedy role to regain perspective. This process appears to represent an attempt at maintaining a homeostatic condition regarding his inner needs and the demands of the situation.

Attempts to maintain dual roles in the state of spontaneity are weakened by the hypnosis as many inhibitions are removed, and the freeing of the creative ego is facilitated. There is an inhibition of the patient's acceptance of the roles of creator and observer, through which he may become critical of the performance. Responses to peripheral aspects of the situation, without integrating the deeper levels of the personality, are curbed. As the patient approaches a deeper and less critical state of spontaneity he tends to reject touching upon many

[2]J.L. Moreno, *Theatre of Spontaneity*, Pg. 445.

emotions without deep involvement. He is more disposed to work out one emotional tone at a time. This results in greater catharsis, further delineation of role range, together with re-evaluation and reorganization of the concept of self. These processes of reorientation occur *in situ* and embody relationships to persons included in the situations portrayed and at crucial points in the situation. Thus they give the therapy more meaning in terms of life outside of the therapeutic setting.

While the more profound spontaneity states may be achieved without hypnosis, in many cases it requires long and arduous training. With hypnosis it is achieved more easily.

Pathological spontaneity states seem to occur more readily in hypnodrama than in psychodrama. Techniques for handling these states will be presented following the discussion of the protocol.

Hypnodrama has the advantage of showing the patient's deeper personality structure early in the course of therapy. He responds verbally and kinesthetically to a situation and carries through the action on his own terms, involving the major portions of the personality. There is a minimum of defensive and evasive behavior. This enables the therapist to make a good estimate of the situation in terms of the patient's present functioning, and to base his plan of therapy more directly on the patient's needs. As the patient is treated in inter-action with his social atom, the therapeutic results will be reflected in his extra-therapeutic life in a relatively short time.

Spontaneity training is aided by attaining the more difficult states early in the course of treatment. As therapy continues, the patient finds that lighter states of spontaneity, which mingle emotions, are made richer and become more in balance with his needs in the situation.

A deep catharsis may be obtained while therapy is in its beginning stages. Through hypnosis the gap between the stage *in statu nascendi* and the achievement of the more creative state is decreased. This hastens the development of the patient's ability to warm himself up and to use this ability to achieve states of spontaneity in terms of the moment[3]. He moves toward a condition wherein he is able to readjust continually as the demands of the situation change.

Action Catharsis

The greater catharsis achieved through action is undeniable. The patient is able to express kinesthetically many feelings for which he has no words. These feelings may be expressed through gestures, changes in posture, more active body movements, and inarticulate sounds. He

[3] J.L. Moreno, *Psychodrama*, Vol. I, Pgs. 104-105.

develops emotional insight regarding himself and his relationships without its necessarily becoming verbalized. This insight is demonstrated through improvement in role function. Deviate behavior becomes more in tune with the situation. In many cases new and more adequate interaction with his social atom becomes evident, even though verbalizations of an insightful nature may be absent.

Extending situations and fulfilling act hungers which become apparent in the action allow the patient to show himself previously denied roles. His concept of self is thus improved. The lessening of inhibition in hypnodrama makes it possible to gain action catharsis on deep levels. The patient's ability to use symbolism in the expression of feelings may be utilized. Often he is able to verbalize the desire implicit in an act while he is still incapable of performance. In this case he may spontaneously symbolize the object of the incompleted act, then attempt to close the tension system through interaction with the symbol. At times it seems advisable for the director to initiate the process of symbolization so that the patient may gain release from specific tensions.

Hypnodrama forcefully brings out the necessity for considering the symbol as an expression vastly more primitive than words; as embodying several ideas at the same time, rather than being expressive of only one theme. Without knowledge of all the meanings which the symbol may have for the patient in a given situation, attempts at interpretation are at best incomplete. Their therapeutic value becomes doubtful, and clues to tense areas of the personality in its environment are passed without recognition by the therapist or the patient.

In hypnodrama the various meanings of a symbol may be brought to light in a comparatively short time. The techniques used to determine symbol interpretations allow the patient to ascribe the meanings, freeing the interpretations from the involvements of the therapist. At times the patient may not be able to verbalize meanings of the symbols but will gain catharsis and insight through his interaction with them. Work with symbols is possible in psychodrama but is made easier by the use of hypnodrama.

PRODUCTION TECHNIQUES

Induction of Hypnosis

In hypnodrama, hypnosis is induced on the stage. Psychodramatic techniques are used to speed the process and to relate it to the patient's everyday experience. The patient is warmed up in a psychodramatic manner to being in his bedroom or some other situation which he associates with sleep. After the setting becomes real to him, the director continues with the usual suggestive technique for the induction of hypnosis. When the patient is hypnotized the situation for beginning action is brought out through a hypnodramatic interview. As action begins the situation may change; therefore, the entire procedure must be conceived as a flow of the warming-up process which is not rigid in its direction but changes with the demands of therapy.

In order to facilitate the introduction of auxiliary egos, it is advisable to warm up the hypnotized patient to the entire group present. This becomes unnecessary after the first few sessions. Auxiliaries are introduced in essentially the same manner as in psychodrama. The only important difference lies in the pre-action warming-up of auxiliaries. This takes place on the stage more often than is common in psychodrama. Hypnosis does not appear to limit the use of auxiliaries in any way, but allows a more rapid transfiguration of the auxiliary into the role.

Direction

In all action techniques the role taken by the director is defined by the situation of the moment. There are many circumstances which demand that the director become aggressive and structure the situation. Other conditions may require greater patient-direction with comparative passivity on the part of the director. He must assume his roles on a basis of the patient's needs. In making his assessment of these needs, the patient's internal tensions, as well as his position and interaction with his group must be considered. Knowledge of the group structure should be used to direct action toward a restructuring of inadequate relationships and the extension of productive ones.

When therapy is being done in a group situation, the inclusion of the group in the director's thinking is essential. This does not imply any restriction as to material dealt with. The arousal of negative feelings from the group toward the patient is rare. When this does occur it is due to inept therapy. The importance of the therapist's knowing the sociometric structure of his group cannot be over-emphasised, for without this knowledge, adequate group psychotherapy is impossible.

The closing of sessions on a high note is a cardinal principle of psychodrama. This applies in hypnodrama. When the patient has enacted frustrating roles, it becomes extremely important that he be warmed up to a pleasant situation which he can handle to his satisfaction before he is awakened. If this is not done, anxiety or depression may result. He must be given an opportunity to act a successful if not heroic role, thus allowing the warming-up process to become reoriented.

When the patient is out of the hypnosis, the director should interview him psychodramatically and analyze the session. The amount and nature of material retained from the hypnodrama will be brought out. Relationships between this and present or past experiences may be discussed.

In order that the process of hypnodrama be made clear, two sessions are presented below. The first protocol is that of an early session with a physically well developed, well nourished male of 24. He presented behavioral and psychosomatic problems in early childhood. Feelings of guilt, inadequacy, insecurity, and ideas of persecution began to crystalize when he was about sixteen. At this time he started making the rounds of social agencies and receiving therapy. This did not alleviate the situation. Within the home his relationship to his father, stepmother, and sisters was poor. His own mother left his father when the patient was an infant. He lived with his father and sisters until the father remarried when the patient was twelve. His sisters had made homes of their own about two years prior to this marriage. During that interval he had been going to school and keeping house for the father. When the stepmother was brought into the household, he resented her. Apparently she and the patient entered into a battle for the love and attention of the father. At nineteen he had his first brush with the law over stealing from the stepmother. This brought on interviews with psychiatrists, the diagnosis of paranoid schizophrenia with psychopathic trends, and further treatment. Still his adjustment became more inadequate and he was unable to hold a job.

He was brought to Beacon Hill Sanitarium. On arrival his behavior fluctuated between mild hostility and indifference. There was a tendency toward withdrawal and underactivity. He was generally apathetic. Intellectually, psychological tests showed him to be below normal. There was autistic thinking and difficulty with verbalization. Persecutory ideas and concern with his body odors were manifest.

In psychodrama, under comparatively passive direction, his performances were characterized by sluggish movements and difficulty with verbalization. When the director became aggressive he showed increased facility in speech and movement. This led to the decision to use hypnodrama since the director could become extremely aggressive in the induction process, and re-assess the relative aggressiveness of his role as the action began.

To understand the protocol it is necessary to state certain events which were taking place in the patient's life at the time of the session.

He had made friends with a female patient and had been escorting her to the movies with some degree of regularity. The friendship suffered a sudden breach about two days before this session. The girl claimed that he had tried to rape her, an act which he denied. In a later session it developed that in helping her up some stairs he had put his hand on her shoulder, and noting the usual maze of straps, was prompted to say: "I don't see how you girls can stand wearing all that in this hot weather." Whereupon the girl ran into the house, firm in the conviction that she had been raped. The following session took place between this unhappy event and its clarification. The audience is composed of professsional personnel and patients, including the "outraged" girl.

Unfortunately the recorder did not pick up the first step of the process. Actually the patient was seated in a lounge chair with his feet propped on a straight chair. The scene was warmed up to the setting of his resting on the bed in his room. When the scene had become real to him the hypnosis began.

FIRST PROTOCOL
HYPNODRAMA SESSION WITH JOHNNY

Jim Enneis: And now you are asleep—sound asleep. Deeper and deeper in sleep. Put your feet on the floor—put your feet on the floor. Now stand up. Stand up! (Johnny stands up.)

Jim: Come over here. Turn around and face the audience. Stand right there. Now when you open your eyes, Johnny, you will see a lot of people—you will see a lot of people in front of you—Open your eyes, Johnny, and you will see them. (Johnny opens his eyes.)

Jim: What are you thinking, Johnny?

Johnny: That there is plenty of talk about me.

Jim: Plenty of talk about you—go ahead tell us what you think.

Johnny: They seem to a . . . About my personality.

Jim: What about your personality?

Johnny: The way I talk—the way I walk—my ah—stature. They seem to despise everything about me.

Jim: (Whispering) Go ahead.

Johnny: That makes me mad.

Jim: Makes you mad?

Johnny: Yeah.

Jim: You're mad, huh?

Johnny: Yeah.

Jim: What are you going to do about it?

Johnny: Tell them to go to hell.

Jim: Well, why don't you tell them? Tell them off, go ahead!

Johnny: Go to hell, you goddamned girls. I don't like girls anyway. They never did any good in this world except make people unhappy. That's all they ever do—just make people unhappy.

Jim: The girls are right here—tell them what you think.

Johnny: Yeah. Make people unhappy—that's all you ever do. I don't

care if I ever get married now. I don't like girls anymore. They
don't understand me.

Jim: They don't understand you?

Johnny: I try to make them understand but they don't seem to understand me. I try to be good and everything but they seem to—they
don't like my—well they like me for a little while and then suddenly they don't like me anymore.

Jim: Why? Why do they suddenly not like you anymore?

Johnny: Maybe because they are traitors—that could be it.

Jim: Traitors?

Johnny: Yeah, Maybe they don't trust me?

Jim: They don't trust you?

Johnny: No.

Jim: (Whispering) No!

Johnny: I don't know what to say.

Jim: What do they think you'll do?

Johnny: They think I'm too forward.

Jim: Too forward?

Johnny: And I don't think I'm any such thing as forward.

Jim: They think you're too forward . . .

Johnny: I like to go around with girls—I like a nice intelligent girl—
intelligent and nice to be with—nice company but when this happens like this and they talk about me like that, it takes all the interest I had before—it takes it all out of me: I get to be a woman
hater. I despise them. I see them on the street and I don't even look
at them. I even despise my own sisters because they're girls. My
stepmother is a woman—she—she practically ruined my life. My
mother left me when I was small—she was a woman. What did I
get from her? Nothing.

Jim: Go ahead, Johnny.

Johnny: (Doesn't answer. Two female auxiliary egos are brought on
stage and pantomime conversation begins.)

Jim: Who is that over there, Johnny?

Johnny: Elizabeth and Yvonne.

Jim: That's your stepmother over there. She's talking to her friend
about you.

Johnny: Yeah, that's my stepmother.

Jim: That's your stepmother; she's talking about you. What's she saying, John?

Johnny: (Intently watching the stepmother and her friend.) That woman will never rest until she knows that my life is completely
ruined. My stepmother—she's old and she's lived her life and she's

got one more thing to fulfill before she dies and that's to ruin my life, and she's making a good job of it, with the help of others— spies she has—so called spies—that's what I call them. They're going around town trying to pick up every bit of information that they can so that they can talk about me.

Jim: What do they report to her?

Johnny: How I act—my speech—that I was seen out on the street at one o'clock in the morning talking to a fellow and that I can't be doing anything worthwhile at that hour. I should be in bed.

Jim: What else does he say?

Johnny: She says that she's going to hang me—someday she is going to bring me in jail—behind bars.

Jim: She's saying what?

Johnny: She's saying that she's going to see me behind bars someday.

Jim: That she's going to see you behind bars someday?

Johnny: In fact she said that that's where I'm going to end up.

Jim: That's where you're going to end up?

(Elizabeth and Yvonne acting as stepmother and friend talking about Johnny in Italian dialect about how he always wants to eat.)

Johnny: She hids every bit of the food and keeps it under lock and key. If I want to eat, I have to ask her permission and when I ask her she says no.

Elizabeth: That's a lie. I've struggled all my life. I hate you. I've had such a hard life. I've suffered all my life.

Jim: What are you thinking, Johnny? Say what you think, Johnny.

Johnny: She always kept saying that she didn't know how she was going to put up with that boy Johnny in the house.

Jim: What are you going to do about it?

Johnny: I want to get the hell out of that house. I can't stand on my own two feet in that house.

Elizabeth: (As stepmother—continuing to argue and talk about him, provoking Johnny as much as possible.) I will throw him out of the house, that's what I will do.

Jim: What are you thinking, Johnny? What are you going to do about it?

Johnny: I can't do anything. It seems all the confidence I had in myself has been all drained out of me.

Jim: All drained out of you? And who drained it out of you?

Johnny: The continuous nagging—it's all been drained out of me. I just want to go in the kitchen and sit down and read a prayer.

Jim: You just want to go in the kitchen and read a prayer?

Johnny: Yeah.

Jim: All right, go into the kitchen.

Elizabeth: That's all he does. (Shouting) He sits and sits all day long.

Jim: You're sitting in the kitchen, Johnny. What are you thinking Johnny?

Johnny: That's what got me, the continuous shouting. I wish the world would just crack open and everything would fall into it—like a—a universal earthquake. That's what I think.

Jim: Yes.

Johnny: I don't like anything. I despise myself—I hate myself—I hate—I hate my father—I hate my whole family. I don't want to be with anybody. I want to be by myself. I want to eat by myself. I have no interest—no love—no interest in meeting new people or nothing. (Johnny looks at the floor.)

Jim: What is that on the floor. Johnny?

Johnny: (Doesn't answer.)

Jim: Well?

Johnny: It seems like it's pulling my left leg—strong—I can't pull it back. (Johnny shows muscular strain in left leg.)

Jim: What is this force? Where is it coming from?

Johnny: It seems to be coming from that direction there but I don't see anything.

Jim: Look harder and you'll see where it is. See? See?

Johnny: It looks like some kind of a thing—what the devil is it? It looks like some kind of a lizard.

Jim: A kind of a lizard?

Johnny: It may be a snake or something. I never saw anything like that.

Jim: How does it look?

Johnny: It has a big long tail—it's got legs . . .

Jim: Well, look at the animal—how does it look?

Johnny: A head like a snake—it looks like a . . . . . It's a lizard. Big feet with nails sticking out, three eyes and it looks like it can get a hold of me and eat me up.

Jim: What's it doing there?

Johnny: It's breathing hard and its mouth is going up and down. He's looking at me—right in my eyes.

Jim: Keep looking at him, Johnny. Tell us what he does.

Johnny: He's making a noise and he has all scales all over his body. All kinds of scales. They seem to be very crusty and hard.

Jim: What sort of features does he have?

Johnny: A snake-like head.

Jim: Snake-like head?

Johnny: And a snake-like body but he has legs.

Jim: Look at his eyes, Johnny. Look at his face.

Johnny: I can't seem to move that leg now.

Jim: Can't move that leg?

Johnny: My left leg. (Makes unsuccessful attempts to move his left leg. His face expresses fear and is half turned away from the direction of the lizard. Both hands are clasped tensely around the calf of his leg. His body is half crouched and bent over.)

Jim: What is he doing to your body? Is he drawing you to him?

Johnny: I don't know. I can't seem to have any strength in my leg to move.

Jim: No!

Johnny: It just wants to stay there.

Jim: Wants to stay there?

Johnny: He seems to be more powerful than my own mind and makes me keep my leg there.

Jim: Yes. What's he going to do? What's he doing, Johnny, look at him!

Johnny: (Shuddering) It makes my blood run cold when I look at it. (Turns his face a little more, stares in horror at one spot on the floor. He is perspiring rather heavily.)

Jim: Why?

Johnny: Because—he must have tremendous strength in his jaws? If he ever grabbed my leg it would sure . . .

Jim: Is he going to grab your leg?

Johnny: No, he seems to know that I won't move and he's taking advantage of it!

Jim: How is he taking advantage of what?

Johnny: He knows he's got me where he wants me and he wants to make me suffer a little, like a cat plays with a mouse before he kills it.

Jim: So, he's playing with you now?

Johnny: Yes. (Turns his head away again.)

Jim: Who is he, Johnny? Look at it! Who is it?

Johnny: That's my stepmother's nephew.

Jim: Your stepmother's nephew?

Johnny: That's right.

Jim: Yes sir, it is. It's your stepmother's nephew! What's he doing?

Johnny: He's looking at me yet.

Jim: What about your leg? Can you do anything about it?

Johnny: Now, I can move. I can move it up and down. (Does this once, then stops.) But I'm afraid to move it because he might make a lunge at me and snap my leg in his jaws.

Jim: Does he look as if he is going to do that?

Johnny: Yes. It seems that he moves his jaws if I move my leg a little and he's very fast and I'm afraid he might snap my leg in half.

Jim: Are you going to stay there all day?

Johnny: (Uncertainly) I don't know!

Jim: Forever? The rest of your life?

Johnny: I want to move but I'm scared. I'm just being cautious. I'm just staying here—I'm just hoping that someone will come in and kill it. Get behind its back.

Jim: Why don't you kill it? You're the one that should kill it!

Johnny: I'm afraid to move. I wish I had a—a gun or something and then I would shoot it right between the eyes. There's nothing here in the kitchen to kill it with.

Jim: No gun in the kitchen?

Johnny: No.

Jim: What else is there in the kitchen that you might use?

Johnny: (With much feeling) There's nothing that will kill that—horrible looking—I don't know what to call it. It's got such thick scales all over its body.

Jim: What are you going to do about it?

Johnny: I yell for help.

Jim: Well, yell for help.

Johnny: It don't do any good.

Jim: Yell and see!

Johnny: I yell for my father. (He makes a feeble attempt.)

Jim: Well, yell for him! Holler for him!

Johnny: It doesn't do any good.

Jim: Try! You never know until you try. Try!

Johnny: He's working, my father.

Jim: He's not there?

Johnny: He's working—he's not in the house. I want to call anybody.

Jim: Well, call somebody.

Johnny: There doesn't seem to be anybody home. The people upstairs are out.

Jim: Well, what are you going to do? You can't just stay there.

Johnny: I'm afraid—I can feel a thud in my chest.

Jim: Watch it. Watch him, Johnny!

Johnny: He's starting to breathe deeper.

Jim: Breathing deeper? He's getting tense, Johnny!

(At this point it was decided to see the effect of a male and female directing together, so Zerka was sent up on the stage.)

Johnny: I know there's no use trying to fight that thing . . .

Jim: Watch his eyes, Johnny!

Zerka: Watch his eyes!

Johnny: His eyes seem to be getting bigger.

Jim: Yes and he's coming closer!

Zerka: Closer!

Jim: He's going to lunge.

Johnny: He's getting tired of playing and he's going to try something.

Jim: Yes, he's going to try something.

Zerka: What are you going to try?

Jim: Watch him, Johnny! Look at him!

Zerka: Look at his eyes!

Johnny: He's going to grab my leg—better to step away than lose my life. If he grabs my leg and breaks it off—I'll run—I'll go in the other room or someplace and close the door behind me.

Jim: Watch him Johnny. He's getting higher and higher. Look at him!

Zerka: Look at him. Watch him!

Johnny: I'll get something and put it between us.

Jim: Watch him. Look at his eyes!

Zerka: He's getting ready for something!

Johnny: He's got me licked. I can't do anything.

Jim: He's getting more and more tense.

Zerka: He's coming closer.

Jim: He's getting ready to spring. Look at his jaws!

Zerka: Look at them!

Jim: Look at those jaws.

Johnny: His mouth is open.

Jim: Yes!

Johnny: He's got a different shaped tooth. Now, he's got me scared, I can't move. I'm paralyzed.

Jim: He's beginning to breathe harder again!

Zerka: Can you see the scales?

Johnny: It's no use—I can't move. I just can't.

Jim: Well, try! He's tired—tired of waiting—tired of playing.

Zerka: He's mad too.

Johnny: I think he's trying to frighten me to death—that's what he is trying to do.

Jim: He's crouching again!

Zerka: He's going to get you!

Johnny: I can't seem to move—I have no will to move. I just want to sit here and be scared.

Jim: He's not going to let you stay there and be scared. He's going to lunge!

Zerka: He's not waiting!

Johnny: I know he'll bite.

Jim: He's going to bite.

Johnny: Even if he bites, I still don't want to move.

Jim: He's still going to bite. Watch him.

Zerka: He'll eat you. What are you going to do, Johnny?

Johnny: I feel like a . . . . I'm so disgusted that I don't care what the hell happens.

Jim: Watch him, Johnny! Watch those jaws! Look at him! Look at him! He's getting his mouth open bigger and bigger as if he's going to bite any minute. He's getting more and more tense. Watch him, Johnny! Watch him close!

Zerka: You just can't sit there! Watch him!

Jim: Watch him! He's looking at your leg, John. Look!

Johnny: He's looking at my feet. That's right.

Jim: Yes. He's looking at your feet.

Zerka: Are you going to let him get your foot?

Johnny: Now, he's making sounds with his throat.

Jim: Yes, hear them.

Johnny: Huh! I don't know whether to laugh or cry or what to do.

Zerka: What are you going to do with your foot? Are you going to keep it there?

Johnny: No, I'll move my foot.

Jim: He's going to get it, John. He's getting ready. See!!

Johnny: The only way I'll escape this thing—the table is in front of me. If I manage to move my other foot behind the table, to distract his attention and with a quick push, push the table in front of him and run away . . .

Jim: And run away? He'll follow you, Johnny.

Johnny: I can run faster than he can.

Zerka: Move your foot away, Johnny.

Johnny: I can move the table in front of him.

Jim: He's getting closer, Johnny.

Zerka: I can hear him now. He's moving.

Jim: Look at those teeth!

Zerka: His breath! His mouth!

Jim: He might bite!

Johnny: (Wincing) He's biting me now.

Jim: Yes, you can feel him on your foot. Feel those teeth sinking in!

Zerka: Deeper! Deeper!

Jim: They hurt, don't they?

Johnny: It's like something that's been after me for so many years and finally got me. He is all the people who have hurt me—my stepmother's nephew, my uncle, my father, my stepmother and all the others. His teeth are right in my leg.

Jim: Where are his teeth?

Johnny: Right here. (Pointing to leg)

Jim: How does it feel?

Johnny: Like a . . . Like a thousand needles in my leg.

Zerka: Can you pull it away?

Johnny: I can't. He bit me and he's got his jaws around my leg. My leg—the pain is terrible. I can't stand it.

Jim: Can you move the leg away?

Johnny: No, I can't move.

Jim: What are you going to do about it, John? Pull him off! Pull him off!

Johnny: I can't. He's too heavy.

Jim: Try! You must try!

Johnny: His teeth are sunk right in my leg.

Zerka: Can't you pull it away?

Johnny: I can't. He's too heavy. The more I try—I can't even move my own leg.

Zerka: Can't you do anything with your hands?

Johnny: It will be useless—His strength is too—He's got a thick coat of scales around him. He's protected in all ways.

Jim: Who is he, John?

Johnny: It's my stepmother's nephew.

Zerka: What's his name?

Johnny: Jerry.

Jim: Has he been turned against you, Johnny?

Johnny: His mind has been poisoned by my stepmother, by exaggerated lies. Other people that know me have told him how exaggerated they were.

Jim: How did he get those scales?

Johnny: I don't know. He's got them.

Zerka: Did he always have them?

Johnny: As soon as I saw that beast or whatever it is, I knew it was something that was out of this world. I don't think it can even be killed with a gun.

Zerka: Does she like him?

Johnny: She does like him. Yes!

Zerka: She likes him better than you?

Johnny: Oh—she even likes the dirt that she walks on, better than me.

Zerka: She loves a miserable animal like that and she doesn't love you.

Johnny: She despises the ground that I walk on—my stepmother does.

Zerka: She loves that beast there (With contempt).

Johnny: She's wanted me out of the way as long as I can remember. I couldn't even communicate with my father during the daytime; she'd be sneaking around listening. One time I was talking with my father and she didn't know I saw her, but she was sneaking there near the doorway listening to what my father and I were talking about.

Jim: The beast looks like her, doesn't it?

Johnny: Yes, it does.

Jim: What are you going to do about it, John? The teeth are sinking in further and further.

Zerka: You won't have any leg left, if this keeps up.

Johnny: I can't help it—I . . . .

Jim: Try to pull him off!

Johnny: I want to move away yet I can't . . .

Jim: Grab your leg and try to pull him off!

Johnny: (Makes a half-hearted attempt.) It's useless—it's useless.

Jim: It's not useless, John. Try!

Zerka: You want to have a leg, don't you? She won't give you a leg to stand on—you've got to keep your own leg.

Johnny: She wants me to be a cripple. She said so, "I wish you were a cripple."

Zerka: Well, don't give them a chance to do this to you. John. Get rid of it! Get rid of it!

Jim: Pull it!

Johnny: (Pulling at it)

Zerka: Harder! That's not the way.

Jim: Use your hands.

Zerka: Push it—push it away. Give it to him!

Johnny: I'm pounding his head and he's making a loud noise but it doesn't seem to hurt him. (Pushes with something in his hands.)

Jim: Try again, John! Harder!

Zerka: More!

Johnny: He's crouching and he's foaming at the mouth—all foam all over his mouth. I'm using the leg of the table to push him away.

Jim: Pull him off!

Johnny: He's getting mad.

Jim: Pull his head.

Johnny: I've tried but I can't.

Zerka: Keep at it—get rid of him.

Jim: Hit him with the table!

Zerka: Harder! Harder! Smash him!

Johnny: I'm hitting him with the leg of the table and it doesn't seem to be making even a dent.

Zerka: Smash it!

Johnny: He's making a sort of "ooooh" noise like that. He's very aggravated now—very mad—

Zerka: Give it to him, John!

Johnny: All foam is coming out of his mouth. His mouth is so—like a . . . . . He seems to be worried now—he seems to know that I'm making an attempt to get away now.

Zerka: What about that leg, John? What about that leg?

Jim: Push him away again, with the table. Push hard, John! Push!

Zerka: Go ahead, Johnny.

Jim: You can beat him off!

Johnny: This thing is powerful.

Jim: Push harder, Johnny, you can get him off.

Johnny: I know I—he knows—he knows that I'm trying to get the courage to fight him back and he knows I'm doing a good job of it.

Jim: Sure you are, John!

Johnny: He's getting madder and madder.

Zerka: What are you going to do, John?

Johnny: I could . . . .

Jim: Push that head away—harder!

Zerka: What is he doing to your leg now?

Johnny: If I want to get away, I'll just get a club and throw it at his mouth. His mouth is burning now.

Jim: Push that thing harder and make him turn loose. Push that table at him and then you can get away. Push!

Zerka: Give him one good push! Go ahead give it to him!

Jim: Push it! Squeeze it!

Johnny: I'll try and crush that skull!

Jim: Well, go ahead and crush his skull!

Zerka: Kill it!

Johnny: I'm getting more power in my hands.

Zerka: More! More!

Johnny: I'll get my teeth together. (Grits teeth.)

Jim: Go ahead and push harder.

Zerka: What about your leg, John?

Johnny: I think his grip is loosening.

Zerka: Good!

Johnny: But there's a deep gash in my leg.

Jim: You've got to kill him before you can do anything else. Get something to kill him with, Johnny.

Johnny: He's thumping his tail back and forth. If I can keep him there and get a heavy object—I'll concentrate on his head.

Jim: Go ahead and give it to him good, Johnny.

Johnny: His head isn't as good and as well protected as his body is. I'll concentrate on top of his head.

Zerka: Go ahead, John! Go ahead!

Jim: Get something to beat him with!

Zerka: Is there a knife in the kitchen?

Johnny: A knife wouldn't be any good. If I try to reach out, he might snap and grab my arm.

Jim: Get a club!

Johnny: It's going to be hard to kill this thing. I'll have to do it with the top of the table. (Pushes table in direction of the lizard.)

Zerka: That ought to do it. Give it to him.

Johnny: The leg of the table is about three-fourths of an inch away from this head. Right now he seems to be going into a fit.

Jim: Give it to him, John.

Johnny: He's jumping all over the place. There seems to be a funny substance oozing out of his head—his brain—that might be his brain. Boy, how I hate this thing and my stepmother.

Jim: Did you step on his head? Is that your stepmother or your stepmother's nephew?

Johnny: That's my stepmother's newphew—that's my stepmother's nephew.

Zerka: Are you going to leave him right there?

Jim: Watch him, John. He might try to escape.

Johnny: I'm going to kill him and he won't escape.

Zerka: Give him a good heavy one.

Jim: Go ahead and give it to him good, Johnny.

Zerka: Go ahead and make it good and strong.

Johnny: I'm pushing this table further and further in his head. (Makes pushing motion again.)

Jim: Yes.

Johnny: I've got it about six inches in his head. (Pushing harder.)

Zerka: Ah, that did it.

Johnny: Oh—all white stuff is coming out of his brain—that's his brain. Oh—it makes me—I could almost throw up—that stuff keeps coming out of his head.

Zerka: Kill it! Kill it! Get rid of it! You have to finish it up.

Johnny: His mouth is all—keeps closing and opening.

Jim: Keep sticking it in him. Tell us what you think—tell us what is happening.

Johnny: I feel good—it gives me a good feeling now. (Keeps making pushing motion with table.)

Zerka: How is your leg, Johnny?

Johnny: My leg is—the pain in my leg—but I forget about that and concentrate on him.

Zerka: Is he still moving John?

Johnny: Not much but he's not dead yet—far from dead.

Zerka: John, what is he doing now?

Johnny: His mouth is opening and closing—he's going like this (Showing Zerka).

Jim: Look at the way he is moving around, Johnny.

Zerka: Look at him, the way he's thrashing. Hit him hard!

Johnny: I spit on him (Spits)

Zerka: Kick him too—kick him hard!

Jim: Go ahead and spit on him some more.

Johnny: I want to kick him but I don't want to hurt my feet.

Jim: What does it look like, John?

Johnny: It's just like a cat . . . . That's been caught by a heavy truck.

Jim: Go ahead and look at him!

Johnny: It's just a bloody mess—his skin and scales all over the place—his head—there's just a white substance that's oozing out of his head.

Jim: Look at it.

Johnny: His eyes are—I can see his eyes—his eyes are open. (Looks with disgust, turns his head away.)

Jim: Keep looking at it, what is it?

Zerka: What are you going to do with all that stuff, John?

Jim: Call the police department and tell them to send someone from the sanitation department to come and pick it up.

Johnny: No, I don't want to call them up.

Jim: Call them up and tell them to come.

Zerka: Come, let's call them up.

Johnny: You call them up.

Zerka: Okay, "Hello, please send over a truck with a hose, we have to clean a mess in the kitchen."

Jim: Well, John, that's all. (John walks away.) Where are you going?

Johnny: Ah—down to the corner.

Jim: Not yet, how do you feel?

Johnny: I feel just the way I felt when I was sleeping in the bed in the house—afraid, depressed, no confidence in myself, no interest in anything. Even after I destroyed that thing, I still have no feeling—isn't that funny?

Jim: What would have happened if you hadn't destroyed that thing?

Johnny: I still haven't destroyed the past, people when they see me, still remember the past—what they heard about me and they're still doubtful about what kind of a person I am. Even though I wiped it out completely, I'll never feel free—I'll still feel depressed and never relieved—I'll always be very dull, unhappy and sorrowful, doubtful. Everyone talks about me—that's what hurts, especially when they don't tell it to my face.

Zerka: What are they talking about?

Johnny: They're calling me names.

Zerka: What are they saying?

Johnny: That I'm—I'm no good. I know that, that's not true and I'm not exactly an angel but that's not true what they are saying.

Zerka: But they talk anyway.

Johnny: They talk anyway. They use me for their gossip at all times.

Zerka: You can show them—you can show them that you are alright.

Johnny: I can show them but still I haven't got the will to do it—I want to do it and yet I can't.

Jim: What can't you do, Johnny?

Johnny: I can't go out and show them what kind of a person I really am.

Zerka: Why not?

Johnny: I know down deep in my heart that I can do it but I can't seem to do it. I feel like there's another million of those things I have to kill first. When I think of the job that I had to kill that thing—to make me discover that I could kill a million of them before I can wipe the past all out.

Jim: Is the pain still there?

Johnny: No, my leg feels swollen. (Presses his hands on his calf.)

Zerka: It's beginning to go away though—just take the poison out—make it bleed a little bit.

Johnny: No, I can't even feel the pressure I put on my leg with my hand—it's completely numb—from the knee down. It seems like it's way in to the bone and like I lost that part of my leg from the knee down. I got rid of that beast but that woman wants me out of the way.

Zerka: Maybe she's one herself.

Johnny: She is one. She's one that has all kinds of power—just like a devil. She seems to be helped by some strange kind of power—she's got a lot of power for a woman her age. She's strong—she's pretty well educated—she can read and write and she understands English and she can read a little English. She's got power, you know. She's very much against me, that woman.

Zerka: What kind of power does she have, John?

Johnny: You know the kind of people that can communicate with people.

Zerka: Yes.

Johnny: She can start a campaign of propaganda in that town and I had to leave Hackensack—Just one person to spread a rumor around and that rumor can ruin my life. That's what she's doing and it actually succeeded and she knows it.

Zerka: Why do you let her get away with it, John?

Johnny: There's nothing I can do about it.

Zerka: You can start a campaign of your own.

Johnny: I've tried that and I've tried everything. I've tried to consult with my father but he wouldn't understand. He opposed me—his mind had been poisoned. Everybody I know had heard this rumor about me. I walk down the street and people look like they are spying on me—watching every move I make.

Jim: Walk up the street, John, and let's see what happens. Walk down the street. Here is the street. (Takes Johnny by the hand. They walk around the stage together.)

Johnny: In fact I'm walking in a lonely part of the town, so I don't have to see any people. I'm afraid to meet people with those rumors floating around and when I see somebody, I cross the street. I walk on the other side.

Jim: Why do you cross to the other side?

(Zerka is called off the stage here and Jim continues directing alone.)

Johnny: Because I—I don't want to meet anybody. It gives me a lousy feeling—a feeling of guilt—I shouldn't have that feeling of guilt but yet I do have that feeling. She saw me cross the street and walk on the other side and I can imagine what she's thinking. She's probably thinking I've got a guilty conscience.

Jim: She's not here now and there is no one here that you are ashamed to meet. You're walking towards the white house. Walking towards the white house. (Drops Johnny's hand and Johnny walks slowly on, then stops.)

Johnny: I see a lot of people.

Jim: But there is no one here that you fear—you can go in the white house and go to bed. How is your leg now?

Johnny: It's better but it still feels numb.

Jim: Your leg is better and it will keep getting better. You will be able in a little while to use it completely. You will be able to use it fully. It feels good now doesn't it?

Johnny: Yes.

Jim: In a little while you will go upstairs and go to sleep. You feel very good and very relaxed. Very secure—very comfortable and very secure. You feel yourself sinking deeper and deeper into sleep. You're becoming more and more comfortable and more and more secure. It makes you feel very, very comfortable and very secure. You're going to sink even more deeply than you are now. You're beginning to feel very very good, very very comfortable. Very very good. You're going deeper and deeper. Deeper and deeper all the time. Now you are asleep. Now you are asleep. Sound asleep. Sound asleep.

Johnny: It's hot and stuffy.

Jim: You are in the woods. You see yourself in those woods. See the trees.

Johnny: I don't want to walk there.

Jim: You don't want to walk there? Where do you want to walk?

Johnny: I don't want to walk.

Jim: What do you want to do?

Johnny: I want to go and stay in my room.

Jim: You want to go and stay in your room.

Johnny: Yes, I want to stay in my room.

Jim: Yes.

Johnny: I don't want to go anyplace. That's all I want to do.

Jim: Why don't you want to do anything?

Johnny: That's where I would be now. (Walks to a chair and sits down.)

Jim: That's where you would be now—that's why you're in your room. Your windows are open. You hear the crickets outside. Now you are going to think about all the things you did yesterday. Remember yesterday afternoon. You were out on the lawn by the tennis court. You are thinking about these things and you are sitting on your bed in your room. Now take a deep breath of that fresh air. As you are thinking of these things. You are going to sleep, deeper and deeper and deeper to sleep. You are thinking about yesterday, you were playing ball. You had a good time yesterday, playing ball. That's a good game isn't it?

Johnny: Yes, I hurt my finger.

Jim: You hurt your finger out there yesterday, playing kick the bat. Do you want to play kick the bat now? You would, wouldn't you?

Johnny: I'd like to break something.

Jim: What would you like to break?

Johnny: Anything.

Jim: Anything. What would you like to break?

Johnny: I'd just like to break things and play tricks on people. To hurt people as much as possible.

Jim: What people?

Johnny: All kinds of people.

Jim: All kinds of people?

Johnny: I want to throw things at them.

Jim: Alright.

Johnny: I want to hurt people because I've been hurt so much and I want to hurt them—I want to hurt people myself. I don't want to kill them, I just want to destroy them.

Jim: You want to destroy them?

Johnny: Yes.

Jim: What do you want to destroy?

Johnny: Everything.

Jim: Everything.

Johnny: Yes. Everything that people have built, I would like to break. Maybe that will hurt them.

Jim: Hmm. Why?

Johnny: It gives me a feeling . . . . ah—that I've hurt somebody. I want to hurt people myself.

Jim: What people?

Johnny: All people.

Jim: You mean the people here too?

Johnny: Everybody.

Jim: Everybody here has hurt you?

Johnny: Everybody—except—but they aren't here. Everybody.

Jim: Everybody here has hurt you. How has everybody hurt you?

Johnny: They haven't hurt me physically but with their talk, and with words.

Jim: What did they say?

Johnny: I don't want to talk about it. They've just hurt me, that's all.

Jim: They've just hurt you. Do you think they meant to?

Johnny: To my knowledge, yes. They might think before they speak. I feel worried and depressed.

Jim: Is that feeling past or is it still with you?

Johnny: Yes, I keep remembering.

Jim: Why? Are you punishing yourself?

Johnny: I am punishing myself.

Jim: Why?

Johnny: Because I keep thinking things over and over.

Jim: What things?

Johnny: I remember July 4th; we were eating outside in the afternoon and I remember seeing my father and my sister with me. Dr. Moreno was there and he spoke highly of me. He said something to my father and my sister. It affected me—I felt like—it made me lose all my trust, I felt all confused. He made me feel like a lazy good for nothing dog. He said there wasn't anything wrong with me. He said that to my sister. There must be something wrong.

Dr. Moreno: I'm sorry if you misunderstood me, John. It was because I wanted to express my opinion that you can get well. I meant that there is nothing organically wrong with you that you cannot make good. I believe that Johnny will get well completely. I want John to understand that as we are here in the treatment room and I believe he will get completely well.

Jim: Do you understand now?

Johnny: Yes, I understand.

Jim: You understand now and it makes you feel better, doesn't it?

Johnny: Yes, it does.

Dr. Moreno: I think Johnny has done wonderfully and that he will get entirely well. He will go home and go to work and show his step-mother and her friends that he is able to contribute something to the world. I believe that someday he will find a girl that will love him and whom he will love and will be able to spend the rest of his life with.

Jim: That sounds good, doesn't it, John?

Johnny: Yes, it does. It seems to put a sparkle of life in my system, just by saying that.

Jim: Of course it does, because you know it's true. Do you know it's true?

Dr. Moreno: We all like John and respect him.

Jim: Makes you feel good, doesn't it?

Johnny: Yes, but I . . . . I want to be fair to everybody but yet people get the wrong impression of me. I do my best for people—I try to be sensible—I try to be good to them and yet it always ends up that people get the wrong impression of me.

Jim: Did you get the right impression of what Dr. Moreno said, John?

Johnny: What do you mean?

Jim: About what he said during the 4th of July.

Johnny: Yes, I understand now.

Jim: Well, then you have to allow other people to make a few errors also. You didn't understand until he explained to you.

Johnny: I understand now that he has explained.

Jim: Well, will you allow other people a few errors then?

Johnny: Yes.

Jim: John, I'm going to wake you up now. (Puts his hand on his arm in a reassuring manner.) I'm going to wake you up. You're going to feel good. You're going to feel more comfortable, more relaxed and more rested. I'm going to count to six and when I finish you will be fully awake. One, two, three, four, five, and six. Get up. Wake up. Get up from there. Let me see. How do you feel?

Johnny: (Stands up) Alright.

Dr. Moreno: Now, perhaps a few words before we close. It explicitly shows that hypnosis working with a psychodrama produces a lot of valuable material. Hypnosis, psychoanalysis and psychodrama are here combined. We have to maintain the unity in the warming-up process. A unity between the director and the actor, the director and the double. If this unity is working then hypnodrama is possible. (To Johnny) Do you remember anything you said during the test?

Johnny: I don't know.

Dr. Moreno: Do you remember with whom you spoke?

Johnny: I spoke to Mr. Enneis.

Dr. Moreno: With whom else?

Johnny: That's all.

Dr. Moreno: Were any other people on the stage besides Mr. Enneis at any time?

Johnny: Yes.

Dr. Moreno: Who?

Johnny: Three other people.

Dr. Moreno: Who were they?

Johnny: Elizabeth, Yvonne and Zerka.

Dr. Moreno: Did you speak with anybody else?

Johnny: No.

Dr. Moreno: Did anybody in the audience try to speak to you?

Johnny: No.

Dr. Moreno: Well, all the people who worked on the stage have a high regard for you. Recently I spoke to your father and sister. Do you remember that?

Johnny: No, I don't remember.

Dr. Moreno: Well, it was out on the lawn. Do you remember that?

Johnny: Yes, I remember that.

Dr. Moreno: Do you remember what happened then?

Johnny: Yes, I remember.

Dr. Moreno: What happened?

Johnny: We were eating our pie.

Dr. Moreno: Yes and they asked me about you. What did I say? Do you remember?

Johnny: You said that you thought highly of me and that there was nothing wrong with me.

Dr. Moreno: Yes, that's right. That's what I said. How did you feel when I said that?

Johnny: I felt this way . . . .

Dr. Moreno: Yes.

Johnny: That you are a doctor and you know your business and you can tell when there is something wrong with a person or not, so if there is nothing wrong with me, let's just say that I'm no good and lazy and that's what I thought.

Dr. Moreno: I didn't mean it that way. I didn't want your family to think that you are so sick that you will never get well. Do you know what I mean? I didn't want them to go home thinking that you are very sick and there isn't any possibility of your getting well. Do you understand now?

Johnny: Yes and I didn't think of it that way.

Dr. Moreno: I want you to understand Johnny that everyone here likes you and that we trust you implicitly. You have been very helpful. Thank You.

DISCUSSION OF SESSION

As the session opens, the patient is made conscious of the audience. He is then asked to give his thoughts *in situ*. The purpose is to try to get him to take the initiative in setting the scene for action. He does this. The effect of the tele between the patient and the audience is shown as he begins to warm himself up to the strained relationship with his one-time girl friend. As the warming-up continues, he moves toward a more basic pathology in his relationship with women through expressing the inadequacy of the roles played by his stepmother and mother in his life.

This constitutes a major problem in his adjustment and it is deemed advisable to give catharsis in this area.

Two female auxiliaries are brought on stage and given the role of the stepmother and friend. They pantomime conversation, waiting for the patient to set the content and emotional tone for their action and audible dialogue. This is an example of the auxiliaries being warmed up on stage, and of the patient's beginning to direct them in their inter-action with him. In this session he uses the auxiliaries to mirror for us and for himself his concept of the stepmother's relationship to him.

As the action continues he verbalizes the effect which he feels the relationship has had upon him. He reacts by withdrawing into the kitchen where he begins to verbalize his own feelings of hostility and inadequacy. The warming-up continues in the direction of aggressive action taken toward him but now, in order to make the catharsis more complete, he spontaneously symbolizes the aggressors. During a solilo-quy expressing the hopelessness of his existence he stares at the floor. First as a force and then as an animal he begins the process of symboliza-tion. In past sessions he has spontaneously brought in snakes under similar circumstances. This is a new beast. The psychoanalytic interpre-tation of the animal is obvious and probably true, but not complete. His action and the actions which he ascribes to the animal show that it has multiple meaning. As the creature teases him he gives it the additional meaning of a specific person. His position becomes one of frightened passivity and hopelessness. He wishes to be rid of his tormentor but cannot take the action himself and rejects the possibility of help from others. He would be content to leave things as they are, but in order to force more aggressive behavior the director begins extending the scene, thus fulfilling the fears of the patient so that overt action will be taken.

As the animal attacks he recognizes it as representing all of the people who have hurt him and names several specifically. He attempts to play a defeated role but the director persists in forcing action on his part. As this continues he accepts the symbol, first as his stepmother's nephew and then as the stepmother, expressing his feelings about the relation-ship between these two, himself, and his father. At this point the director becomes more insistent in pushing the patient toward aggressive action rather than allowing him to accept what he considers to be the inevitable.

The degree of the patient's involvement after having killed the beast can be seen through his revulsion at the sight of the symbolic mess on the stage. Immediately after killing the animal he experiences a feeling of well-being for a short period of time. As the direction of the warming-up continues toward a job which he has considered completed, this feeling begins to dissipate. When it becomes necessary for him to have someone else's aid in cleaning up the mess, we observe the development of pathology in the warming-up. It would appear that a cooling-off process had already begun, reached a plateau and reversed itself to a warming-up in a new direction, that is, toward himself. He reverts once more to withdrawal and feelings of hopelessness. This brings him back to the situation with the girl.

Attempts at warming him up to further action in terms of the stepmother or the symbol are largely unsuccessful. As he shifts the scene of his action he begins to take over the direction more and more but his warming-up is more diffuse and he begins to warm up toward the symbol audience, past action and himself in a spotty manner. He resists suggestions of the hypnotist and tries to attain a state of immobility. Gradually he warms up to the group structure within the audience and brings out new material concerning his relationships within the institution. Here the action begins to take place between the patient on the stage and Dr. Moreno in the audience. As this new action progresses it begins to take on pleasant meaning for him, thus arriving at a point at which the session, under hypnosis, may be closed.

It seems advisable to use hypnodrama in conjunction with psychodrama so that we have a constant check on the patient's functioning level in the waking state.

Since this paper purports to describe a technique rather than a case history, no analysis of the psychopathology will be made. It may be of interest to the reader, however, to know that this patient has left the institution, obtained a job and has been getting along well for several months.

SECOND PROTOCOL
PSYCHODRAMA SESSION WITH SUSAN

(The subject, a young negro woman is hypnotized and the drama begins.)

Jim: What are you thinking, Susan?
Susan: I am thinking of mother and me back when I was twenty-two.
Jim: Where are you?
Susan: At home with mother sitting on the porch.
Jim: Just you and your mother?
Susan: Yes, I was reading and talking.
Jim: Where is home?
Susan: Baltimore.
Jim: Address?

Susan: 501 East —— Street.

Jim: Stand up Susan and set up the scene.

(Susan stands and moves to the lower level of the stage.)

Susan: This is the house here (points toward the rear of the stage, hesitates).

Jim: What kind of house is it? Wooden, brick?

Susan: Brick. This is the porch. (Moves on stage, begins to set up porch.) This is the swing and there is a chair here and another one over here. This is a pot of geraniums. Mother is sitting in the swing. I am in the chair.

Jim: Is there anyone else with you?

Susan: No. Just the two of us.

Jim: Mother is in the swing and you are in the chair. Would you like to be your mother?

Susan: Miriam could be my mother.

(Miriam comes up.)

Jim: (To Susan) Look at Miriam. What is her name?

Susan: Mattie Frank.

Jim: How does she look?

Susan: Just like that. Mean and resentful.

Jim: How does she sit?

Susan: She sits like this. (Shows. Miriam sits in position illustrated by Susan.) I am sitting over here like this.

Jim: What are you doing?

Susan: Reading.

Jim: What is the name of the book?

Susan: *Gray's Anatomy.*

Jim: You are reading what?

Susan: The chapter on reproduction.

Jim: Look at the book! Look at the book! What chapter are you on?

Susan: Fifty-one.

Jim: You are twenty-two years old?

Susan: Yes.

Jim: Do you have a boy friend?

Susan: Yes. I go with a boy.

Jim: What is his name?

Susan: Bob Fulton.

Jim: How long ago did you meet him?

Susan: About three months ago.

Jim: What do you do? Do you work or go to school?

Susan: I work with my father. I help him in the shop.

Jim: Where did you get *Gray's Anatomy*?

Susan: In college.

Jim: In college. Do you go to college?

Susan: I did.

Jim: What happened?

Susan: The money ran out.

Jim: And you are reading *Gray's Anatomy*?

Susan: Yes.

Jim: What is your mother doing?

Susan: Sitting in the swing. She's sitting in the swing listening to me read.

Jim: Are you reading aloud to her?

Susan: Yes, and talking.

Jim: Go ahead.

(Long pause.)

Susan: The woman's womb is a pear shaped organ which contains the embryo and when she gives birth it is an extremely painful procedure.

Jim: Does she answer you?

Susan: Yes.

Jim: What does she say?

Susan: She tells me about when she had her first child. She says . . . .

(Then Jim points to Mattie.)

Miriam: I remember when my first child was born. I was so happy and didn't really mind the pain.

Susan: No! No! That isn't what she said at all. That isn't like her.

Jim: You take both roles. When you are here in the swing you are Mattie, when you are in the chair, you are Susan.

Susan: Oh honey, don't ever have any children. With that first child I thought I would die. It was just terrible. I thought I would be split wide open.

(Inaudible)

(Susan goes back to her seat and soliloquizes her thoughts.)

Susan: I was just fearful. I was fearful especially because it had said it was painful in the book.

Jim: Soliloquize what you think! Soliloquize what you think!

Susan: I was just fearful. I don't see how I could ever have a child. I had a figure like a pear. I don't see how I could ever come out. I'd like to talk to her about it but she thinks I am just dumb. I don't see how it could ever come out but it does.

Jim: I'm going to get you a double to help you soliloquize. Here is your double. You are Susan number one, you are Susan number two.

Double: A girl like me. How could I ever have a child.

Susan: I'm skinny, I'm not built like other girls. I begin to think I'm a boy. Just a boy who's lost his penis.

Double: I know there is something wrong with me.

Susan: The more I eat the skinnier I get. I look like a fly. I'm just so skinny I know that I would die, and I'm so shy that probably I would never have a chance.

Double: No one loves me. I just can't stand all that pain. Mother always loved Nattie my sister best. She thinks I am so weak. I was sixteen years old. I didn't even know what the world was about. I didn't know what had happened.

Jim: What did happen? Look at your mother sitting over here.

Susan: I didn't know what I was thinking. I didn't know what Kotex was and I didn't do it anyway. I came in at night and the toilet was stopped up and ran over. Daddy had been working all afternoon trying to get it fixed. It was stopped up with a Kotex. They said I had put it in there but I didn't do it. I didn't know what a Kotex was. I didn't do it. I didn't!

(Inaudible.)

Susan: About that same time I went to see the doctor. I thought I had tuberculosis. I was so skinny. My wrist bones just stuck out. It wasn't a real doctor; he was just an interne. When he looked at me he kinda laughed. I didn't have any clothes on. He called another interne. They were looking at my bejinie and they both laughed. They knew I was funny looking. I was built funny. I wasn't like other girls. I couldn't understand what they thought was so funny though. Then my sister wanted to take my boy friend. She wasn't skinny like me. Everybody loved her best. No one loved me. Mother always thought that I was doing all kinds of things. She accused me of everything. She accused me of trying to take her home away from her and her husband. My father worked like hell and lived in a living hell.

Jim: All right, Susan, I am going to change the roles. You are Mattie Brown. What is your husband's name? How old are you?

Mattie: Fifty-three.

Jim: What do you do?

Mattie: Nothing.

Jim: How many children do you have?

Mattie: Six.

Jim: Where is your husband?

Mattie: He is at work in the Tailor Shop.

Jim: What do you do all day?

Mattie: I clean the house and cook and look after my children.

Jim: Where is your daughter, Susan?

Mattie: She is in Washington.

Jim: You don't have to worry about her so much?

Mattie: No. I don't have to worry about her so much. She is doing all right there.

Jim: She is coming to see you. Mattie, Susan is coming to see you.

(An auxiliary comes in as Susan coming to visit Mattie.)

Jim: Where does she find you, Mattie?

Mattie: In the living room.

Jim: All right Mattie, this is Susan. She's come all the way from Washington.

Susan: I would like to take both roles.

Jim: How do you feel Mattie?

Mattie: Oh, I feel about the same. I don't feel any too good.

Jim: You don't feel any too good. You want to see Susan?

Mattie: Yes. I want to see her.

Jim: How do you think she will greet you when she comes in?

Mattie: I think she will be happy to see me.

Jim: What do you want to talk to her about Mattie? Mattie, Susan's coming in.

Susan: Hello, Mother.

Mattie: How are you dear? Are you feeling better?

Susan: Oh yes. I'm feeling much better.

Jim: Louder. I can't hear you.

(Inaudible)

Mattie: Oh my God!

Jim: What is it Mattie? Why do you say Oh my God? (No answer). Alright.

Mattie: Hello Susan, honey. Let's start again.

(Auxiliary comes in as Susan.)

Susan: Mother, what's the matter? What's the matter Mother?

Mattie: Nothing. Nothing, child.

Susan: Tell me what's the matter Mother.

Mattie: You ought to know what's the matter.

Susan: Mother, tell me.

Mattie: Don't act to me like you're a damn little fool. Susan. You're no fool.

Susan: I want to know.

Mattie: You are no fool.

Susan: What is it? What have I done?

Mattie: You're just trying to act so damn innocent.

Susan: Why do you always talk to me like that?

Mattie: Don't just stand there. You know my feelings about your father.

Susan: Mother, it's not true!

Mattie: Get out of here! Get out of here! Do you expect me to believe you? You've broken up my home. You've taken my husband away.

Susan: It's not true! You've always believed that, but it's not true.

Mattie: I don't believe a word you say.

Susan: Mother, you're wrong.

Jim: Tell her what it is, Mattie.

Susan: What is it, Mother? Tell me, what have I done?

Mattie: You're not fooling me. Don't pretend that you don't know. Your father is never at home. He never comes home any more. I've stood for just about all I can stand. Your father talks like I'm going crazy. I'm not crazy! If I haven't gone crazy in all this time, I'll never go crazy!

Susan: You always blame me. You always blame me for everything. You always make me feel like I'm dirt.

Mattie: You don't love me. You never have loved me.

Susan: You blame me. You blame me for everything.

Mattie: I never make you feel like anything.

Susan: You're always blaming me.

Mattie: Go on. Go on upstairs. Get out of my sight!

(Susan goes upstairs with Mattie screaming. "Get out! Get out of my sight"!)

Jim: Here comes Dennis. He's coming in to see you, Mattie.

Dennis: Hi Mattie. What happened to Susan?

Mattie: Get out of here!

Dennis: What's the trouble, Mattie. What's biting you now? I want to see Susan. She's my gal. She's my girl.

Mattie: You go back to that woman next door. Get out!

Dennis: Now wait a minute, dear. I don't like to see you act like this. You act like a crazy woman half the time.

Mattie: No, I'm not half crazy. You've been telling me that all my life.

Dennis: I don't blame Susan for going half out of her head. You're enough to drive anyone crazy. Course I got a woman next door. Do you think I want to to sleep with you? Do you think I want to sleep with something like you, nagging and fighting all the time?

Mattie: I've birthed seven kids for you.

Dennis: Seven kids, to feed, huh! I'm not even sure they're mine. How can I ever be sure they're mine, the way you act.

Mattie: I've never had another man but you. You know that.

Dennis: Oh, I don't know how to talk to a woman like you. I'll have to go see the woman next door. I have to get out of this house. You always drive me out of this house. Where do you think I can go?

(Dennis walks off the stage.)

Jim: Where is he going, Mattie? Where do you think he is going?

Mattie: To the shop.

Jim: To the shop. Does he have a woman next door?

Mattie: Yes.

Jim: Who is she?

Mattie: Bell Moody.

Jim: Are they in love?

Mattie: No.

Jim: What do they do together?

Mattie: They meet and I don't know what they do.

Jim: Mattie, Mattie, why does he have to go next door? Why does he have to go see Bell? Why isn't he happy with you? (Long pause) Why does he have to go there? (Pause continues) Do you know Bell well?

Mattie: Yes. She's my next door neighbor.

Jim: Mattie, come here. You take the part of Bell. How do you look and talk. Black hair, brown eyes. Are you married?

Bell: No. I'm divorced.

Jim: What's your last name?

Bell: Moody.

Jim: How many times have you been married?

Bell: Once.

Jim: What happened?

Bell: He died.

Jim: How did you get along with your husband?

Bell: We got along well. We had one boy.

Jim: Your boy is how old?

Bell: He's nineteen and he's in college.

Jim: You are Bell Moody?

Bell: Yes.

Jim: Tell me, Bell, do you have any boy friends now?

Bell: Yes, I have a boy friend.

Jim: Is he married?

Bell: Yes.

Jim: Does he have any children?

Bell: Yes. He has seven children.

Jim: What's his name?

Bell: Dennis Brown.

Jim: Where does he live?

Bell: Next door.

Jim: How old is he?

Bell: I don't know just how old he is.

Jim: How old are you? (pause)

Bell: I'm in my late forty's.

Jim: Bell Moody. That's a rather nice name. How did you manage that? Were you born with that name or did you marry that name?

Bell: I married that name.

Jim: Oh, It's rather a nice name, isn't it?

Bell: Oh, I don't know.

Jim: You sound sort of doubtful.

Bell: No, I just never thought of it.

Jim: Bell, you're having an affair with Dennis. Where does he meet you?

Bell: Oh, we don't meet any one place. We're too smart for that.

Jim: Oh. Well, suppose you walk around town and Dennis will meet you. You run into him. Go ahead. You'll meet Dennis somewhere along the way.

(Bell walks around the lower level of the stage. Dennis walks up.)

Dennis: Hi Bell, how are you? What's the matter Bell, don't you know Dennis? How are you, Bell?

Bell: Don't you know we can't be seen together? I just went by your house and saw Mattie sitting on the porch.

Dennis: Well you know, oh, I'll tell you. I'm having a hard time with her. Bell, I really don't know what I'm going to do. I'm living in hell.

Jim: Move to the front of the stage.

Dennis: Let's go sit down. Let's sit down over in the park.

Bell: All right.

Dennis: Here's a park bench. You know Bell, I'm very fond of you.

Bell: Yes, I'm very fond of you too, but it doesn't seem quite right somehow, all those children and you already married.

Dennis: Bell, you know what pure hell my life is there.

Bell: But isn't there something you can do about it?

Dennis: I don't like to run out on it but I just can't stand it. My poor Susan came to see me today. You know, I wish I could better understand what goes on between those two women, Susan and Mattie.

Jim: Dennis, get in the role. You are the lover of Bell. You love Bell. That's the important thing now.

Dennis: You know, Bell, I love you very much. You can give me things that Mattie has never given me. You know I haven't slept with her for over seven years. You seem to understand me and that's why I want to be with you.

Bell: I feel sorry for you but I can't have your wife coming over there annoying me and making a spectacle for the neighborhood.

Dennis: It doesn't somehow seem fair to you, Bell.

(Inaudible)

Jim: All right, Bell, come here. Susan, now you are Mattie again. What do you think about Bell?

Mattie: I know she has my husband. I know she's got him.

Jim: You know she's got him?

Mattie: Yes. She's got him.

Jim: She seems like trash to you?

Mattie: Yes, of course she does.

Jim: Just like trash to you.

(Mattie moves to the center of the stage in swing.)

Jim: You are sitting on your porch, Mattie?

Mattie: Yes, in the swing.

Jim: Look in the street. What do you see? Look at Bell. She's going to walk by. (Bell walks by humming in a seductive tune.) Soliloquize what you think, Mattie!

Mattie: She has no husband to keep a woman like that. She's taken my husband. A woman like that!

Jim: Look at her, Mattie. Look at Bell Moody. It looks as though she's coming on your porch.

Mattie: She'd better not come on my porch!

Jim: There she is.

Bell: Hello, Mattie. How are you?

Mattie: Get off my porch. She's got her nerve coming on my porch. A woman like that. Get off my porch! I'll get you off my porch.

Bell: What can you do about it?

Mattie: Get off my porch! I don't want to see you. You know you've got my husband. Get off my porch.!

Bell: All right, all right. (Leaving) I'll take him away anyhow.

Mattie: It takes a woman like you to do it. Just one of your type.

Bell: I'll catch him. I'll see him tonight.

Jim: Soliloquize what you think, Mattie.

Mattie: She will. She will take him. She'll get him. There's nothing the matter with her. She's not a decent woman.

Jim: You are a decent woman, Mattie?

Mattie: I am. I've lived all my life being decent. I've birthed seven children.

Jim: What are you going to do about it, Mattie?

Mattie: There's nothing I can do about it.

Jim: Mattie, how old was your daughter Susan when she first began to wonder about sexual things?

Mattie: She was very little.

Jim: How old was she?

Mattie: About six years old.

Jim: About six years old.

Mattie: No, it was younger than that. Between three and four years old.

Jim: Between three and four years old she began to ask you about these things?

Mattie: No, I caught her.

Jim: You caught her? Doing what?

Mattie: I caught her playing in the woods.

Jim: With a boy or a girl?

Mattie: A boy. She was playing doctor.

Jim: She was playing doctor?

Mattie: Yes. She had his peter in her hand, and she was playing around. It was her little boy cousin.

Jim: Just where was this, Mattie?

Mattie: In back of the house.

Jim: Just she and her little boy cousin. Just how old was she.

Mattie: Between three and four.

Jim: Between three and four. How old was the boy cousin?

Mattie: About her age.

Jim: Were they sitting on a hill?

Mattie: He was lying on a hill.

Jim: Oh, he was lying on a hill. And where was Susan?

Mattie: She's standing up over him.

Jim: Standing up over him. How do you mean?

(Auxiliary comes in to play Susan.)

Jim: This is Susan. She's here as Susan should be. (Auxiliary playing the cousin lies on hill.) How does she stand?

Mattie: She doesn't stand exactly, she kneels and she's got that thing in her hand. She's got his peter in her hand and she's sticking a few little sticks over it.

Jim: And where are you, Mattie?

Mattie: I'm in the back yard and I'm running.

Jim: Run! Run, Mattie!

(Mattie runs over to Susan and begins to push her away. Susan begins to cry and Mattie to scream.)

Mattie: You'll ruin that boy! You'll ruin that boy!

Jim: What does she do, Mattie? What does Susan do?

Mattie: I don't remember what she does.

Jim: You do remember, Mattie. Mattie, what does Susan do? What does she do?

Mattie: I really don't know.

(Director reverses roles.)

Jim: You are Susan. This is Mattie. You are in the back yard on a hill. You are with your little cousin. What are you doing? How are you standing? Stand over him.

(Cousin lies on back. Susan sits on his thighs. Susan sobs, tries to open the fly of the auxiliary playing the little cousin. He gets panicky and gives her a thumb. She clutches and makes motions as if sticking twigs around. Auxiliary playing Mattie comes out screaming.)

Mattie: What are you doing? You'll ruin that child. Oh, you bad wicked child. You'll ruin that boy.

(Susan lies on the ground sobbing.)

Mattie: You get up from there, you bad child!

Jim: What does Mattie do next, Susan?

(Susan trembles and is broken out in perspiration. The role is reversed again. Susan is playing in Mattie's role in order that the action be continued.)

Jim: You, Mattie, this is Susan, go ahead. Action! Go ahead, Mattie. (Susan and Mattie both sobbing.) Mattie, Mattie, look at her. There is Susan, Mattie. What are you going to do, Mattie?

Mattie: I'm going to beat the hell out of her!

Jim: Here or somewhere else?

Mattie: Here. I'm going to wear her out good. There's a little tree over here.

(Mattie breaks switch and begins beating. Scene becomes very intense as Mattie beats Susan. Susan screaming, "Stop, stop Mother." Director decides to cut scene as he is afraid auxiliary will actually become hurt. Cut! Cut!)

Jim: Mattie, Mattie, Mattie, (In soothing tones to cool situation which has become overheated. Mattie begins sobbing more quietly.)

Mattie: I wore my hands out.

Jim: You wore you hands out? And what did that ungrateful girl do? (Pause) And what did that ungrateful girl do? (Repeated softly.)

Mattie: She is over there sitting in the corner.

Jim: Did you talk to her, Mattie?

Mattie: No, I didn't. I don't know how.

Jim: Would you like to talk to her now?

Mattie: Yes, I think I might, but I don't think it would do any good.

Jim: Why don't you talk to her Mattie? There she is. Talk to her, Mattie.

Susan: You hurt me, Mother. You hurt my feelings.

Mattie: A mother has to do that sort of thing. A mother has to have some way of teaching her daughter what is right and wrong.

Susan: I didn't mean to do anything wrong.

Mattie: But you did. You are a very wicked girl.

Susan: (Crying.) I want to be your baby.

Mattie: But you are not a baby.

Susan: But I want to be a baby.

Mattie: But you can't be a baby.

Susan: But I am a baby.

Mattie: I know you're not.

Susan: I didn't know I had done anything wrong.

Mattie: But you did. You are wicked now. I hope you understand that you mustn't do that sort of thing.

Jim: And so, Mattie, you might have talked to your daughter like that. Do you think that might have helped her, Mattie?

Mattie: No. I just didn't know how to talk to her, to any of the children. There's no way I could help them.

Jim: What were you afraid of when you saw Susan in the yard with the cousin?

Mattie: I don't know. I was just afraid it was the wrong thing.

Jim: Mattie, what are you afraid of? (Mattie holds stomach with an expression of pain.) Are you afraid you are going to become pregnant?

Mattie: I am just so ashamed. Somehow, I've never been able to do anything with my children. (Jim cuts session and awakens Susan. Susan, still in role of Mattie, begins a discussion with group.

DISCUSSION

The second session illustrates hypnodramatic action which deals directly with traumatic situations, whereas the first protocol is that of a highly symbolic production.

Hypnodrama has been found useful in cases where the patient is unable to express himself through other techniques sufficiently well to gain catharsis and therapeutic success. It has especial value in conversion hysteria and psychopathic states. It has been found to have some success with schizoid personalities. When used in conjunction with psychodrama, it speeds up the therapeutic process without loss of values attributed to therapy given on conscious levels.

Directorial Aids

The handling of pathological states of warming-up or spontaneity, such as the one illustrated in this record, may be facilitated by the following techniques: (1). A double may be sent in. (2.) An aggressive auxiliary ego may be fitted into the action and change its direction. (3.) The director may force the patient into a new channel. (4.) It may be necessary to cut a scene and to set up a new one.

The following techniques are useful in determining symbol meanings: (1). Soliloquy *in situ*. (2.) Detailed description of the symbol by the patient. (3.) Observation of the action which the patient takes toward the symbol and of the action which he ascribes to the symbol. (4.) Observation of inter-action of patient and symbol. (5.) Extension of act hungers.

Dual Direction (See first protocol)

It was decided to investigate the effect of using a male and female director in this situation. In view of the patient's feeling toward women this attempt cannot be called wholly successful. In this session it was tried spontaneously and the two directors had not had an opportunity to warm up to each other in the situation. Therefore, the direction of the movement in the hypnodrama lacked unity. In later sessions dual direction was more successfully used, giving the opportunity to note the effect of mother and father figures directing the patient.

Memory and Hypnodrama

In other techniques of hypnotherapy many workers have found a lag between the patient's presentation of material under hypnosis and acceptance of it into consciousness. In general it has been felt that presentation under hypnosis speeded this acceptance and resulted in more rapid integration due to the partial catharsis which occurs under the hypnosis. Perhaps tension surrounding the event is released in sufficient quantities to make this conscious recall less painful. While work in hypnodrama is yet too meager to be conclusive, it appears that memory for action taking place under hypnosis is greater. This could be accounted for by the greater release of tension occurring in action. Memory for events occurring in hypnodrama seems to depend more upon the amount of tension surrounding the scene rather than the depth of the hypnosis.

Learning and Hypnodrama

Retraining which takes place in psychodrama has the advantage of adding the kinesthetic senses to those which are usually used for education. It becomes possible for the organism to learn as a whole and in situations which are not too different from those encountered outside of the therapeutic setting. Hypnodrama allows us to extend learning situations toward the upper limits of the patient's level of function. The ceiling of his upper limit is probably raised due to the lessening of inhibition and the achievement of deeper states of spontaneity. By forcing him to function closer to the upper limit, we bring out factors which have been inhibiting his production and enable him to approach this level in a waking state. Catharsis, spontaneity training, and improved warming-up processes allow him to realize new and more productive roles. These changed concepts readily transfer to the waking state.

Dreams

Dream work may be done with ease in hypnodrama as in psychodrama. It is interesting to note that the dream as told by the patient prior to his production on the stage is usually very incomplete. In hypnodrama the patient gains insight into the meaning of the dream without the therapist necessarily giving an interpretation. This insight may be considered an action insight and may or may not be verbalized by the patient. Hypnotic dreams may be produced in the patient and acted out on the stage. Such procedures afford cathartic value as well as allowing the patient to realize the roles which he has previously denied to himself.

SUMMARY

In this paper the technique of hypnodrama has been presented with some theoretical considerations. Technical information of use in direction is also given. Some of the uses of the technique have been pointed out. Two verbatim protocols of hypnodramatic sessions have been presented and discussed. Characteristics differentiating hypnodrama from the usual hypnotherapeutic techniques and psychodrama are pointed out.

Further work is needed before any definite conclusions concerning the full scope of the application of hypnodrama can be drawn.

16
Training of the Unconscious by Hypnodramatic Re-Enactment of Dreams*

Rolf Krojanker

J.L. Moreno has repeatedly stated his conviction that the unconscious can be trained to overcome emotional trauma and hidden conflicts. Desoille and Bjerre have used "directed dreams" to resolve conflicts. In these techniques, Desoille leads the patient into the visualization of situations full of Jungian symbols, carrying with them the portent of resolution of conflicts. These techniques are based on Freud's findings, that dreamers use symbols to highlight, condense and generally report conflicts they are dealing with in their minds at the time of the dream. The meaning of such symbols is much clearer to the dreamer in the sleeping or dreaming state, that is, at a time when unconscious processes are only inadequately checked by the conscious, the "censor." Desoille and others then argued that therapists could address their interventions to the unconscious by using symbols germane to conscious understanding as equivalent for the resolution of a patient's conflicts and suggesting such symbolic situations while the dreamer reclined on the couch with his eyes closed and his conscious effort reduced to listening to the therapists' "directed dream." Desoille and Brachfeld reported decrease in anxiety sometimes after just one such session.

The value of symbolic gratifications has been known to other

*Reprinted with permission. *Group Psychotherapy* (June 1962) Vol. 15, No. 2.

workers in Psychiatry, for instance Mme. M. Sechehaye has used "symbolic realization" successfully with schizophrenic patients in the waking state.

However, Moreno has initiated the use of action techniques, such as hypnodrama and dream enactments, to demonstrate that the understanding and correction of one or more dreams of a single night is a good therapeutic maneuver. Much like conscious attitudes can improve by role training, it is possible to modify unconscious expectations and behavior through training, e.g., let a dream conclude with a "happy end" instead of a catastrophe, learn to experience pleasant feelings when looking down from high buildings, gazing at one's step-mother, facing one's boss, etc.

The present report will deal with a series of connected dreams of "Norma," as well as their re-enactment and correction in situ. The dreams were experienced during a three week workshop in 1961 at Beacon and were dealt with in the presence of all its participants.

NECESSARY INFORMATION

Norma is pregnant for the second time, and in the third month of pregnancy. She has a three-year-old boy. In the first pregnancey, Norma was ambivalent about having the child while she was pregnant, but changed her attitude to one of frank love of the child at its birth. In her current pregnancy, her ambivalence is again manifest.

Norma is otherwise a quiet happy housewife. Her ambivalence with regard to assuming the added responsibilities of a mother in the future, changing to self-confident love upon finding herself adequate to handle the new job, can often be observed in modern mothers.

In other words, we are dealing with a fairly common attitude regarding pregnancy. Prior to this first dream, Norma had suffered two or three minor falls during social activities at Beacon, which were of no consequence; that is, she never really hurt herself when falling. She seemed just to glide down and sit comfortably on the floor, yet a fleeting air of fear and anxiety would appear on her face whenever she lost her balance this way. Usually this happened in front of bystanders who would be quite solicitous in helping her up again.

FIRST DREAM

In the second week of the seminar, Norma offers a recurrent dream to Dr. Moreno, who directs this session. Dr. Moreno suggests that Norma go to sleep on her bed (mattress) on stage. Norma stretches out on the mattress, closes her eyes and tries to warm up to sleep. Moreno then continues:

"Now you are back at the house, asleep." (Bends over her, softly strokes her hair, soothingly, while talking suggestively to Norma.) "Breathe deeply, deeper, deeper, that's right. And now, you are starting to dream. Don't tell me the dream. I want you to reenact it, after you have first visualized it in your mind. While you are there, sleeping, you have that same dream all over again. Do you see the dream? Can you visualize the first part, then the middle, and then the end?"

Norma: (keeps eyes closed, is relaxed, nods her head affirmatively).

Moreno: "And now, as you see the first part, what do you see first in the dream?"

Norma: "I am on the stairs of the house."

Moreno: "Then get up. Are you with someone?"

Norma: (Stands up) "No, I am alone. I am paralyzed and cannot walk down the stairs because I am going to fall down and lose the baby."

Dr. Moreno then insinuates, "You say you are paralyzed; is that true? Try to walk."

"I can't." (She stands as if frozen, on one spot).

"Try!"

"I just can't," says Norma; "I'm afraid to fall and lose the baby!" and begins to cry.

"I'll help you," says the therapist, and does so.

Norma can now walk a few steps but stops when reaching the three stairs of the stage. No amount of persuasion convinces the panicky Norma to negotiate the three stairs. Dr. Moreno then commands Norma's double:

"Go—you walk the stairs down with her!" Even that does not seem to be enough protection.

Dr. Moreno then exclaims, "I will help you too, let us go!"

Hesitantly, Norma follows the two auxiliary-egos, and to her surprise, she succeeds without falling. Her panic eases, but Dr. Moreno gives her no rest; she has to walk those stairs down again and again, first with the double, and then alone. Norma is then urged by Moreno to not fear such a dream again, even to expect to dream that she is negotiating the stairs sucessfully, helped by Dr. Moreno or the auxiliary ego. She is ordered to sleep again on stage, and is then re-awakened.

In the following general discussion, Dr. Moreno explained his interventions in modifying the actual dream on stage as *"Dream Correctives,"* in which Norma was helped to overcome her paralyzing fears of falling; it was important to overcome these, not only once on stage, but to go through these motions repeatedly, so that the acts started to carry with them a positive conviction of success; a positive conviction of NOT falling in the future. In this way, during the hypnodramatic trance, her unconscious attitudes toward falling, as well as the motions necessary in order not to fall, had been trained with her.

Note

As we shall see soon, unconsciously Norma was not sure whether she wanted that baby really and whether she was able to take care of a helpless infant around the clock, waiting patiently for months and years for it to grow up and become self-sufficient. A fall, followed by an abortion, might indeed have provided a natural remedy for this predicament.

Another possible meaning of walking safely downward with a pregnancy suggests itself, namely, the symbolism of giving birth to a baby between one's legs. So Dr. Moreno helped Norma *and her child* down safely and alive; he rehearsed with her symbolically not only not to fall, but also to give birth to the baby aided by another doctor in the future.

Norma does not report any recurrences of this dream in the succeeding days. Dr. Moreno has departed for an international convention. Toward the end of the Workshop, a second opportunity to be a protagonist is offered to Norma who has had three other dreams. She is put into a trance by me on stage, and re-enacts the following brief dream:

"Dr. Moreno has died." (Weeps.) "I cannot look at him; it is so terrible."

"Go and look at him; there he is lying in the casket."

"I can't."

"It is all right; you can." She finally looks at the auxiliary ego embodying Dr. Moreno.

Therapist: "You see, you can look at him. Do you want to talk to him?"

"Yes."

"You can talk to him; he will be able to hear you."

She finally does so and is urged to talk to him as a first corrective.

"Dr. Moreno, I hardly can believe it; it is so terrible; we miss you so much." Therapist: "You see, you can talk to him. Now if you want to bring him back, you can! Go ahead and pull him up—go ahead!" She does so and sighs with relief from an anxiety state, bordering again on panic in its intensity.

"Dream Corrections"

This dream was corrected in two phases. The dreamer at first accepted without hesitation that she could "talk to Dr. Moreno" and expressed very positive affect toward him. In this fashion, she had already tacitly accepted that "Dr. Moreno" was not really dead, only absent or paralyzed, as it were.

In the second phase of dream correction and training, she not only talked to him, but with physical effort, lifted him up, saved him from death or paralysis. What a "reversal of roles" from the session with Dr. Moreno! As a result of "dream training" she now saves Moreno from death as she saved herself from falling.

With regard to the death, I felt that this was a symbolic dream picture to explain the master's absence from the Workshop, and many participants of the Workshop were indeed missing him. Since, however, there are often ambivalent feelings toward father figures in general and toward the father in Norma's pregnancy in particular, Norma was allowed to resuscitate the dead to rid her also of any guilt feelings.

Yet Norma had in this dream willed Dr. Moreno a combination of husband, father, doctor and teacher, also dead. Her crying gave evidence of positive feelings toward him as well as of anguish and guilt concerning her death wish. What the therapist allowed here was to undo that murder. Undoing is one of the frequent mechanisms of defense. He then allowed her to change from a murderer into a saviour, thus to over compensate for her death wish. Since all this was done in a trance state, these corrections were not addressed to the consciously functioning Norma, but to her subconscious, as it were. One might ask here: When is a corrective used in hypnodrama and in psychodramatic interpretation of dreams? Even though that cannot be answered categorically, manifest anxiety of the dreamer on stage often calls for a corrective, since it is indicative of a conflict. Oftentimes the associations of the dreamer with regard to the dream will give a clue for the need for a corrective.

Another question is more difficult to answer: Is this repressive therapy? Yet it seems evident, that no emotional conflict with a basis in reality was repressed here. Instead more acceptable solutions to the issues weighing on the dreamer's mind were suggested and rehearsed, but only *after* the dreamer had had a chance to first give her version of her solution and had obtained the understanding without criticism of the therapist.

She next reports the second brief dream of the night, dreamt after she awoke to overcome Dr. Moreno's death-dream. Again she re-enacts it as follows:

"Isn't it dreadful, Manuel, the head of our Half-Way House, has become sick, crazy. They put him into a straight-jacket, because he acts so wild."

No further associations can be elicited from Norma.

Correctives

Norma is urged to change Manuel's fate by her intervention. She goes to the auxiliary ego enacting Manuel, gets him out of the straight-jacket, berating the attendant on stage, talks soothingly to Manuel, whom she believes to have become sick from over-work. She then reports the straight-jacket incident to another doctor, rejecting me as having "nothing to do" with the straight-jacket. The "doctor" warns the "attendant" on stage to destroy all straight-jackets, or else to suffer consequences.

Norma is visibly relieved by this outcome.

Note

We observe here that the second dream of that night carried with it evidence of some "dream work," since the hero of the dream was not anymore "dead," only "mad." In correcting this dream on stage, the dreamer had a chance to save the hero from the sickness she had dreamed up for him, and as a result of which she felt quite distressed. She also had an opportunity to express her concern about her husband's overwork. Finally, she could enlist the help of another father figure, the "doctor," to help her patient.

Norma is put to sleep again, and then re-enacts the following, third dream which she experienced actually three days after the above reported ones.

"My second child is born. I give birth to a beautiful son, much like my first son. His name is Craig. The delivery was quite different because I get up from the table right away, 'take the child away to my mother', and, we both *walk* to her home. Craig is very mature, walks and talks like my first one, but is not toilet-trained. We have a wonderful relationship." Norma has actually written down this dream in order not to forget it. She seems depressed now.

Re-Enactment with correctives

Norma is asked to go into any detail of the dream as she re-enacts it on stage. She may tell anything she would wish to change in the dream and we will try to modify the dream accordingly on stage. She now talks to Craig after the delivery about how much she loves him. Then she cries about her own impatience in wanting to see him grown up; she accepts him anyway, but, much rather, would like to see him unable to walk and talk, just a normal new-born baby. She can wait for it, and as to toilet training, she does not mind at all. This is re-enacted on stage, and Norma's love for her child moves the audience and she feels pleased with herself. Norma holds her baby's face and cuddles it in her arms while the baby acts helpless, immature, yet ready to be loved. Baby does not talk or even sit yet. Norma feels visibly happy and relaxed. She is then put to sleep again and finally taken out of trance altogether.

To close this hypnodramatic experience, Norma declares that she now feels she is emotionally ready to bear a child and not make excessive demands upon his capacities:

"He does not have to walk and talk yet from the start; I can wait."

Note

Since both the dream and the notes taken of it seemed to end on an expression of denial of a conflict, namely, a "wonderful relationship," some preliminary explanation was needed to recognize the need for a corrective. True, this dream showed the fulfillment of a wish; namely, to give birth to an exceptional son, yet the happy end of this dream did not seem to correlate with Norma's affect in the previous dreams. So Norma was given a free hand in this correction; one might say, she was asked to freely associate to it. Indeed, she soon showed the underlying conflict and frustration and broke out in tears. Now, the corrective was applied and she was allowed to have a child that acts like a normal baby, cannot talk, or walk, etc.

Final Discussion Period

I then asked for a discussion on the following thoughts about change of emotional attitudes toward the coming child as evidenced by the dream sequence itself, and the correctives designed to train unconscious attitudes.

In the dream of the first session, a clear fear of losing (accidentally killing) the child through a fall was expressed, and the phobia was corrected in situ by descending steps successfully, with disappearance of a panic state while in trance. In the highly charged atmosphere of the Workshop, her following dreams gave evidence of training and dreamwork.

The next dream showed Dr. Moreno, the "father," dead instead of the child. The dreamer brought him back to life again. Indeed, the dreamer evidently wanted to save both father *and* child; this was the reason why she worried about her dreams.

A dream followed in the same night, where the "father" of the Half-Way House is not dead, but mad; or, as one of the discussants pointed out, "half-dead." The dreamer volunteered to help the father. On her own request, she now made sure the father would get well.

A final and later dream shows a successful birth with a prematurely developed baby. Mother again volunteered to correct this dream; she wanted a "normal" baby all the way.

It was evident to all participants that Norma really wanted to have that second baby, and would be a wonderful mother for it.

The presentation of this hypothesis was accepted eagerly by the persons present and ended this session.

Note

This discussion was designed to highlight only the positive actions of Norma in order to bring closure to this session. A final discussion should tend to reassure the protagonist and the group. This was probably a reason for the group's ready acceptance of exclusively positive statements regarding the dreams in the final discussion.

The final discussion of a psychodrama session is often of great importance, since it helps to obtain a group consensus regarding the value of the issues presented by the protagonist, and how these affect the lives of the other members of the group. In hypnodrama, however, and in dream interpretations, issues are dealt with, which a patient might not like to tell the group, or take responsibility for, in the waking state; therefore, care must be taken to present the dreamer's conflict in a face-saving manner. In this final discussion, this was done by mentioning only the noble instincts of the dreamer, namely, her urge to save husband and child. No mention was made of the other side of the coin, namely, that the dreamer wanted to save a husband and child as well as the therapist *from her own death wishes.* This in itself was a positive suggestion, a corrective maneuver, this time aimed at the protagonist and the group in the waking state. Such a final maneuver will not always be necessary with an ongoing therapy group, but it is safer to tie up loose ends this way in a training group as ours was, where one endeavors not to leave emotional scars unnecessarily exposed. Just as during the hypnodramatic session, the emotional catharsis of tears and drama occupied a preeminent place in the experiences reported here, the final discussion avoided dramatic action and substituted catharsis with insight.

DISCUSSION

Sequential dream analysis has been reported by various authors. Most of the authors do not show such a rapid shift toward resolution of conflict as this sequence showed under the influence of hypnodrama, nor was such progress witnessed by concurrents to a Workshop.

Hypnodrama stands alone in adding to subconscious experience the third dimension of space, i.e., while conscious experience or interference is reduced to a minimum. In so doing, hypnodrama excels over the ordinary hypnotic state, where muscular tensions or movements have to be suggested. Here they are actually felt, the person is moving, hitting, falling, talking in reality, in space. In moving about, something of the helpless submission of the hypnotic trance is also removed; the hypno-dramatic protagonist does not move about like a robot, but, rather like a cooperative partner, and the main actor is the patient, not the therapist.

Dream work in hypnodrama requires a thorough understanding of psychodynamics from the director of the sessions, as well as sufficient previous experience to be able to give a sufficiently plausible interpretation of the dreams "on the spot" to himself in case the protagonist is unable to volunteer dream correctives, so that he may guide or induce correctives to the dream almost while the dreamer "dreams."

Hypnodramatic dream interpretation again brings into dream analysis the action techniques which are not offered in any other approach. In this dimension, it even exceeds the original dream itself, makes it more concrete and adds to it. This is a very creative instrument when further expanded by the use of correctives. This time the dreamer has the unheard-of opportunity to redream, to remodel his dream as if he were an artist with his masterpiece.

One might here add the influence of the therapist. In a sense he has made the dream his own work too, by witnessing it, and even though he wants to help, his unconscious is set in motion too; hypnodrama even more than hypnosis is a process of *inter-actions*, with a co-unconscious experience once therapist and patient interact around a common ground. Even as the group shares that dream, they enter the co-unconscious experience, as it happened in the here reported sequence. So, e.g., the participant who acted as Norma's child in the dreams, felt quite wanted and loved in the final corrected version of the dream, as she reported in the final discussion. In many other scenes during this workshop, she had indeed tried to relive an unhappy childhood and "dream up" a happy one, like being a wanted and loved child!

Freud sees wish fulfillment as the dynamic basis for dreams, and he distinguishes between their manifest and the latent content. The latent content of our dream sequence was certainly only barely touched, since we dealt with a quite delimited and specific issue: an ambivalent attitude toward a pregnancy which had shown up also in the patient's waking hours. The manifest dream content showed only barely concealed gratification of Norma's impulses (death for the child and/or the father), with an amendment or revelation of underlying fears in the final dreams (sickness or abnormality of father or child). Our dream correctives were designed to "undo" these dire results and so alleviate Norma's guilt feelings in the waking state. We then trained Norma's unconscious to expect a normal childbirth which would preserve father's health as well as the child's health.

If we follow C.G. Jung, we need not worry about "wish

fulfillment." Instead, we observe the relevant, yet vague issue the dreamer tackles with and help her clarify and think about this issue. The dreamer oftentimes will guide us to the solution she really wanted. Norma, e.g., when free to choose, wanted Dr. Moreno alive, and her child a healthy strong baby.

We follow Dr. Moreno's conviction that anxiety-producing results in dreams can and should be corrected. Anxiety is indicative of a conflict between impulses and their controls and if insight cannot be obtained by free association about the dream, a symbolic correction of this conflict can be effective.

Such a correction is held to be more effective in the dream state, since along with diminished consciousness one can expect a decreased willingness to resist therapeutic suggestions. If this is true, it would follow that the training or the reconditioning of attitudes would have a better chance of success while the patient is in a state of decreased consciousness.

In our particular case demonstration, we are glad to report that Norma's pregnancy continues uneventfully through the months; she has stopped falling and has developed a confident air about her condition.

When starting to work with hypnodramatic re-enactment of dreams, it would be safer for the new director to use the classical approach (see monograph by Dr. Moreno and J. Enneis on hypnodrama), namely, to have the protagonist and his auxiliary egos re-enact the entire dream in the original version, then let him go to sleep again, and now dream and re-enact a corrected version of the dream. However, a more abbreviated procedure has been demonstrated by the writer in the present sequence.

REFERENCES

MORENO, J.L.   Interpersonal Therapy and the Psychopathology of Interpersonal Relations, Beacon House, Beacon, N.Y., 1937.

MORENO, J.L.   Psychodrama of a Dream in *Psychodrama Vol. II,* Beacon House, 1958.

MORENO, J.L. and ENNEIS, JAMES.   Hypnodrama and Psychodrama, Beacon House, Beacon, N.Y., 1948.

17
Hypnodrama,
a Synthesis of Hypnosis and
Psychodrama, a Progress Report*

Leonard K. Supple

Herewith follows a brief description of the origin of the Hypnodramatic Technique. Hypnodrama is a synthesis of psychodrama and hypnosis. The idea of hypnodrama came to Dr. Moreno through an accident. In the summer of 1939 the late Dr. Bruno Solby brought a young woman for treatment. She suffered from paranoid delusions accompanied by nightmares, every night the devil came to visit her. She was unable to get into a psychodramatic re-enactment of the incident. After trying the self-directed technique and methods of mild prompting without results he became highly directive; this put the patient unexpectedly into a hypnotic trance. Dr. Moreno decided to try a psychodrama under these novel circumstances. With the aid of two male auxiliary egos the patient was able to portray two meetings with the devil, one as it had happened the night before, one as she expected it to happen the following night. Apparently hypnosis operated as a "starter" and spurred her spontaneity.

Several years later Dr. Moreno made a number of hypnodramatic experiments in association with James Enneis, the results of which they published in a monograph.[1] Enneis describes the technique as follows:

"In hypnodrama, hypnosis is induced on the stage. Psychodramatic

*Reprinted with permission. *Group Psychotherapy* (March 1962) Vol. 15, No. 1.
[1]*Hypnodrama and Psychodrama* by J.L. Moreno and James Enneis, New York: Beacon House, 1950.

techniques are used to speed the process and to relate it to the patient's everyday experience. The patient is warmed up in a psychodramatic manner to being in his bedroom or some other situation which he associates with sleep. After the setting becomes real to him, the director continues with the usual suggestive technique for the induction of hypnosis. When the patient is hypnotized the procedure continues with the psychodrama, using all its well known techniques."

"The closing of sessions on a high note is a cardinal principle of psychodrama.[2] This applies also in hypnodrama. When the patient has enacted frustrating experiences, it becomes extremely important that he be warmed up to a pleasant situation which he can handle to his satisfaction before he is awakened. If this is not done, anxiety or depression may result. He must be given an opportunity to act a successful if not heroic role, thus allowing the warming-up process to become reoriented."

Since last May we have on various occasions used this combined mode of therapy with different types of patients. It has been quite successful and has allowed the patients to go deeper into their portrayal in the psychodrama while in the hypnotic state than they would without the hypnosis, at least in some cases. In several instances this has been a revelation and in fact, some of the patients who in the usual form of psychodrama did not give their all, once they were in the hypnotic state would eagerly participate in hypnodrama for two hours or more and reveal much deeper levels than in the psychodrama. To explain this more fully, allow me to state that I have seen patients in psychodrama who have revealed themselves on very deep subconscious levels, and in fact, I have seen cataleptic patients respond to the psychodrama where mirror technique, role reversal, auxiliary ego methods and other modalities were employed.

Perhaps it would be well if at this juncture I were able to give some details of one particular case in which hypnodrama worked very well. The subject, a young lady, is a teacher in the southwest and holds a Master's degree in Science from a recognized university. Clair came to the Moreno Institute in Beacon to study at a summer seminar held there under the direction of Dr. Moreno. While a group member there, she stated that she herself had problems which had been bothering her for quite a number of years. She had two sessions of psychodrama. I was present at one of these although I did not participate at this particular session. During these sessions, she reenacted certain situations in her past experience at home and elsewhere and was given considerable

[2]*Psychodrama* Vol. I and II, by J.L. Moreno, Beacon House, Beacon, N.Y.

insight into some of her problems but felt that she had not completely conquered the entire situation. At Dr. Moreno's suggestion, I saw this young lady who had entered into a light hypnotic trance on one previous occasion for her Dentist at home. I proceeded to induce a light trance in privacy in this student. The following day, with very little difficulty, I induced her into a medium trance, which I helped her to make much deeper. While in this particular trance, she reacted well to my suggestion that Dr. Moreno would now take over the Psychodrama or Hypnodrama session. Dr. Moreno, together with Mrs. Moreno and others who were present at the teaching seminar, then entered into the Hypnodrama and this session continued for approximately 1½ to 1¾ hours. During this time, I reinforced hypnosis on two or three occasions although I was not certain this was necessary. However, it did quite well. Clair reacted very well and went through several intimate scenes in her past life, especially in childhood without any fear whatsoever of going into the intimacy of these details. At the end of the drama, I awakened her from the hypnotic trance and she stated that she felt well and she was satisfied with what she had presented.

The following day, I was able to induce Clair into a trance by the mere use of one of Dr. Erickson's more streamlined and more dramatic techniques, raising her hand in mine and having her look at her hand without knowing it, holding it closer to her face and eyes and as it came closer, she automatically went into a deep trance. With this, I then had her sit down and deepen the trance until it became very deep. I then made the statement that she could, if she desired, open her eyes and stay in a state of a very very deep hypnosis and walk around or talk, ask questions, answer questions or whatever else she chose to do but meanwhile staying at all times in this very deep hypnotic trance. On this occasion, Clair remained in a trance for a period of approximately 2½ hours. During this time, she walked about the Psychodrama stage, she literally circled the lowest step on the stage countless times, followed by her auxiliary ego, and she responded beautifully to the suggestions of her auxiliary ego, to those of the Director and the other participants in the session. During this session, she reenacted a scene from her early childhood in which she lay down upon the stage and at the time she lay down was back to about two years of age in her mind, in the hypnotic state. She could see two other participants in the Psychodrama who were taking the roles of her Father and Mother and who were lying upon a mattress which represented a bed upon the stage. She immediately registered all the reactions of horror and fear. She stated that "Daddy is beating Mommy up." It soon developed that what she had seen at this early stage both physically many years ago and also in hypnosis on this occasion was an act of intercourse between her Father and Mother, but at the age when she saw this, she interpreted it as physical abuse of the Mother by the Father. It was interesting that she was able to regress in the hypnotic state on only the third session which I had with her to a state where she could once again visualize this act of aggression as she interpreted it. There is frequently the question raised what regression means in dynamic terms. According to Moreno's hypothesis, regression is a "psychodramatic" regression, not a "physiological" regression. This hypothesis can be empirically tested. This interpretation of regression may not change the therapeutic effect of the re-enactment of past episodes. Later on when she was out of hypnosis, we discussed the matter. She had an entirely different interpretation of what she had seen. She now was able to discuss it at the adult level and understand that what she had seen was not what she thought she saw when she was two years of age. It is extremely interesting to note that one not versed in hypnosis but versed in Psychodrama can accomplish age regression in a subject who has been put in hypnosis by another individual. Clair discussed many areas of her life, her associations with men, her associations with superiors of the faculty and of her students with complete freedom from embarrassment or difficulty of any kind. She was able to give of her innermost self during this entire period of time and we believe that she did better with this technique than she would have with either Psychodrama or hypnosis alone.

At the end of this session, several of the group who were observing the technique asked me if Clair was still in hypnosis. In order to show them, perhaps one might say "dramatically" the answer to their question, I asked Clair if she was awake or in hypnosis and she said she thought she was awake but she wasn't sure. I therefore asked her if she would not sit down, which she obligingly did. I told her that if she wished to, she could go even deeper into hypnosis by just closing her eyelids. Being a very gracious subject, she closed her eyelids and went into a much deeper trance than she did 2½ hours previously. I then suggested to her that when she awakened from hypnosis, both of her upper extremities would be in a catatonic position and she could not put them down till such time as I snapped my fingers. I then aroused her from the hypnotic state and immediately both of her upper extremities went into the catatonic position very comfortably. She sat there and talked to me for a period of about five minutes after which I snapped my fingers and Clair's arms became relaxed and the upper extremities returned to a normal state.

We do not feel that this is a panacea or cure-all for *every* patient who comes to us for therapy. However, we feel that in some selected cases this can be a very advantageous type of treatment. We feel also that there has not been enough work done in this particular field to fully outline the type of patient who is best treated by this combined technique. Further research should allow us to more accurately determine which type of patient would benefit most by this method.

There are several other cases with which we have worked in this, we believe, new and certainly different technique. We feel that much progress can be made in this direction by a combination of hypnotic and psychodramatic techniques. However, there is much still to be learned and therefore we intend to continue with the research in this field. We feel it is extremely interesting to note that two techniques can be combined so successfully. Dr. Moreno, of course, has done hypnosis in the past but has not specialized in this particular therapy. I have done other things myself but have gone more and more toward the hypnotic technique. It is interesting also to see how easy it is to transfer the patient from the one who induces hypnosis to the one who carries on the Psychodrama. I feel that if the Psychodramatist were someone not versed in the hypnotic techniques this could present problems. However, this still remains to be proven. Personally, I believe that by the combination of hypnosis and psychodrama, it may be possible entirely to achieve much more brilliant results. There are certain patients whom I have observed in Psychodrama and Psychotherapy who are somewhat reticent or one might say, bashful in giving their all. They seem to withhold something from the group or from the Psychodramatist. In the particular cases which we have studied in the combined form of therapy, this reticence or bashfulness or withholding has been largely overcome. These patients seem to *want* to give all of their innermost and subconscious thoughts for their own benefit and that of the group with whom they are working. Naturally, one can envision the much greater benefits from this type of situation than from one where the patient withholds even a small part of the information which is present in his conscious or subconscious mind. In more recent sessions of hypnodrama, we have observed that the patients have told us that after each session they have been very active at home and have established, in most cases much better rapport with their families or at least several members of each family than had been possible in the past. Since we envisage our program to be one of establishing rapport of the patient with his or her family, we have been encouraged greatly by the reports from the patients. We feel that ours is a teaching situation. In other words, we are teaching the patient to better establish relationships with all members of his or her family and with the others with whom he or she comes in contact. Apparently we are succeeding in this respect.

Part V

HYPNODRAMA:
The Group Approach

18
Hypnodrama and Group Hypnosis

Ira A. Greenberg

Introduction: Creation and Development

Hypnodrama and Moreno

Hypnodrama, which combines the power of psychodrama with the sensitivity of hypnosis, is an action therapy that very quickly helps the one in treatment, the protagonist, get in touch with repressed material and gain insights following the deep and meaningful emotional experiences undergone. As in psychodrama, the protagonist in hypnodrama deals with a problem in which he uses other members of the group to play the parts of people involved in the problem. The process enables the protagonist to go through both age and emotional regression to get at, deal with, and work through forgotten experiences of a traumatic nature. It is not only an outgrowth of psychodrama but also the fruit of the personalities and experiences of the two individuals who were responsible for its creation and development. They are the late J.L. Moreno, M.D., the psychiatrist who fathered psychodrama, group psychotherapy, and sociometry, among a multitude of other modalities, and psychologist James M. Enneis, M.S., one of Moreno's principal disciples following World War II and today among the giants of psychodrama who are continuing Moreno's work.

Moreno, as noted in the first and last chapter of the previous section, invented hypnodrama in 1939 in conjunction with some trained medical hypnotists working with him. It is more likely than not, however, that Moreno created this method of treatment at a much earlier date. I make this speculation through personal knowledge of Moreno the man and the creative giant, as well as through having some close involvements with him during which I experienced the force of his personality and the impact of his presence. It is highly conceivable that through the influential effect of his manner and the action and emotion he tended to stimulate around him, especially when directing a psychodrama, that many of his protagonists and possibly some audience members slipped into the hypnotic state, entranced as they may have been by the movement, shouting, and gesticulation of this magnetic individual. This may have been the beginning of hypnodrama, but when I questioned Moreno about it in the spring of 1973, a year before he died at the age of eighty-four, he would neither confirm nor deny it.

Enter Enneis

Enneis, while working with Moreno, invented hypnodrama in 1948 independently of Moreno. An army lieutenant during World War II who served as a psychologist with the Medical Corps, Enneis discovered psychodrama while in the midst of a doctoral program at Duke University and soon dropped out in order to study with Moreno. As a classicist might say, Enneis simply exchanged the Apollonian calm and reason of academia for the Dionysian spontaneity and theoretical eruptions of this living legend, the innovator who could not sit still, the genius who fought fiercely for his ideas, the intellectual street brawler who upset the applecarts of psychiatric complacency and left his enemies strewn about behind him in his march toward the goal of treating all of mankind. He left them battered and bruised but ready to retaliate, as many did over the years, in ambushes and attacks scattered throughout the scientific journals and occasionally in books. In any event, Enneis, though of a much quieter and reserved nature, was quick to see that some of the things he had learned in the treatment of shell-shocked or battle-fatigued soldiers, so that they could be returned quickly to active duty, might serve as a useful complement to psychodrama. Military psychiatrists during the Second World War had achieved notable success in treating withdrawn and even catatonic servicemen by having them relive the traumatic events that had triggered their psychoses. To achieve this revivication quickly the psychiatrists administered drugs to induce hypnosis or they and the psychologists working with them delivered verbal hypnotic inductions, and in this state the patients were able to relax the defenses that had kept the traumas from conscious awareness and so were able to reexperience the feelings and thoughts that had accompanied the original events. Enneis had been involved in this form of short-term therapy on numerous occasions as an army psychologist and the dramatic results of this treatment made him see the possibilities for enlarging the scope of psychodramatic therapy by adding this new dimension to it. He presented his ideas to Moreno and was much disconcerted[1] when Moreno casually replied, "Oh, yes, I was just doing that last week."

The two combined their efforts in this direction and conducted many exciting hypnodramas, together or individually, adding their findings to the literature of psychodrama and group psychotherapy (see chapters 14 and 15). However, as interesting and exciting as hypnodrama proved to be, it drew few adherents over the years simply because its practice required more of the director than many were willing or able to bring to it. In conducting a psychodramatic event in which the protagonist is in a state of hypnosis, it is incumbent upon the director to be both a capable psychodramatist and a capable hypnotherapist, and the acquiring of these capabilities entails a considerable amount of training, study, supervision, and experience. While there are many competent psychodramatists available, few had the interest or training opportunities to become skilled hypnotherapists, and for the hypnotherapists even fewer had the interest or incentive to leave the confines of their offices to venture upon the psychodramatic stage and risk failure before a public or professional gathering. Thus, while both psychodramatists and hypnotherapists were aware that such a thing as hypnodrama existed, few knew much about it and even fewer employed it.

Wright Questions

Such was the state of affairs when hypnodrama developed in a new direction. M. Erik Wright, Ph.D., M.D., professor of psychology and psychiatry at the University of Kansas and past president of the American Society of Clinical Hypnosis, was addressing a group during the annual convention of the Society of Clinical and Experimental Hypnosis at Palo Alto, Calif., in October, 1969, when the subject of hypnodrama was brought up. Wright, who had just read my first book, *Psychodrama and Audience Attitude Change*, which I had given him that spring in appreciation for his advising me on a hypnotherapeutic procedure, thereupon tossed the question to me. "Ira, just what is hypnodrama?" he asked. "Is it the protagonist who is hypnotized or the auxiliary egos or

---

[1] I had a similar experience. In 1963 I invented Simulated Psychodrama, in which an actor is employed to replace a patient in order to affect the audience, but Moreno had published an article on this procedure in 1942. (Greenberg, 1968, pp. xxv, 55-57, 108.)

the audience or the director or what?" "It's only the protagonist who is hypnotized," I replied from my seat at the rear of the gathering. "In hypnodrama usually the director or a hypnotherapist does the induction. This," I continued, "is done either privately, and the protagonist is then brought before the group, or it is done in the presence of the group. But as I said, the way Dr. Moreno does it, only the protagonist is under hypnosis."

Wright thanked me for my comments and resumed his address to the audience of professional and research hypnotherapists. And while Wright continued talking, my thoughts remained with my own last statement and with Wright's question. "Only the protagonist is under hypnosis," I thought, as I recalled the articles I'd read on Moreno's work and the two brief hypnodramas I had directed the past summer with student volunteers at Camarillo State Hospital in Southern California. "But why not the others?" I asked myself.

It seemed to me then that greater *telic* (empathetic) bonds between the protagonist and auxiliary egos might be developed if the auxiliaries were also under hypnosis during the hypnodrama. "And why not the audience, too?" I continued to myself. "And even the director?" I resolved to put this idea of hypnodrama and group hypnosis in practice at my first opportunity, and as it turned out I was scheduled to present my first professional workshop in hypnodrama and the group induction process (for teaching participants self-hypnosis) the following month, November 1969, at a growth center just south of Los Angeles.

First Attempt

The workshop extended from Friday evening through Sunday afternoon, and the hypnodramas were scheduled for Saturday night, to serve as the emotional and interactional high point of the weekend, with Sunday designated for follow-up work as well as for the introduction of some new and comfortable hypnotic experiences. During Friday evening and Saturday, the group members went through some brief encounter-type sessions, learned to go into hypnosis as a group and learned some techniques of self-hypnosis. During the afternoon they also learned about and experienced psychodrama, so that by the evening the some dozen participants were looking forward with enthusiasm, and some anxiety, to the hypnodramatic experiences. I also recall having some slight anxieties since this was a new experience for me as well as for the others. Because I had been directing the psychodramas in the afternoon and was set to direct the hypnodramas, I asked one of my associates, Bernard Greenblatt, D.D.S., Ph.D., a dentist-turned-clinical-psychologist, to give the group hypnotic induction. I then lay down on the floor along with many of the others to better prepare myself for the group hypnotic experience by making myself as comfortable as possible.

At the conclusion of the hypnotic induction, I rose to my feet and with my eyes open I began addressing the group on the subject of hypnodrama and on some of the things we might explore with this modality. The others, also with their eyes open, were sitting in a semicircle about me, some on chairs but most on the floor. Two of the women present indicated they wished to be protagonists and began setting up their tape recorders after I gave them permission to do this, explaining I would permit people to tape their own sessions but not those of others because of the confidentiality factor. I had felt very slightly disoriented and my face seemed somewhat wooden when I first stood up, but as I proceeded with directing the two sessions these feelings wore off, and I felt as awake and alert and involved with the protagonists as is usually the case when I direct psychodramas. The hypnodramas[2] dealt with a middle-aged psychology professor who relived an experience that had occurred when she was seven and was criticized by her mother for not being able to carry a tune, and with the boyfriends and ex-husband of a thirty-year-old psychiatric nurse and with a dream concerning them and several other aspects of her life. The first protagonist's session lasted thirty minutes, while that of the second protagonist, involving several relationships and a lengthy dream, lasted for more than an hour. Through the use of the Cheek-LeCron (1968) ideomotor responses[3] with each protagonist, I learned from their subconscious minds that it was in their best interests to remember all that had occurred during their hypnodramas. I then took each protagonist by the hand, and I had the three of us sit down on chairs close to each other. As I did this, I said aloud, "Close your eyes; that's good," as I closed my own, saying to myself, "Oh, no, Greenberg, this is too much," in mock disgust at the way I seemed to be overdramatizing the experience. I then counted to three.

The next thing I remembered hearing was Dr. Greenblatt saying something like, "Wide awake now, and open your eyes." I opened my eyes, and then knew for certain that I had been in a state of deep hypnosis. I thereupon asked the others present, as is usually done in

[2]The hypnodramas are described in more detail in "Psychodrama and Hypnosis Workshops," by Ira A. Greenberg, in a chapter, *Workshops of the Mind*, edited by Bernard S. Aaronson, Doubleday Anchor Books, 1976.

[3]A technique of getting responses from the subconscious through finger movements, detailed in *Clinical Hypnotherapy*, by David B. Cheek and Leslie LeCron (1968).

psychodrama, to share with the protagonists some of their own feelings and experiences that were evoked or brought to mind during or as a result of the hypnodramatic enactments. All reported having been very strongly moved by having been able to identify and empathize with the protagonists during the courses of the hypnodramas, and several persons reported having gained insights into some of their own feelings through having participated in the hypnodramas either as auxiliary egos or as audience members. At the time, I did not feel that what I had done was any different from what I normally did when directing psychodrama sessions in 1969. But those present who had seen me direct elsewhere maintained that they saw a considerable difference, saying that I seemed more attuned to the protagonists than before. Such were some of the events involved in the creation and development of hypnodrama, both that in which an individual protagonist is under hypnosis and that in which many individuals representing the various types of personnel in psychodrama or hypnodrama (i.e., protagonists, director, auxiliary egos, audience) are brought under hypnosis.

THEORY: CHOICE AND PARTS

Hypnodrama or Psychodrama?

Where there is a choice between directing a hypnodrama or a psychodrama—meaning that a director-hypnotist or other clinical hypnotherapist is present—it is, according to my experience, usually the psychodrama that is done. This is because most problems presented lend themselves more easily to psychodrama than to hypnodrama. Being the powerful therapeutic modality that psychodrama is, a good director can help a protagonist to get quickly to the core of the presenting problem and then get to and deal with the cause of this fundamental aspect of the problem. For example, suppose a protagonist sought to deal with a problem involving his never satisfied boss. Through psychodramatic interactions, including role-reversals between the protagonist and auxiliary egos, it might be determined that the core of the problem is not so much that the boss is difficult to work for but that the protagonist's perceptions of his boss are the main source of the problem.

And getting at the cause of the misperceptions might, in the specific hypothetical case, lead to the protagonist's recalling and reenacting some childhood events in which he had to interact with or try to relate to a father he found awesome. The spontaneity of the interaction of action and emotion during the enactment could be expected to lead to catharsis and insight, which concepts, among others, will be dealt with subsequently. Thus, despite the protagonist's having experienced age and emotional regressions during the enactment, he dealt with material involving conscious cognitive recall, and psychodrama could prove highly adequate for the purpose.

Had the protagonist needed to deal with repressed material, which would of course be beyond immediate conscious recall, then a hypnodrama that might include hypnotic age regression would be the preferred therapeutic vehicle. For example, a protagonist at one weekend workshop told me he had been in therapy for a number of months but seemed only to be dealing with peripheral causes for his inability to relate meaningfully with marriageable women; he wondered if there might be an event or events in his childhood that he was unaware of that was causing his problem. In a hypnodrama, he relived the anger, fear, rage, and guilt he had experienced at the age of six when his mother told him he could no longer play with the girl next door because she was of a different religion. This was an incident he had successfully repressed and one that he had only been able to reexperience by means of hypnotically induced age regression.

Hypnodrama also is helpful in enabling an inhibited protagonist to break through many of his defense mechanisms and get in touch with and express fully some of the feelings of fear and frustration, anger and despair, and the often-not-expressed need for love and understanding, hope and happiness. A third important use of hypnodrama is that through the hypnotic warm-up, both in individual and group hypnodrama, potential protagonists may let their subconscious minds bring forth specific problems that are appropriate at that time and place for the individual to deal with in a hypnodrama. Therefore, as may be noted, there are specific purposes for the employment of hypnodrama over psychodrama, but in most instances psychodrama has been found sufficient for the need.

Basic Parts

Warm-up The three basic parts to a hypnodrama or a psychodrama are the *warm-up,* the *enactment,* and the *audience sharing.* In the warm-up the director will discuss psychodrama or hypnodrama or talk about current personal and societal problems or talk about what has been happening to him explaining where he is at at the moment or do or talk about whatever he may feel is appropriate to help those assembled become a cohesive psychodrama group that is open to or ready for a strong emotional and possibly insightful experience. He moulds them into a group that is able to empathize with and support the needs of whichever protagonists present themselves or are selected by the director or by the group. The director thus *warms up* those present to becoming a group and some individuals in the group to becoming protagonists. The director also warms himself up to the intellectually and emotionally demanding task of directing a psychodrama or hypnodrama. In a hypnodrama, the individual or group hypnotic induction occurs during the warm-up, but subsequently during the one-hour or three-hour or daylong or weekend period of that particular group's existence, the director may lead an individual or individuals or the whole group in and out of hypnosis. These subsequent inductions and arousals may occur during the enactment, which follows the warm-up or in the warm-up preparatory for another enactment.

Enactment It is in the enactment that the protagonist works on his problems with the assistance of trained auxiliary egos (assistant therapists) or auxiliaries chosen from the audience, and these auxiliaries play the parts of people involved in the protagonist's problems. At the same time, one or more may serve to help the protagonist be more himself by playing various aspects of him, by *doubling* for him. These *doubles*, who sit or stand to the side of the protagonist away from the audience and slightly to his rear, serve to help him gain insight into his behavior through helping him get in touch with feelings he may be unaware of, throwing ideas his way by means of verbal asides, and helping him escalate and intensify the expression of his thoughts and feelings through subtle and later not-so-subtle exclamations in the role of the protagonist and in his behalf. The most important technique employed in the psychodramatic or hypnodramatic enactment is the *role-reversal*, which Moreno devised in the early 1920s when he created psychodrama. The role-reversal occurs most often under the director's orders, and he gives these instructions at crucial moments in order that a) the protagonist may instruct all those present as to what are his perceptions of the "important other" he is interacting with, which may or may not have a relation to reality, b) the protagonist may experience the world of this important other, particularly how this other individual sees the protagonist, and c) the protagonist, as the important other, may answer any important questions that he, the protagonist, may have asked the other during the height of the spontaneous action and emotion of the moment.

Some other important techniques a director may employ during an enactment are the *mirror*, in which an auxiliary portrays with slight exaggeration the protagonist's behavior while the protagonist observes this from the front row of the audience; the *soliloquy*, in which the protagonist either alone or with the help of a double walks about that stage and thinks his thoughts aloud, usually in response to a specific interaction or statement that had just occurred; the *high chair*, in which a protagonist achieves a sense of stature and power by standing on a chair or other object so as to be able to look down upon and deal with those who had tormented him in the past from this new position of strength; *empty chair*, in which the protagonist interacts with a *phantom other* who is perceived in the empty chair, a Morenean technique taken over by the late Dr. Fritz Perls and used as a principal tool in gestalt therapy; the *split protagonist*, in which various auxiliaries play specific aspects of a protagonist and thus enable him to interact with these aspects, and finally, the *multiple protagonist*, in which others in the group who have or have had problems similar to that of the protagonist are called to the stage and given the opportunity individually to interact with the auxiliary ego portraying a particular role, such as, boss, parent, sibling, teacher, or whatever; this calls for a very strong, i.e., talented and trained, auxiliary ego in order to be able to quickly and effectively interact with one emotionally distraught individual after another, adapting the role in order to meet the needs of each of the often half-dozen or more protagonists who come at the auxiliary with unusually intensified feelings. Many other techniques are available to the experienced director, some of which he will occasionally invent during the high state of spontaneity-creativity that occurs in all well directed psychodramas or hypnodramas.

Audience Sharing The final part of the psychodrama or hypnodrama is the audience sharing, in which the director, sitting close to the protagonist and often holding his or her hand or with an arm around the shoulder, depending on the protagonist's need, will conclude the session by inviting audience members to share personal experiences with the protagonist and with the others present that may have some bearing on the protagonist's problems. The director is responsible for specifically pointing out to the audience that the protagonist has shared some strong feelings or a very meaningful part of his life with those present, and following the enactment it then becomes incumbent upon audience members to share with him from their lives and most emphatically they are not to question, criticize, explain, or interpret to the protagonist. Occasionally, these directions have to be repeated when an audience member may attempt to use this opportunity to give vent to his own needs and to then play at "being doctor" at the expense of the protagonist.

Postsession Rapping There is a fourth part to a psychodrama or hypnodrama that takes place at the Psychodrama Center for Los Angeles, Inc., and at other psychodrama centers. At the Los Angeles Psychodrama Center, a federally tax-exempt training and community service institute, which has been influenced by sociologist and psychodramatist Lewis Yablonsky, Ph.D., in this respect, participants are invited to remain following the final psychodrama to have coffee and tea and cookies and to talk to people they did not get a chance to talk to during the sessions and to generally descend from the emotional heights they may have achieved before returning to the world outside the Psychodrama Center facility. This makes for a pleasant transition from the inner reality of the individuals present and the group reality they had created to the other reality beyond the doors.

THEORY: CONCEPTUAL COMPONENTS

Spontaneity

The most important concept in the Morean therapeutic-philosophic system, as I see it[4] is *spontaneity*, otherwise known as *spontaneity-creativity*, with the other basic concepts being, *situation* or the psychodramatic stage, *tele, catharsis*, and *insight*. These concepts are well presented in Moreno's most important work, *Who Shall Survive?* (1934, 1953), and in another important work, *Psychodrama, Vol. I* (1946, 1964, and reviewed and presented in my book, *Psychodrama and Audience Attitude Change* (1968), and in my anthology, *Psychodrama: Theory and Therapy* (1974), and so not too much space will be devoted to them in the present chapter. When Moreno discusses spontaneity, he concerns himself with it as a human trait, such as intelligence, and he sees its importance in terms of its high positive correlation with survival. Just as intelligence and learning ability have been important determinants of success and survival among the cave dwellers and in modern society, so it is with those having a high degree of creative spontaneity: they are able to adapt to new situations and succeed. Others as intelligent if not more so may fail through lack of situational flexibility and the ability to size up a situation and act appropriately—"to keep your head while all about you are losing theirs," says Polonius, or to "keep your cool," says modern youth.

Spontaneity, as defined by Moreno, is an adequate response to a new situation or a new and adequate response to an old situation. Because it sounds so simple, it bears repeating, and I invariably do this in my lectures. An example I often give to audiences goes something like this: "Here we are talking about psychodrama and psychotherapy, and a wild-eyed man rushes in waving two forty-five automatics and yelling, 'I hate all you mental health type persecutors, and I'm going to get you!' What do you do?" Audience members can give a multitude of responses, and some show exceptionally good spontaneity-creativity in their responses. The usual criterion is the pragmatic one, "Does it work?" If it

---

[4] See Chapter 10 (Greenberg, 1974), for key concepts as seen by Moreno and Bischof.

does, the person survives—unless he chooses to sacrifice himself for the group—and displays good spontaneity. Should he get himself killed or maimed in the process of seeking to subdue the wild-eyed one, he is credited with having made an *inadequate* response to this new situation. As to the new and adequate response to the old situation, I simply describe a situation that might be improved through a new input—such as an unhappy marital situation in which one of the partners changes his or her behavior which requires a change in that of the other if the relationship is to be maintained—and then I usually challenge my audiences to come up with their own examples.

Situation

The psychodramatic situation or the psychodramatic stage is a place where everything occurs in the *here and the now,* a term Moreno first used some fifty years ago. The psychodramatic stage may be a section of the floor in front of the audience, it may be a raised circular or square platform, or it may be the Moreno-designed psychodramatic stage that consists of three concentric levels, each smaller than that below and each about eight inches above the other, over which is a balcony, which may be used for many purposes, including depicting scenes of heaven and hell in an individual's private world. Some psychodrama directors confine the action to the stage, while others, when they feel it is called for, will turn the entire psychodrama theater, audience area and all, into the psychodrama stage, bringing the action and interaction to whatever part of the facility they feel to be appropriate. The psychodrama situation is one that transcends the barriers of time and distance, as well as those of states of existence. In the latter situation an angry or frightened protagonist may be given the opportunity to kill his antago-nist or in other instances give life to the dead and give life to their fantasies; they thus have the opportunity to make myths come alive and to live the legends they may have dreamed of. All this and more may be found in the psychodramatic situation, with the only limits being those of the director's spontaneity, as well as the spontaneity factors of all others present. It is in the psychodramatic situation that the protagonist is invested with what Moreno call *surplus reality,* in which his experi-ences are augmented on the stage to greater-than-life size and in which a moment of his real-world time is enlarged (i.e., taken from its linear context and expanded horizontally) so that he might deal with it in many ways and in many degrees of intensity. The psychodramatic situation is a magical, timeless place in which reality is turned inside-out and in which all may occur.

Tele

Moreno uses the Greek prefix, *tele*, to designate the concept of "feeling-into distance," and he sees it as a two-way event or transaction in which those connected by telic bonds are able to get inside each other's skins and see and experience the world from their respective viewpoints. It is, stated Moreno in 1914, "a meeting of two: eye-to-eye, face-to-face. And when you are near I will tear your eyes out/and place them instead of mine/and you will tear my eyes out/and place them instead of yours,/then I will look at you with your eyes,/and you will look at me with mine." (Moreno,1964) A somewhat weaker equivalent of tele but much easier to deal with is *empathy*, a two-way type of empathy, in which an audience member might feel for and identify with a protagonist who in turn will be able to reciprocate with the audience sharing. Many persons have tried to explain tele in terms of the Freudian concept of *transference*, and Moreno has sought to correct this confusion by explaining (Moreno, 1964) that transference and *counter-transference* are merely unidirectional phenomena that represent negative tele in that the former represents a neurotic need of the patient, which Freudians see as a part of all successful therapeutic relationships, while the latter represents a neurotic need of the therapist, and where it occurs it must be dealt with by the therapist in his own personal therapy or in supervision or in the consultation he should seek from senior therapists. Moreno sees tele as a healthy event and sees transference and counter-transference as unhealthy; whereas, Freud sees transference as an important part of good psychotherapy and sees counter-transference as unhealthy.

Catharsis

Moreno uses the term catharsis in the Aristotelian manner in which the tragic actor on the Athenian stage through *hubris*, the character flaw of extreme pride that brings about the hero's great fall, evokes in the audience pity and fear and the sense of relief and cleansing when these and other strong emotions are purged, and the audience departs in a more peaceful frame of mind than on entering the theater. Such also occurs in psychodrama, but not only does the audience experience the catharsis that accompanies great drama, but so do the auxiliary egos, the director, and especially the protagonist, who in his psychodrama is not reciting lines written by another but who in most instances is living his life, or segments of it, much more intensively in the psychodramatic situation than in his everyday experience. By the very nature of what is involved in the interaction of spontaneity, situation, and tele, all good or well directed psychodramas must bring forth catharsis to some degree among those present; if catharsis has not occurred, what took place on stage and among the audience members was either inadequate or not psychodrama at all.

Insight

Although Moreno does not deal definitively with the concept of insight, it is implied throughout his writings as a phenomenon that may be expected in many good psychodramas, but not necessarily in all good ones. The concept dealt with here is that of *cognitive insight,* as formulated by the gestalt psychologists of the Berlin School, prior to and during World War I. In this concept insight is achieved through the restructuring of the perceptual field by the individual concerned. Excellent examples of the achievement of insight, as opposed to learning through random responses, are given in Wolfgang Kohler's famed work, *The Mentality of Apes* (1959), in which he reports experiments he conducted during the First World War. A typical experiment involved the placing of a basket of fruit outside a chimpanzee's cage, just beyond arm's reach. Insight was achieved in an average of seven minutes when the chimp made the connection between a stick he had played with earlier and its use as an extension of his or her arm. What had occurred was that the chimp had restructured his perceptual field, enlarging it to encompass both the stick and the fruit, which earlier he had seen separately and had seen as being independent of each other. Sometimes the insight that occurs in psychodrama is startling and spectacular, while at other times it does not seem to occur. Often it will spring forth unexpectedly the following day or during the days or weeks subsequent to the psychodrama, usually when the individual is thinking of something else. As psychodramatists are often heard to declare to protagonists and to audiences just prior to concluding the session. "The psychodrama doesn't end here, though we are ending the session, but it will continue in your head, and you may continue to gain from it."

REPORT: DIRECTOR IN HYPNOSIS

What is it like to direct hypnodramas while the director himself is in hypnosis? On the basis of my own experience, I would say that it is very much like directing psychodramas if one begins while in a light or medium state of hypnosis. In cases of this sort, I find that I simply and spontaneously come out of hypnosis during the course of the hypnodramas. When I am in deep hypnosis, as was the case in the hypnodramas mentioned previously, then the matter is somewhat different, and from the viewpoint of the director—and, I have been told, also from the viewpoint of the audience—the sessions can indeed be exciting. Although I had directed hypnodramas previous to the two mentioned, which occurred on the night of November 22, 1969, these were the first I had ever directed while under hypnosis myself. It may very well be that these two sessions marked something of a first, in that there are no known reports of this having been done by others prior to that time, and Dr. Moreno has told me that although he had directed many hypnodramas since inventing this approach, he never directed any while he himself was in the hypnotic state. (To many of Moreno's disciples, myself included, the idea of anyone being able to put Moreno into a hypnotic trance seems utterly inconceivable.) Therefore, I will try to describe something of what I was experiencing while directing the middle-aged psychology professor and the thirty-year-old psychiatric nurse in their hypnodramas.

I had been sitting slumped in the chair when Dr. Greenblatt, who had given the hypnotic induction, asked me to take over the group and proceed with the scheduled hypnodramas. I stood up quite easily, opening my eyes as I did so, and proceeded toward that part of the large room I had previously designated as the stage. Although I did not feel hypnotizied, I noticed that I was walking somewhat sluggishly, as the rear foot dragged each time I took a step forward with the other. However, this feeling lasted only a few seconds and then it seemed that I was walking no differently than usual, setting the stage, calling for a protagonist, and then getting the auxiliary egos involved. I felt very much in tune with what was occurring in this and in the subsequent hypnodrama, which at the time I felt was no different from what I usually experienced while directing psychodramas or doing hypnodramas without myself being under hypnosis. I remember having been very much involved with all that was happening on the stage, being on top of the situation throughout, and being little concerned with what was going on in the audience. In directing psychodrama, however, I usually try to be fully aware of the audience at all times.

At the conclusion of the second hypnodrama, I brought the first protagonist back on the stage and had the two protagonists, one on either side of me, sit on the chairs that were there and close their eyes. To repeat what I'd noted previously in this chapter, as I told them to sit down and close their eyes, I did the same, and as I did this, I seemed to chuckle to myself and silently say, "Oh, no, Greenberg, this is too much," meaning that this was much too theatrical. I seemed to grin sheepishly, as these words went through my head. Nevertheless, I continued addressing the two women protagonists and myself, suggesting that we were going back into hypnosis before being brought out of the trance by the man who earlier in the evening had done the induction. And as I was saying these things I was quite certain that I was not under hypnosis nor that I had been under hypnosis throughout most of the two-hour period. It was only when the hypnotist reminded the group of a suggestion he had given during the induction, which I had no recollection of, that I was convinced that I had been hypnotized the entire time; this reminder came while he was counting us into the alert waking state. It was not until quite a while after this experience, however, that I recalled something else which differentiated it from other psychodramas and hypnodramas I directed. In almost all until then, besides being much aware of the audience throughout the sessions, a common factor was that at least once and sometimes more often there would come a time when I would ask myself, "Well, where do we take it now?" or "What do I do next?" These questions seemed to arise in spite of my having had a fairly solid background in personality theory, in unconscious mechanisms that may relate to developmental problems, and in psychodramatic techniques, as well as having had a number of years of experience working as a clinical psychologist. The fact that these questions had often arisen in my mind while directing psychodramas, as they do to many highly skilled directors, some of whom have reported this to me, makes me accept the questions as a part of the process involved in the cognitive aspects of directing psychodramas. Nevertheless, as far as I can recall, the question of "Where do we go from here?" did not come up at all while I was in deep hypnosis directing the two hypnodramas.

CASE REPORTS: HYPNODRAMAS

Since the initial combining of hypnodrama with group hypnosis in 1969, I have directed numerous group-type hypnodramas, mostly at professional conventions and at experiential weekend or daylong workshops.[5] In almost all instances the vehicle of hypnodrama combined

[5]These include the Association for Humanistic Psychology, where in 1970 I began directing hypnodramas at each national convention and at subsequent regional conventions, and the annual conventions of the California State Psychological Association, the American Society of Group Psychotherapy and Psychodrama, and occasionally at conventions and gatherings of the Psychotherapy Division of the American Psychological Association, the Southern California Society of Clinical Hypnosis, and professional consultations for staffs of such hospitals as Napa State Hospital in Northern California, the Psychiatric Department of the San Bernardino County (Calif.) General Hospital, Forest Hospital in Des Plaines, Ill., and at growth centers and institutions in this country and abroad.

with group hypnosis quickly enabled protagonists and would-be protagonists to get in touch with problems that were appropriate for them to deal with at the time. The hypnodramas enabled them to effectively and in a fairly short time work through the problems and emerge with meaningful insights. Some of these hypnodramas have already been reported (Aaronson, 1975), and some half-dozen or so more will be recounted here.

The Reluctant Pianist[6]

Marjorie Turner, thirty-two-year-old psychiatric social worker who was excited about her work in a private mental hospital and in love with her husband, a clinical psychologist, was among the half-dozen individuals who stepped up to the stage of the large hotel ballroom that had been designated for the hypnodrama presentation. It was at an annual convention of psychologists and professional psychotherapists, and Marjorie was one of the some two dozen people who had gone into a deep medium or a deep state of hypnosis during the group induction. There were about eighty to one hundred persons present, and about half of them chose to experience the hypnotic state. Those on the stage had indicated during the hypnotic state that they had some personal problems that would be safe and appropriate for them to explore during the hypnodrama demonstration. They also had accepted the fact that because of the limitations of time only one would be chosen as a protagonist and that the remainder could expect to get whatever insights they were ready for in a dream or while going about their daily lives. Normally, a regular stage would not be desirable, since it is too high for there to be good contact or tele between audience and actors. In this case, however, the stage merely was a platform upon which the head tables at a banquet were set, and so it was suitably close to the audience to be used in a psychodrama or hypnodrama.

With the exception of those on the stage and some trained auxiliary egos, everyone had been brought out of hypnosis. The director turned to the people on the stage who were slumped in their chairs and asked them to let themselves go deeper into hypnosis, intending then to interview each of the persons and then select a protagonist for the hypnodrama. This was not to be, however, as the protagonist was self-selecting. The woman we were soon to learn was Marjorie suddenly burst into tears and cried out defiantly, "No, I will not practice the piano, I won't, I won't." As she let herself go into deeper hypnosis, she had spontaneously

[6]The names and some details in each case have been changed to maintain confidentiality.

regressed to the age of ten and had begun shouting to her mother some of the things that she, as the good little girl she had been brought up to be, had occasionally thought about but had never dared verbalize. As a little girl, Marjorie was discovered to have musical talents and her musician mother and minister father had wanted her to become a concert pianist. It seemed to this little girl that she was not loved for herself but was valued simply as the possible fulfillment of her mother's ambition and as the epitome of good behavior that one would expect of a minister's daughter.

Auxiliary egos were quickly brought to the stage to portray Marjorie's parents, and in the enactment that followed Marjorie poured forth in vehement denunciation much of the frustration, despair, and rage that she had experienced while growing up, but which she had never vented, either verbally or emotionally. Toward the end of the enactment she took advantage of the opportunity to punish her parents through verbal and physical actions, for having treated her as a pianist rather than a loved daughter, but when given the opportunity, she forgave them for not knowing how to be otherwise with her. At the conclusion of the session, following the audience sharing, Marjorie turned to the director and said, "You know, my husband's been wanting to buy me a piano for quite some time, but I've refused to consider it; now I think I'll let him buy it." About a year later, when the director was conducting a professional weekend workshop for staff members at Marjorie's hospital, Marjorie held an informal party for the group that Saturday night, and as soon as the director entered her home she intercepted him with a surprise. "There's something I must show you," she stated and led him by the hand to the music room, a beautifully planned and furnished room, with the focus of attention being the gaily decorated and obviously much used upright piano.

A Blow for Freedom

Thad Calhoun, a thirty-eight-year-old psychologist employed at a local counseling agency, had attended the monthly meeting of the Southern California Society of Clinical Hypnosis in Los Angeles because he had heard there was going to be a hypnodrama demonstration and was curious about this unusual modality. He was among some forty physicians, dentists, psychologists, and their guests, who had just finished dinner in a meeting room of the Los Angeles County Medical Society Building. He was also among the some two dozen who entered hypnosis, following the director's group-induction procedure. After taking part in the guided fantasy trip that the group had experienced, Thad was among the eight persons who indicated they wished to be protagonists in the hypnodrama, and his presenting problem was his sense of being intimidated by a female colleague at his agency. The director chose Thad as the protagonist because first his problem seemed appropriate for a hypnodrama (although it might also have been dealt with in a psychodrama), second it seemed simple enough to deal with in the confined space of the meeting room where the group had just dined and where the tables were not completely cleared, and third Thad appeared to be very much involved emotionally in what would become the situation in the hypnodrama. Other would-be protagonists were not selected because their problems could easily be dealt with in regular hypnotherapy or psychodrama sessions or because the problems involved concepts and there were not enough trained auxiliary egos present to deal with them or because one problem seemed too intense and could be too overwhelming for the protagonist to handle within the time and space limitations of that setting.

An auxiliary ego (Maurica Anderson, M.A., a humanistic counselor) was brought onstage to portray Thad's colleague, and from the tentative manner in which he was interacting with her, the director hypothesized the possibility of an overbearing parent and brought forth another auxiliary (Walt Anderson, Ph.D., political scientist and social psychologist), also under hypnosis, and the two interacted very force-fully after the "father" quite critically interrupted the conversation Thad was having with his colleague. In the exchanges and role reversals that followed, Thad got so involved in the interaction and so caught up in his heretofore repressed anger that while standing on the high chair he struck the father auxiliary very forcefully in the face. Anderson, who had come out of hypnosis by this time, accepted the blow and continued the action, sustaining the situation, without interruption. The scene ended with Thad in the role of an adult rather than in that of an angry little boy, and in this new role he spoke with assurance telling the father he could deal with his current life situation. He found his father no longer threatening to him, and without being aware of it he stood taller on the stage. The director then had him end the scene with his father, getting the father off the stage, and then the director returned Thad to the original scene at the counseling agency. Just as the world had suddenly become less threatening following the enactment with his father, so did his professional involvement with his colleague, and in-stead of finding her awesome, he perceived her to be an attractive single woman and felt enough self-assurance in the hypnodrama to ask her for a date. The auxiliary playing the woman psychologist was noncom-mittal in her response, but several weeks later Thad reported that he had dated his colleague several times and found her company most enjoyable.

The loss of control Thad exhibited when he struck the auxiliary playing his father—or rather, letting go and being then ready to give up control, which is often a part of the hypnotic condition—apparently was what was needed to help him break through the bottleneck of personality constriction and to free himself from the fears of the past. Actual physical attacks upon auxiliary egos are of course strongly discouraged in psychodrama or hypnodrama. Thick leather or naugahyde covered cushions are used as targets upon which a protagonist is encouraged to vent his anger, and protagonists are helped to reach the peaks of anger necessary to find expression in the spontaneous pounding of the pillow through the efforts of the director who sets up the pillow-hitting scene, through those of the auxiliaries who provoke his anger, and through the double or doubles who help him escalate and intensify his feelings to the point where the anger bursts through. This is a part of psychodrama or hypnodrama; it is sought where appropriate and effective when the feelings are real, rather than assumed (as some protagonists do) to follow the instructions of the director. However, in hypnodrama and psychodrama, the unexpected is a condition that also is a part of the modality, and since Walt Anderson was not seriously injured, although the blow obviously hurt, and since it was not struck with malicious intent, he carried on to Thad's great benefit. Had the session been stopped when the blow was struck, Thad probably would have been apologetic and might again have learned that being oneself, bursting free from tight emotional reins can be dangerous.

Missing Husband and Multiple Protagonists

In another situation, Walt Anderson, a highly skilled psychodrama director, carried on a *tour de force* in the role of the angry, frustrating, small-minded, game-playing, insincere, bullying, insensitive, cheap, inconsiderate, and inadequate husband to a dozen or so women participating as multiple protagonists in a hypnodrama conducted several months later in 1971 at a national convention in Washington, D.C. The hypnodrama began immediately following a guided fantasy and the psychodramatic crib-scene,[7] created by Doris Twitchell Allen, Ph.D., some dozen years before, and which involved about one hundred persons

---

[7]In the crib-scene, one person will play the loving mother and another the needy baby, and even without hypnosis the spontaneous regression that often occurs is impressive; when participants are in hypnosis, especially when large numbers of dyads are involved, the results are even more impressive and the rewards to the participants are multiplied many times because of the emotional contagion that occurs and is manifested by the sobbing going on in various parts of the room.

in varying states of hypnosis. As the director was interviewing various hypnotized persons as possible protagonists, a woman stood up and announced to all: "I have something to work on. When I went home this noon, I found all of my husband's things were gone. Without any warning, he suddenly took everything of his and left. I don't know what to think. He just disappeared, with no warning at all." A number of individuals gasped in shocked empathy at this disclosure, and, although this was something that might have easily been handled in a psychodrama, the director called the woman to the stage area, and commenced to direct her in a hypnodrama. Anderson, in the role of the husband, charged her with being unable to meet his needs, and the woman accused him in turn of being impossible to please, and on many occasions found, because of his constant complaints, he was not worth the effort to please. The hypnodrama gave her the much needed opportunity to vent her anger, not only because of her husband's sudden desertion but for many past problems that she had not confronted him about. As she was shouting at Anderson and hitting the pillow furiously, other women in the room shouted their encouragement, and as they did this the director called them up to the stage area, having them line up behind the protagonist and her double, Fred A. Moore, Ed.D., a counseling psychology educator, who was helping the protagonist express some of her feelings. When the protagonist had gone as far as she was able to at the time in attacking her husband, the director had her stand aside and then had each of the dozen women lined up behind her express some of the held-in hostility to their respective husbands. Anderson smoothly shifted roles for each protagonist, responding as needed and challenging and counter-accusing in turn, while they, assisted by Moore in the role of their double, grew more angry so that they were able to pour out long repressed or suppressed thoughts and feelings. The original protagonist was then brought back into her enactment so that she could get some closure by having her end the scene with her husband and by having her, while in a high state of spontaneity, make a general declaration concerning her future courses of action. As has been noted, the hypnodramas with the multiple protagonists might just as well have been psychodramas, but the would-be protagonist and other members of the group were in states of hypnosis and the would-be protagonist's need was desperate. So without delay the director helped her set the scene for hypnodramatic enactment.

The Washroom Lady and Multiple Protagonists

A year later, at the annual convention of the Association for Humanistic Psychology in Squaw Valley, California, Anderson had the opportunity for a repeat performance (see the chapters immediately following this). In brief, after a group hypnotic induction and guided fantasy experience that some eighty persons participated in, the director called for potential hypnodrama protagonists, and one young lady arose saying that in her fantasy she found herself in the high school lavatory, where the lady in charge sat and had little to say to the girls. The protagonist, Diane Zimberoff, a counselor, stated the woman looked very kind and that she often had felt a need to talk to her, but did not. An auxiliary ego, sociologist Mary K. Moore, M.A., was called to the stage, and in the interaction Diane complained about how hard and unfeeling her father was. Anderson, of course, was called to the stage to do one of the roles he does well—though it should be stated that he in actuality is a very kind and loving father to his son Dan and a kind and loving husband to Maurica. Again, the protagonist, with the aid of Fred Moore as her double, got quickly into her feelings, and other women in the group, also in a state of hypnosis, easily identified with her, and some half-dozen of them were called to the stage. Each then had her turn tearing into her parent for his many acts and omissions. This was one of the largest hypnodramas the director had been involved in, with at one point three different scenes or interactions taking place in different parts of the stage simultaneously. A more detailed description of this session is to be found in the chapters that follow.

The Unfinished Dissertation

Frank Rubin, a slight, kindly, balding, young man approaching his thirtieth birthday, revealed himself to be a concerned psychologist who was enthusiastic about his profession but had some misgivings about his future in it because for the previous five years, he carried the title, "ABD," which in the academic community means "All But Dissertation." He had completed all of his work for the Ph.D. degree and had completed almost all of his dissertation, but for some unknown reason he had for five years been unable to write the final chapter although he knew the material well. And this was the problem he sought to deal with during the hypnodrama presentation at the 1973 annual convention of the Association for Humanistic Psychology in Montreal. He got into an interaction with some important people in his life, including his parents, and dealt with some aspects of their need for him to succeed gloriously, as well as some aspects of the failure they had programmed into him as a little boy. After concluding the scene with these important others, he again declared that he knew what he wanted to say in his final chapter, knew how to say it, but just couldn't get around to doing it. Anderson, who this time was doubling for the protagonist—in the previous hypnodrama he had again protrayed a tough, unfeeling father—conferred with the director, and the director told him, "Go ahead, and do it."

The director then turned the session over to Anderson, who, standing behind the protagonist, placed his hands over the hypnotized protagonist's eyes and said, "I want you to see your dissertation as it is," and when the protagonist said that he did, Anderson said, "Now I want you to see the last chapter added to it." Again, the protagonist said he was able to see it. "Now," Anderson continued, "I want you to sit down and write that chapter," and the protagonist began making typing movements with his fingers. The director had earlier instructed the protagonist in time-contraction in hypnosis, and so time sped past much more rapidly for the protagonist than for everyone else, and in a comparatively short time, the protagonist broke into a big smile and announced with a sense of pride and relief that it was finished. The session was concluded shortly, with the protagonist being given the posthypnotic suggestion that he would get to work writing his final chapter shortly after arriving home and that he would complete it in an appropriately fast time. On coming out of hypnosis, the protagonist talked with assurance about finally finishing his dissertation, stating he knew just how he was going to do it and knew for certain that he could. He said he was enjoying the convention but could not wait to get home and be done with the dissertation.

Sonovabitch Suicide

Sally Winter, Ph.D., a blonde, thirty-year-old mother of two, is a clinical psychologist who signed up for the weekend workshop on self-hypnosis, group hypnosis, and hypnodrama specifically to learn something about hypnodrama; she wanted to use some of the techniques in her private practice. Saturday she had been in a group encounter experience with a dozen other workshop participants and had gone in and out of hypnosis several times to take part in such communal activities as doing artwork under hypnosis and getting feedback from others on her drawings, as well as reacting to the drawings of others, going on a guided fantasy trip while under hypnosis, and then taking part in the sharing of experiences and observing some additional clinical work as the leader taught the group self-hypnosis and provided those who wanted it with motivating suggestions to help them be better able to deal with problems involving eating, smoking, sleeping, and studying. However, interesting as these were, they were nothing new to Sally, having been a good hypnotic subject before attending the workshop, as well as having had some training in hypnotherapy and self-hypnosis. She enjoyed the experiences and the interacting with other members of the group, but her principal interest so far as the workshop went was to learn the techniques of hypnodrama and add them to her psychotherapeutic armamentarium. She decided that when the hypno-dramas were presented that Saturday night she would be one of the active participants, although she was not sure of what traumatic material she had to deal with that had been left over from her childhood.

Following the group hypnotic induction that evening, Sally, in a state of deep hypnosis, moved to the stage area of the large room in the New England mansion where the workshop was being conducted and sat quietly as other hypnotized potential protagonists arranged them-selves about her. Each individual was then asked what he or she would deal with if chosen to be a protagonist, and when it came Sally's turn she spat out, "That sonovabitch husband of mine, that selfish, no good sonovabitch." And she burst out crying. An auxiliary was selected, and Sally began interacting with her "husband," whom she presented as a very brilliant young internist who was inundated with feelings of inade-quacy and who suffered extreme feelings of depression. Besides bearing him two children, which he had not wanted, and taking care of the house, Sally also had been involved in her own career. Until she received her doctorate the year before, she had been a graduate student majoring in clinical and social psychology at a major university. She was also playing mother to her husband; getting him up in the morning, assuring him that he was fit to go to work, that he needed to go to work, that she would always be there for him, and that she did indeed love him and need him. All of this emerged during the first fifteen minutes of the enactment in which she explored her relationship with her husband from several perspectives, including those involving her own needs and the rewards she was getting from the relationship. Then without warning, she exploded. "You sonovabitch! You no-good sonovabitch fucking bastard, why did you do it. Why did you have to go ahead and kill yourself. Why did you have to desert me like this. You no-good, rotten bastard!" And she continued interacting with her husband, while the auxiliary ego playing the role quickly shifted viewpoints so as to pres-ent the husband as one who is dead but still involved with those he had left behind. The auxiliary of course was assisted in this by the director, who while directing also served at times as an auxiliary ego to the protagonist.

Sally dealt with her feelings about her husband's behavior while alive and then got in touch with some repressed feelings and thoughts involving the hurt and outrage she felt for his having deserted her through his suicide. Later, while explaining the meaning of her husband's death or his refusal to live for her children (portrayed by auxiliary egos chosen from among the workshop participants), she was able to reveal her anger in terms her children would understand. In trying to help them to understand the reasons behind the suicide—that neither they nor she was to blame but it was something their father had to do because of his own needs—she found to her surprise that she was not only able to forgive him for what he had done against her and others close to him, but to symbolically bury him and much of the pain that had been a part of her life. During her interaction with her children she found herself planning a new life for the three of them that included a change in location and in her professional direction. She then expressed an interest in an academic and research career as opposed to being a psychotherapist and talked about a university offer she had received a few weeks before but which she had not seriously considered. Following the audience sharing, Sally returned to her seat in the group, and, still under hypnosis, remained in a quiet state during the hypnodrama that followed hers. She said on coming out of hypnosis she had simply let her mind drift and let herself be open to whatever insights might be forthcoming during that period. The following day, at the conclusion of the workshop, she told the leader, "I came here simply to learn about hypnodrama, and I can't think of all that I'm leaving with."

Others

At one psychology convention the initial session concerned a middle-aged woman's choice between remaining in that city to care for her needy mother or pursuing an exciting career opportunity in California as a college counselor. During the enactment, she experienced a range of emotions which she might have done in a psychodrama except the hypnotic state made her more open to her basic feelings. She came to her decision: to remain where she was until she could arrange for her mother to be cared for but determined to accept the new position when the fall semester began. This was followed by a short hypnodrama dealing with a man's anger at his wife, who was not too interested in his career as such but only in the prestige it brought her. The presentation concluded with a very intense session in which a thirty-year-old school teacher reexperienced her having been raped and beaten by the sixteen-year-old son of the local plumber while at a summer resort. She gave full expression to the fear and fury she had contained within her since the attack occurred. At the conclusion of the session, the fear had left her and she had gained some insights into the fact that her casual open friendliness should be reserved for those who could appreciate it. She understood she had to be somewhat cautious in her behavior with those who might see it as an invitation, rather than the cheerful, generous friendliness that it was.

At a weekend workshop in self-hypnosis and hypnodrama, one obese woman interacted with her one hundred pounds of excess weight, portrayed by an auxiliary ego, and saw quickly how it had served as a protective wall behind which she could hide from the world. She then became involved with her ideal self, portrayed by another auxiliary ego, and after several verbal exchanges, and role reversals with both the excess weight and the ideal self, she found herself strong enough to push the excess weight from her life and see herself as closer to her ideal self than she could have imagined previously. On emerging from hypnosis, she told the group that she knew within herself that she could and would lose the excess weight in order to be the person she felt she was meant to be. She promised that within one year the director would see the results of the resolutions the hypnodramas had helped her formulate, but unfortunately, the director lost contact with her and so was unable to learn the outcome of the session. Interestingly enough, however, one of the audience members had become so moved by the enactment that she resolved to lose the fifteen pounds she had been wanting to lose for some time, and this she was able to do, as the director observed each time he met her at a professional gathering during the next two years.

At one of these gatherings, another young woman found while undergoing a guided fantasy in hypnosis as a warm-up to hypnodrama that she was being blocked in her many efforts and aspirations by the "black rage" that she had for years kept confined within herself. A husky male auxiliary in the role of the rage refused to leave her when she requested this during the hypnodrama, and when she sought to push the Rage from her, the auxiliary fought back and the two wrestled furiously until, at the director's instruction he permitted himself to be defeated. The woman arose, panting and exultant after her strenuous encounter and after having experienced a full catharsis that led to the sudden insight of what the Rage represented, a previously unexpressed reaction to the burdens of duty and the strictures of conformity that her parents had placed upon her.

Another expression of rage and fear emerged at a weekend workshop in which the hypnodrama protagonist age-regressed to the five-year-old boy he was in Berlin toward the close of World War II and living in abject terror during the seemingly unending daytime and nighttime raids by American and British bomber squadrons. He clung to the auxiliary portraying his mother and begged her to take him away from this, and at the peak of the experience his anger and hatred toward his mother burst forth for her not protecting him from this terror as a good mother should. The director then sought to get him to express whatever feelings he might have toward the American and British bomber crews and others who were the enemies of his country, but apparently those bombing him were too distant or too conceptually abstract for him to respond to; but his mother was close, and he could relate to her, so he could make her the enemy, which he did and then immediately repressed so that the memory that did come up at the time of his hypnodrama was not previously available to his conscious awareness.

And so it goes, the uncovering, the age-regression, the spontanteity engendered interactions, the catharsis, and the insight, that together with the establishment of telic bonds among all participants make up the dynamics of hypnodrama, the therapeutic modality that delves deeply into the unconscious to bring forth into the healthy brightness of awareness, acceptance, and understanding the hidden, the dirty and the dangerous, the forbidden and the frightening, the sick and the sorrowful. All could emerge in the hypnodramatic situation to be confronted, attacked, and vanquished.

CASE REPORTS: OTHER HYPNODRAMATISTS

Calvert Stein, M.D.

Dr. Calvert Stein, president of the American Society of Clinical Hypnosis for 1971-72 and a psychiatric colleague and close friend of Dr. Moreno, had employed hypnodrama on many occasions over the years in his private practice in Springfield, Massachusetts, as well as at professional gatherings throughout the country. As useful as he himself finds it, he does not feel it is for every therapist. "Effective psychotherapy, with or without hypnosis, is sufficiently psychodramatic for most therapists without the added responsibility of managing several patients in the somnambulistic trance state at the same time." (Stein, 1968, p. 174) Stein, who also for many years has been a consulting neuropsychiatrist at Westover Air Force Base and at Springfield Hospital in Massachusetts, often works closely with his wife, Lucille, a psychiatric social worker and a trained psychodramatist, and utilizes other auxiliary egos where necessary. He writes of hypnodrama as follows:

> Psychodrama that is done under hypnosis is fundamentally no different from acting out scenes with other characters without hypnosis. In practice, there is often much more spontaneity without hypnosis predirection than with it. Warm-up under hypnosis may be simpler, however, because a single word or

gesture, the suggestion of an odor or color, the sound of a name or a prearranged signal can bring on a series of successive responses. If the subject goes into a somnambulistic trance and relives his hallucinations via actual regression, his behavior may turn out to be unpredictable and must be supervised carefully. Amateurs frequently conclude that the patient has become hysterical but a slap on the face or a dash of cold water isn't always effective as a remedy. (Ibid, pp. 175-76)

This writer had the privilege of participating in a hypnodramatic session Stein presented before a gathering of some five hundred or more persons in Los Angeles in 1971. After giving a short lecture on hypnodrama, Stein invited a half-dozen volunteers to come up on the stage—a theatrical rather than a psychodramatic one. After a short exchange with each, he put us under hypnosis to get in touch with whatever we might be ready to deal with. One woman in our group told of a recent dream in which she was King of England and wondered about its meaning. He had her enact the dream, exploring what it meant for her to be the monarch of a great kingdom, and as she did this, a young woman in the audience, who had slipped into hypnosis during the induction of the volunteers, screamed out that she did not like what was happening, yelling, "What is that man doing under my bed!" Without the slightest loss of aplomb, Stein called her to the stage, where she entered the fantasy being enacted. Mrs. Stein, as a court lady, immediately interacted with the second protagonist, whom we will call Miss Stacey, when she got up on stage; she was upset with the king for being unfaithful to her. The first protagonist, whom we will call Mrs. Smith and who was the king, was no longer actively involved in the session but simply remained in the passive hypnotic state. Mrs. Stein thereupon assumed the king's role. During the enactment that followed, it came out that Miss Stacey's boyfriend had not kept a date with her. She was angry with him, jealous of the young woman she presumed he had dated, and she was unhappy at the break-up of the relationship. He, of course, was the man hiding under the bed. After venting her feelings, Stein asked her to remain quiet and await whatever insights she was ready for while he worked once more with the original protagonist. Mrs. Smith's session indicated that she had been frustrated at the lack of control she was exercising over her life, and the dream and subsequent hypnodrama indicated that she was ready to be in more command and that this was appropriate for her. Although the action was kept to a minimum, both protagonists seemed to get much from the verbal and emotional interchanges, as did we volunteers. We had remained passive and somewhat attentive sitting alongside (in facing rows of three or four persons) the protagonists, the auxiliary, and the director, and had remained in pleasant states of hypnosis. At the conclusion of the enactment Dr. Stein gave some positive, useful, and acceptable suggestions to those on the stage and then brought the group out of hypnosis.

George D. Warner, Ph.D.

Dr. George Douglas Warner, a clinical psychologist at the Brock Lane Psychiatric Center in Hagerstown, Maryland, and at the Maryland Psychodrama Institute, called for volunteers to participate in a hypnodrama during the annual convention of the American Society of Group Psychotherapy and Psychodrama in March 1975 in New York City, and again this writer was among the half-dozen who stepped forth. Prior to this, Warner had given a detailed explanation of hypnodrama and how he employed it at his institution. So when the volunteers came forth and were seated in the center of the room, surrounded by some forty or fifty persons, they had a fair idea of what to expect. First, he gave a brief general hypnotic induction and followed this by working with each volunteer individually to help him or her enter a deeper state. Second, he had the individuals conjure up a fantasy, and again he questioned each with the intention of helping make the scene or fantasy more vivid and meaningful. Then he gave the specific suggestion that they would get whatever insights they were ready for as a result of the experiences they had just undergone. He had by this time selected a young woman to be the protagonist, and so he brought the others out of hypnosis and then helped her deepen the trance.

He next had her list the people who were important in her life and designate various audience members to portray them. Warner thereupon had her place each person chosen in various parts of the stage area—one of whom she placed almost out of the room—in accordance with where they were in her life, both physically and psychologically. This done, she was told to interact with them as she saw fit. Her first move was toward her father, who she begged not to die, not only because she loved him but because almost every other member of her family would expect her to take over the responsibility of the family, a task she did not want. She interacted with each member in turn, expressing deep-felt thoughts and emotions and moving the family members to different parts of the stage, or ending their scene and getting them off stage. She had some intense interactions with her younger brother, and then she declared that she wanted to be free. When the director had various auxiliaries attempt to hold her down, she broke away and again declared that she had her own life to lead and her own needs to meet and could not be burdened any longer with the needs of others clinging to her. She eventually saw that what was most holding her back was her own need to be responsible for the others, and she found to her great joy that she was ready and willing to give this up, hoping that in the weeks ahead she would indeed be able to give it up.

Warner's hypnodrama, though more physically active than Stein's, still was not as active as hypnodramas reviewed earlier; nevertheless, both Stein's and Warner's sessions were highly productive and of obvious help to the protagonists. Therefore, whether there is little or much stage movement, exciting things can happen in hypnodramas, providing the directors create the suitable climate for the hypnodramas to be cultivated and then to be fruitful. The director always sets the stage for what happens in hypnodramas or in other action modalities.

SUMMARY AND CONCLUSION: FUTURE PROJECTION AND PRESENT CONDITION

This chapter covered the creation and development of hypnodrama by Moreno and Enneis and this writer's employment of hypnodrama with group hypnosis as a further development of the modality. The basic parts of psychodrama and hypnodrama, namely the warm-up, enactment, audience sharing, and postsession rapping, were described, as were such conceptual components as spontaneity, situation, tele, catharsis, and insight. These descriptions were followed by a description of what it was like for one director to work while under deep hypnosis. The choice of psychodrama over hypnodrama as the preferred vehicle in many instances, other than cases where age-regression and other hypnotic phenomena are called for, was discussed. A number of hypnodrama case reports were given, as were descriptions of the work of such other hypnodramatists as Calvert Stein, M.D., and George Douglas Warner, Ph.D. Where does this leave us in terms of the hypnodramatic tools we now have, in terms of how we might use them, and in terms of how Moreno, the great creator, the great giver, the great demander, might have us use them?

"A truly therapeutic procedure cannot have less an objective than the whole of mankind," Moreno declares in the opening sentence of his most renowned work, *Who Shall Survive?* (1953, p. 3). Even in 1975 this concept that Moreno first gave voice to some forty years ago* has the grandiose ring to it that tells us it is still ahead of its time. Only when such a challenging declaration is accepted matter-of-factly as a part of everyday life can we assume its time has arrived. However, with the

---

*This was in the first edition of the work, published in 1934.

sociometry of nations being what it is, namely a situation of several contending *star* nations, each with its cluster of satellite countries, and the few *isolate* nations, all involved to some degree with each other in terms of telic bonds and negative tele, and with individuals in their specific spheres living in similar sociometric turmoil, it seems hardly likely that mankind is ready for Moreno's grandiloquent objective. But our sages tell us the world had better come to its senses soon or it will be no more. Should the day come when goodwill and the generous gesture will replace the power plays of nations or the need for individual oneupmanship, then Moreno's time will have come and gone. For when the world is at peace and individuals are comfortable with each other, there is no longer a need for a therapeutic procedure. But since the need at present is as great as it ever was, perhaps one might surmise that Moreno's time has indeed arrived and that the only problem is that we, our nation, the world, may not be ready for it. And one of the ways of getting ready for it may be found in the growth that individuals and organizations can achieve through therapeutic procedures, with psychodrama, which through television can reach large audiences, and with hypnodrama, which through the group hypnosis approach can reach many individuals, as among the principal procedures. When Moreno's goal is reached there will be no need for such methodologies as organizational analysis,[8] for competition will have been replaced by cooperation and the power ploys will be replaced by all of the large and wealthy nations seeking to fulfill the needs of lesser nations, to the benefit of all. But that time is not yet at hand.

BIBLIOGRAPHY

1. AARONSON, BERNARD S. (Ed.) *Workshops of the Mind.* New York: Doubleday Anchor Books. 1976.

2. CHEEK, DAVID. B., and LECRON, LESLIE M. *Clinical Hypnotherapy.* New York: Grune & Stratton. 1968.

3. ENNEIS, JAMES M. "The Hypnodramatic Technique." *Group Psychotherapy*, III, 1, (1950), 11-54.

4. GIBBONS, DON *Beyond Hypnosis: Explorations in Hyperempiria.* South Orange, N.J.: Power Publishers, Inc. 1973.

5. GREENBERG, IRA A. "Audience in Action through Psychodrama." *Group Psychotherapy*, XVII, 2&3 (1964), 104-22.

6. _____ *Psychodrama and Audience Attitude Change.* Beverly Hills, Ca.: Behavioral Studies Press. 1968.

7. _____(Ed.) *Psychodrama: Theory and Therapy.* New York: Behavioral Publications. 1974.

[8]See chapter 23.

8. _____ "Psychodrama, Hypnosis, and Hypnodrama Workshops." Chapter in *Workshops of the Mind.* Edited by Bernard S. Aaronson. New York: Doubleday Anchor Books. 1976.

9. KELLY, GEORGE A. *The Psychology of Personal Constructs* (2 Vols.). New York: W.W. Norton & Company, Inc. 1955.

10. KOHLER, WOLFGANG. *The Mentality of Apes.* Translated from the 2d rev. ed. by Ella Winter. New York: Vintage Books. 1959.

11. KROJANKER, ROLF. "Training of the Unconscious by Hypnodramatic Re-enactment of Dreams." *Group Psychotherapy. XV,* 2 (1962), 134-43.

12. _____. "Some New Techniques in Psychodrama and Hypnodrama." *Separata de 'Archivos de Criminología, Neuro-Psyquiatría y Disciplinas Conexas.'* Julio-Stbre. de 1963, Vol. XI, 43. Editorial Casa de la Cultura Ecuatoriana. 411-32.

13. MORENO, J. L. *Das Stregreiftheater. (The Theater of Spontaneity.)* Potsdam: Kiepenheuer. 1923.

14. _____ *Who Shall Survive?* (first published in 1934.) Beacon, N.Y.: Beacon House, Inc. 1953.

15. _____ "Mental Catharsis and the Psychodrama." *Socimetry.* 3 (1940), 209-44.

16. _____ *Psychodrama, Vol. I.* (1946) Beacon, N.Y.: Beacon House, Inc. Revised, 1964.

17. _____ *Psychodrama, Vol. II.* Beacon, N.Y.: Beacon House, Inc. 1959.

18. _____ *Psychodrama, Vol. III.* Beacon, N.Y.: Beacon House, Inc. 1970.

19. _____ "Hypnodrama and Psychodrama." *Group Psychotherapy,* III, 1 (1950), 1-10.

20. (MURRAY, HENRY A., et al.) O.S.S. ASSESSMENT STAFF. *The Assessment of Men.* New York: Rinehart & Co., Inc. 1948.

21. NARUSE, GOSAKU. "Recent Development of Psychodrama and Hypnodrama in Japan." *Group Psychotherapy,* XII (1959), 258-62.

22. STEIN, CALVERT. *Practical Psychotherapeutic Techniques.* Springfield, Ill.: Charles C. Thomas, Publishers. 1968.

23. SUPPLE, LEONARD K. "Hypnodrama, a Synthesis of Hypnosis and Psychodrama: a Progress Report," *Group Psychotherapy,* XV, 1 (1962), 58-62.

24. VOGELER, EDWARD JEROME, JR., and GREENBERG, IRA A. "Psychodrama and Audience with Emphasis on Closed Circuit TV." *Group Psychotherapy,* XXI (1968), 4-11.

19
Hypnodrama at the
Humanistic Convention*

Leo Litwak

The road to Squaw Valley crosses the Sierra summit and passes the site where in the winter of 1846 the Donner Party cannibalized itself. Now one can travel the path of the Donners by an all-weather superhighway. There is every safeguard for the traveler. The mountains are domesticated. Lakes Tahoe and Donner are safely hemmed in by drive-ins, motels, gambling casinos, subdevelopments and pristine acreage owned by the rich.

The ski, introduced by early Norwegian settlers, has proved to be the instrument of civilization. It was the 1960 Winter Olympic Games which finally tamed Squaw Valley, still isolated and unsettled as late as 1930. As the official program for the 1960 games put it, "Before it became the site of these games the valley was remote from large populations. Thanks to the improved roads and increased transportation services, Squaw Valley is accessible to thousands of persons." So, a history which began in dire tragedy ends happily. Within a few minutes of the place where the dead were once cast into stew pots, there is ready access to gambling parlors and hamburger joints.

*Reprinted by permission of the author and his agent, James Brown Associates, Inc. Copyright© 1972 by Leo Litwak. First published as a much longer article entitled, "Rolfing, Akido, Hypnodramas, Psychokinesis and Other Things Beyond the Here and Now," in the *New York Times Magazine* (Dec. 17, 1972), Vol. 122, No. 41966.

The valley is a natural amphitheater, two and a quarter miles long, three-eighths of a mile wide. The surrounding ridges rise to 9,000-foot peaks. The ski facilities are at the far end of the valley. In summer, the improvements of civilization show up as wounds. The cables of unused ski lifts hang from the slopes like harpoon lines from beached whales. Squaw Creek, which divides the valley lengthwise, is bone dry and the ripped-up banks are visible. Ski trails cross the slopes like scars. Snow cures all that.

Yet fun and business don't wait for winter. Summer is convention time at Squaw Valley. The lodge facilities are in full use. Last June, hundreds of pom-pom girls arrived to attend pom-pom school. They were followed by Job's Daughters, a Masonic women's auxiliary. The facilities were then stretched to accommodate Dr. Armstrong's Radio Church of God, attended by 9,000 conventioners.

And finally, after the summer but before the arrival of the snows, the Association for Humanistic Psychology convened in Squaw Valley, far off the beaten academic track. It may have been an appropriate setting for an organization that many academic psychologists refuse to acknowledge as belonging in the ranks of reputable psychology. They might be willing to consign it to the domain of religion. They would certainly agree with the characterization of a recent magazine article which condemned humanistic psychology as an outgrowth of "squishy California thought." But for an increasing number of academics and nonacademics who have participated in its programs, the A.H.P. represents the wave of the future, boldly advancing the range of human potential.

More than 950 delegates registered for the 10th annual meeting of the Association. A $25 fee entitled them to a full sampling of a long and varied program called "Beyond Here and Now: Bridging Boundaries." There was no simple way of characterizing the delegates. There was a mix of young and old, of academic and nonacademic, of male and female. Dress, manner, physical bearing all had a decidedly California cast. The clothing was exuberant, the manner informal and straightfor-ward, the bearing athletic. Swimmers braved the pool in the chill morning hours and during the cold nights. The tennis courts were in constant use. Yoga practitioners meditated on the lawns. A few of the young unfurled sleeping bags near the Olympic Village dormitories, avoiding the room tab and making use of the dormitory plumbing. Families arrived by camper and set up in the parking lot. In the meetings, it was not unusual to observe a nursing mother calm a wailing infant during a crowded session. No one could have mistaken the Squaw Valley meeting of the humanistic psychologists for an academic conference.

A mere glance at the program was enough to distinguish the A.H.P. from the official academic organization, the American Psychological Association. The A.P.A. membership consists to a large extent of professional psychologists with college or university affiliation. In contrast, a substantial number of humanistic psychologists have no academic connections. Of those who do, many belong to departments other than psychology. Humanistic psychology was until recently practiced mainly off-campus at such "growth centers" as the Esalen Institute. It is a movement that, in the past, defined itself in terms of opposition to certain dominant tendencies of traditional psychology; in particular, Skinnerian behaviorism and Freudian psychoanalysis.

I noticed in the program a category of meetings concerned with transcendental states of being and altered consciousness. Evidence that life energy extends beyond physical boundaries is of considerable interest to those humanists who have taken a mystical direction and urge the notion of a transcendental mode of being. I chose first to attend a session in parapsychology, a report by Stanley Krippner of the Maimonides Medical Center in Brooklyn concerning Soviet research in telepathy, psychokinesis, acupuncture and "Kirlian photography."

The basic commitment of humanist psychology is to what is called the "experiential." As a spokesman of the movement expresses it, "The most significant part of education is the experience which involves the head, the gut, the whole man. The mind is not in the head. It is in the whole body." The detached, impersonal view is rejected and the notion of a totally objective science is criticized. A.H.P. officers feel that their organization has received a bad press from reporters who have failed to participate in the events they reported. Encounter groups of various kinds, employing such methods as psychodrama and fantasy trips, remain a crucial part of the program. As the association's executive officer, John Levy, said to me, "You can't understand any encounter from the outside."

The insistence upon active audience participation keeps the meetings from becoming dull. I attended a hypnodrama session at the Hofbrau, an A-frame, chalet-type building, with scripted placards advertising the menu hanging from the walls ("Hier gibts fondue"). The Hofbrau was jammed. We were to be hypnotized, and were then to participate in a hypnodrama. We encircled the fieldstone fireplace in the center of the large dining hall as Ira Greenberg of the Camarillo, Calif., State Hospital led the session. He described hypnosis as a "control of our controls." It was a technique, he said, that enabled us to concentrate deeply and regress to forgotten states; once these states were recalled, hypnodrama could be used to act them out, enabling us finally to gratify the unsatisfied nurture needs of infancy.

We removed our shoes and lay on the floor flat on our backs. We were instructed to relax. We began with the toes and very gradually worked up to the head. We were reassured that the process was pleasant. We were asked to imagine a yardstick within our minds. We slowly counted down the yardstick until we came to the number which we felt represented the depth of our hypnosis. We tried to sink beneath this number. There were a few snores. We were urged to stay awake. We then began a fantasy trip. We flew up the mountain that was behind the. Hofbrau; we were told to soar above the crest and enjoy the flight. We then settled down near the crest by a cave; entered inside and walked down a corridor passing several doors, stopping at that one which enclosed a place we had always wished to enter. We passed through this door, looked around, left the cave, descended to the Hofbrau and then awoke. We assembled in groups of five to discuss the experience. An elderly couple, a trifle disgruntled, denied that they were hypnotized and were skeptical that anyone else was. I myself felt quite relaxed and refreshed. A good many of those in the audience said they had been in deep trances.

A hypnodrama was then staged, based on a young woman's fantasy. When she had been asked to pass through the door to her special place, her fantasy was that she had entered her highschool lavatory; a woman attendant sat at the threshold and refused to acknowledge her; she felt deeply disturbed. Roles were assigned to volunteers. The young lady was returned to hypnosis. She again passed through the door and confronted the impassive woman attendant. She burst into tears, and begged for a demonstration of affection. The attendant rose to comfort her. At the moment of revelation I had to leave for an appointment with A.H.P. officers who were to brief me on the current state of humanistic psychology.

The president of the A.H.P., 43-year-old Lawrence Solomon, is a clinical psychologist and dean of students at the San Diego campus of the California School for Professional Psychology. The outgoing president, 46-year-old Fred Massarik, is a professor in the Graduate School of Management at U.C.L.A. Intense, articulate, academically rooted, they feel that the humanistic movement has gone too far in its opposition to traditional psychology. Massarik fears that "the overcommitment in the experiential direction has produced a growing tide of anti-intellectualism in our movement. There is too much of the attitude, 'All you gotta to do is feel.'

On the final night of the conference, everyone assembled in the Olympic Village cafeteria for a barbecue dinner, followed by a women's guerrilla-theater production. It was a parable about the education of a woman to subservience and her final liberation. It included song and dance and a comic retelling of the Snow White story. At one point a woman was raised on a cross made of a broom and a mop. Two women bongo drummers set up a persuasive beat. At the conclusion of the parable, the players brought the audience on stage. Soon the entire convention was involved. The cafeteria floor vibrated like a drum skin. This spontaneous demonstration was halted at its climax by a woman announcing the next event—a party, set for the lodge bar in 20 minutes. At the bar we were handed leaflets: "Welcome, people-lovers. You are invited to participate in SERIOUS SCIENTIFIC RESEARCH BY HAVING FUN at this rare experiential event: a humanistically oriented party for Making Friends With All The Sexes!!" There followed a detailed prescription for encountering members of the various sexes. The high mood was quickly deflated and, as often happens, the spontaneity that was calculated didn't materialize.

It was clear that this had been no mere association meeting. The delegates were members of a coherent organization with shared values and common attitudes. There wasn't the politicking that goes on at academic conventions. There surely was no sense of rank requiring its proper deference. Unlike those at academic conventions, the meetings were jammed. The insistence on an "experiential" format was a guarantee against dullness. Many programs obviously disregarded the obligations of a rigorous science; but, in consequence, they weren't confined to trivial precision. The Association for Humanistic Psychology is a movement. Its objectives are messianic; its language spiritual. The actions it sponsors are often pure fun.

20
Addenda 1:
A Protagonist's Report

Diane Zimberoff

Out of the many workshops offered at 11:00 A.M. at the Humanistic convention, I decided to attend the one on hypnodrama, mainly because I knew it would be experiential rather than some lengthy lecture. Of course I never expected to participate; I mainly thought it would be exciting to watch.

The room was filled with many more people than most of the other workshops and my first impulse was to leave. But then I decided to stay since nothing else sounded interesting to me. I certainly am glad I stayed since it turned out to be one of the "highlights of my therepeutic experiences."

I was feeling in a very good place, not in touch with any "heavy spaces" and certainly not feeling as if I would participate as a protagonist in a hypnodrama. Dr. Greenberg said he would like everyone who wished to experience hypnosis to follow his directions. "Well," I thought, "I do want to experience as much as I can today, but just for fun." I followed his directions and wasn't certain that it had worked or not—I was aware of feeling very relaxed. One of the directions was to see a door and then to open it up and see what was there. Well, I did this and it turned out to be the door of the girls' bathroom in my high school. I saw this lady in there who I referred to as the "toilet lady." Then I thought to myself what a strange place to go to. I didn't like it at all, so I decided to try it again, hopefully finding something more sufficient behind the door. I started the experiment again and saw the door and opened it and it was the same place. "O.K., I guess there is something here that I am needing to deal with." Pretty soon I started feeling a whole range of emotions which I had not previously been in touch with. He asked for volunteers to be in a hypnodrama, and I found myself raising my hand. At this point I wanted to get at what was happening, and if this was the way to do it, I was willing to try. I only knew I wasn't wanting to leave that room without dealing with what was emerging from within me.

At this point I definitely felt hypnotized. It seemed as though I had been transposed into a different state of consciousness.

I was now sixteen years old and feeling that adolescent pain that I had tried to push away for so long. So there I was again in the girls' bathroom of my high school talking to the lady who was there faithfully every day (no one ever knew exactly what she was supposed to do—we just called her the "toilet lady"). Well, it seems as though she had some significance to me although I had previously only been subliminally aware of her importance. So there I was, crying and screaming at her, wanting attention, love, concern, caring, emotions, reactions etc., but all she did was sit there day after day watching the toilets. Well, you guessed it, all of sudden she changed into my mother. That was obviously where my real pain was coming from, and then I began to deal with that with the aid of alter egos (doubles) and other people playing members of my family.

The whole experience was quite incredible to me and was extremely intense. I was also surprised that the hypnosis seemed to totally transplant me back to that period of time in my life. It was pure feeling, reacting, and experiencing. There did not seem to be any head-trips or mind-games at all. I found it to be an extremely important experience for me and it opened up places in me which had previously been untouched.

21
Addenda 2:
An Overview of the Enactment

Ira A. Greenberg

It was unfortunate that Leo Litwak had to leave the hypnodrama session at Squaw Valley when he did because what he thought was the high point of the session was simply a warm-up to one of the biggest hypnodramas I have had the good fortune to take part in. It also was one of the least taxing or demanding, so far as my directorial skills were concerned, though good things were happening throughout the session and in many parts of the stage. It was less demanding because so many professionals were involved in the hypnodramas as auxiliary egos, and therefore, I had people I could count on to handle their roles well so that I could concentrate on working with the protagonist or protagonists.

When Diane Zimberoff burst into tears as she vainly sought to get a response from the lavatory attendant, Mary Moore (in the role of the attendant) arose not so much to comfort her as to challenge her, demanding to know what it was Diane wanted from her. As Diane herself reported (in Addenda 1), the attendant suddenly became her mother, and Mary Moore thereupon assumed the role of an unyielding, ungiving mother. Walt Anderson then was brought on stage to portray Diane's father, so that she could experience her feelings in this part of her life, and she immediately denounced her father for being cold and unfeeling toward her, for wanting her to get good grades and achieve in other areas, rather than simply loving her for herself. She accused him of being, as she perceived it, concerned more with his own strivings and goals than with her tender needs and concerns.

Anderson of course responded in a strong, direct, and critical manner, pointing out that Diane was not being logical in her demands, that she was acting like a child, and that she herself had a number of shortcomings and was something of a disappointment to him. Just as Diane was wilting under Anderson's counterattack, Fred Moore, as her double, interjected himself and told the father very forcefully to "just cut out the bullshit," and to begin dealing with the real matter at hand, the lack of a meaningful relationship, as Diane saw it then, between him and his daughter. Diane immediatele straightened up and returned to the attack, and a number of young women—and a few not so young— stood up in sudden, strong, telic identification with Diane and vented their own anger at this "unfeeling father."

These some eight to ten women were quickly called to the stage, first to join Fred Moore in serving as Diane's doubles and then, each in turn, getting the chance to be the protagonist for intense periods measured in many seconds or in a few minutes, and turned on Anderson, who in the role of the tough, rational, unresponsive but demanding father, hurled their accusations back at them as he found fault with each, the way he perceived the father of the specific protagonist might. While this was going on, Mary Moore turned into a comforting mother to several of the women who had already vented their anger toward their respective fathers, and Irv Katz was called to the stage to portray a kind and loving father to one or two of the women who had already interacted with the cold, authoritative father, as presented by Anderson.

The actions and interactions on the stage were carried out with varying degrees of intensity, according to the needs of the particular protagonist and according to whom she was involved with at a particular time and in a particular place on the stage. I also found myself totally involved and moving about the stage from one scene or enactment to another. At one point I might be directing an angry encounter between Anderson and one or more of the multiple protagonists, all of whom were given strong support by Fred Moore, and then I would move to another part of the stage to direct an interaction between Mary Moore and one of the "daughters," and later I might be at the opposite end of the stage where Katz was comforting another of the "daughters." And as I moved from one interactional scene to another, I found myself being quite comfortable about it all, knowing that as I left one scene the professional psychodramatists would continue it. I also knew that I did not have to push myself to be at any one place to fill in for an inarticulate auxiliary, as often happens when one works with inexperienced people.

After all the protagonists had said or shouted what needed to be expressed, I called Diane back to center stage and had her conclude the scene with her parents in any way that seemed appropriate for her at that time. She sighed heavily, stated she had needed to get "it" out of her system, and then hugged her parents fiercely, telling them how much she loved and appreciated them but also chuckling as she observed while still hugging them that there had been times they too had been "a disappointment" to her.

All of the protagonists, the auxiliary egos, and others who were still under hypnosis were then brought back to the alert, waking state. The audience members and auxiliaries were then asked to share feelings and events from their lives with the various protagonists. About half the group then left to go to lunch, but the rest of us remained for the postsession rapping, which I have always found to be a rewarding way to wind up—or wind down—an intensive psychodramatic or hypnodramatic experience.

I felt then and later that it was a good session for all of us who participated in it, whether actively on the stage or passively as an audience member. It was a fairly intense session, although by no means the most intense one the other psychodramatists or I had directed or taken part in. However, it was most certainly the largest and busiest, so far as simultaneous action on the stage was concerned, that I have had the pleasure of directing or being involved in, and it was to me one of the most enjoyable and rewarding experiences.

22
Hypnodrama and Symbolization*

Rolf Krojanker

The work of Hanscarl Leuner clearly bears the marks of cross fertilization between psychodrama, Jung, and the psychosynthetic movement. It guides the patient through various highly meaningful symbolic situations for diagnostic and therapeutic purposes. Since many individuals have undergone these standardized situations, the psychodramatist can benefit from comparisons with other protocols, when he invites his patients to visualize and enact such situations, and when he later on modifies the patient's productions as described in the "training of the subconscious by hypnodrama."

The therapist asks his patient to relax, using either a light trance state by suggestion or has the patient induce such a state himself through his knowledge of autogenic training, and then the therapist suggests that the patient visualize himself in each of the situations given below. In psychodrama we often work with a simple suggestion to close one's eyes, relax, and visualize certain situations. Indeed, the psychodrama stage and its atmosphere seem to exert a fascination, even hypnotic effect on patients with their eyes wide open once they have been "warmed up"

*Reprinted with permission of the author. From, "Some New Techniques in Psichodrama and Hypnodrama," in Separata de *"Archivos de Criminología, Neuro-Psiquiatría y Disciplinas Conexas,"* Julio-Stbre. de 1963, Vol. XI, No. 43, pp. 411-432, Editorial Casa de la Cultura Ecuatoriana, Quito, 1963.

by the experienced therapist. I doubt therefore that the psychodramatist will have a difficult time in transposing the initiated symbol projection test into his medium. But now let us take a look at the test.

It consists of these situations: 1) a meadow, with the patient in it; 2) climbing a mountain; 3) following the course of a stream; 4) visiting a house; 5) the ideal personality; 6) affective relationships symbolized by animals; 7) unconscious attitude toward sexuality; 8) pool of water in a swamp; 9) waiting for a figure to emerge from a cave; 10) eruption of a volcano; and 11) the lion.

It is beyond the scope of this paper to discuss the I.S.P. test in detail. The point being made is, that ever since Desoille used directed dreams in treatment, it has been very beneficial to many patients to experience these symbolic situations and find their way through them. However, I propose to my audience to bring these symbolic situations alive through psychodrama, or rather hypnodrama. For instance, in the scene waiting for a figure to emerge from the cave, I obtain the patient's description of whom he expects to see, and then have a role reversal, in which he would be that suddenly appearing figure; a double helps him express his real feeling in the often aggressive situation. One of my overly passive patients, however, saw a "sick bear" emerging from the cave, who just stared at him for a while and then sauntered back into the cave. I certainly wished then that I would have had a double at my disposal to let at least the bear become more aggressive: This cave-figure situation also furnishes a nice spontaneity test on a symbolic level, in which the auxiliary ego emerging from a cave has a firm set of behavior and only the protagonist patient varies in accordance with his character patterns. If one reduces the I.S.P. to about eight cardinal situations with fixed spontaneity-test like stimuli, one has an easy means of projective testing of a patient group at the beginning and during the course of psychodramatic treatment. One important point being made by Leuner is that the above-mentioned symbolic situations increase their therapeutic effect by insisting on the patient's repeated confrontation with the basic problems presented through them. Analysis is not necessary, treatment ends usually with the successful confrontation through the phylogenetic scale ending in the important human or archaic figure emerging from a swamp, at first worms or fishes might emerge; they next give way to birds, to mammals, and finally to primitive and not any more primitive human figures. In accordance with the fixated effect to such a situation, anxiety, panic, hostility may be manifested to this figure. A very interesting warning to the therapist is issued by Leuner, namely to not allow the scene to end on a hostile note, such as killing the beast, which might speed a sick person into a panic or psychotic episode; rather the patient must be moved towards friendly behavior with it. Similar findings appeared in J.L. Moreno's and also in our experience with suicidal patients in psychodrama; the suicidal enactment must find a positive closure or correction so as not to result in a tragedy later on in real life!

In my instance given above, that is, the patient and the sick bear, the reason for such a warning becomes quite clear. The patient himself was the sick, passive, and ugly "monster", and killing the "bear" could have unchained self-destructive impulses. Only during the course of psychodramatic shock therapy might one dare to allow this symbolic way of overcoming the "bad me", following it up, however, by having the "good me" emerging alive and victorious.

The symbolic situation with a figure coming up from a swamp incorporates the important findings about movements upward and downward in space made by Desoille. They represent repressed stimuli of the sexual sphere as well as development on the phylogenetic scale. In turn, the figure emerging at the same level from the cave facilitates the emergence of other mythological figures, probably more symbolic of interpersonal relations. It seems only logical to proceed from these considerations towards representing the upward, downward, and on the level dimensions in space, such as J.L. Moreno has done in psychodrama. Our new psychodrama stage at St. Louis State Hospital is especially suited for such psychodramatic situations, since it is built like an amphitheatre, with stages at different levels.

I shall still describe in some detail a few of the symbolic situations of the I.S.P. which are well suited for representation on stage.

No. 7 The walk: The test especially for female subjects consists of visualization of themselves walking home along a road at dusk after an exhausting walk through the countryside. Then an automobile is to be seen coming along on the road behind them, stopping upon reaching them and the driver asks if they want a lift home. The sex and appearance of the driver, color and size of the automobile have "demonstrated diagnostic significance regarding the sexual development of most feminine subjects." Especially significant are signs of resistance, such as when a subject can visualize the road, but no car appears, or the car disappears into the air as she enters it. We have used a similar situation at the State Hospital with Leon Fine, as a spontaneity test. However, I feel that this situation can be equally well employed on stage with a male patient, and only after he has visualized the car and the sex of the driver, be offered by auxiliary egos on stage according to the patient's description. On the other hand, the sex of the driver might be deliberately changed to test the homosexual leanings or conflicts.

No. 11 The lion: This projective situation consists of having a lion confront any one of the persons our patients may have difficulty with in real life. The lion may overcome the patient's adversaries or submit to them or run away from them, in accordance with the patient's visualization, giving us an idea on how well the patients can express themselves and their hostile feelings. In hypnodrama, this attitude may then be corrected in a somewhat deeper trance, and the patient can be trained to achieve symbolic victories over his adversaries without any ensuing guilt feelings.

Next to the above proposed dramatization of some of the I.S.P. test situations it could be mentioned that some of our standard and routine psychological tests offer a similar opportunity for exploitation through psychodrama, e.g., some of the T.A.T. responses, Rorschach responses, make-a-picture-story test responses. Aside from enriching the results of these tests and making this effort work for the patient in therapy as well as for the diagnostic interviewer, such a technique would give a valuable point of departure for future research and standardizing of the stimuli presented to the patient. By that I mean that it would give us further understanding if healthy people would for instance always overcome the "giant" of the global response of Rorschach card IV, whereas sociopaths would kill it without much compassion, etc.

Another situation used in psychosynthesis for visualization of affective states is:

The technique of the door: In it, the patient visualizes a door in a high wall or home, with a label on it reading in accordance with the therapist's suggestions, an affective state, such as "anxiety", "depression", "love", "hate", or "hope". The patient is to open the door and report what he meets on the other side.

This technique reminds me somewhat of the psychodramatic technique of the "auxiliary chair or chairs", in which the patient is to act on each chair with a different part of his present or idealized personality. The DOOR technique can be easily transposed and refined on stage, and the patient may be made to choose between different doors and labels, e.g., in such an event, this leads to a similarity with the modified "magic shop" techniques of Hannah Weiner. The DOOR technique can also be made to serve future projection, for instance with the labels "death", or "old age" on it, or serve for value analysis in axiodrama, with labels "heaven", or "hell" on the doors, or "success". Instead of the doors, one might use trains or busses with different "destinations" on them.

The technique of the heart: The patient may be asked to enter through a door into an oversized heart, describing what she finds inside. It is probably safer to have the patient first visualize the heart and some of the symbols she encounters on its inside, before trying to provide the stage and cast for the re-enactment. Naturally, one would not like to use this technique, let us say, with a medical student who knows anatomy, but with people in whom one expects conflicts around love and in whom the symbolism of the heart as the seat of love and/or other emotions is maintained. Instead of the heart, one might choose the symbol of the moon (before our rockets land there), an unknown world, etc., in accordance with the situation.

The technique of the inner dialogue: I would rather like to rename this technique, as the dialogue with the ARCHETYPES: In it the patient visualizes a personified symbol, such as the wise old man, or wise old woman, the sorcerer, etc. It has been surprising to me to observe how subjects usually animate or populate their "magic shops" with archetypes. We are usually not so aware of this fact, because when this happens, we feel that the subjects only appeal to a potential therapist wanting to "buy his goods". However the case may be, the patient is then encouraged to ask this wise person for guidance in fundamental questions, for instance, goals in his life, its meaning, satisfaction of their longings.

Let me explain here that the term "archetype" has been coined by C.G. Jung, who has explained its meaning fully. C.G. Jung's influence is quite marked in the thinking and clinical work of meditative psychotherapy. For psychodramatists in the U.S.A., it is mainly important to remember these types: The wise old man, the wise old woman, the shadow, the animus and anima. The first two of these terms might be understood for us pragmatically as the "wise old counsellors" in our society, such as Bernard Baruch, still giving advice to our Presidents; Winston Churchill still being a magic symbol in England. The shadow in each person is the devil in us, the negative side of us personified, such as the "ideal ego" might be our most noble aspirations personified. The animus personifies the idealized male strivings in every female, the anima the idealized female strivings in every male subject. More precise information is available in Jung's writings. For the psychodramatist it is only important to master these ideas for his clinical work with patients, if he intends to work on the symbolic level. The Psychodrama director can then dramatize situations on stage, in which archetypes appear and influence the protagonist, or affect him in one way or another. Let me take the example of a soliloquy in psychodrama, which consists, as we know, in having the patient be alone on the stage, at most accompanied by one or more doubles. The psychodrama director can then instruct one double to act as the patient's shadow, and the other one as the patient's anima or female component, if the patient is of the male sex; the patient will then interact with his two doubles in a set form. He might next use the technique of the inner dialogue as mentioned above, and have the patient face an unknown old man, asking him to act as a referee in the patient's "inner" conflict with his doubles. At this moment the director may want to effect a role reversal between the patient and the "old man", so that the patient will have to give advice to himself.

At the present time, Leuner has proposed five therapeutic principles for treatment on a symbol basis, which he classifies as "Symboldrama." Leuner worked out these principles based on clinical experience, and feels they are open to modification. Nevertheless they seem to fit therapeutic interventions in Psychodrama and Hypnodrama, which we have applied for years without looking for a common denominator, wanting to avoid a rigid technique or a therapeutic conserve. We shall give them here some detailed consideration because of their relevance to psychodrama. We should know in advance that Leuner is in dynamic struggle, namely the pole representing the neurotic-regressive principle versus the pole representing the therapeutic-progressive principle.

The therapist will influence this dynamic conflict following five principles or techniques: 1) The principle of destruction and reduction 2) The principle of nutrition and enrichment 3) The principle of reconciliation and tender embraces 4) The principle of conjunction and incorporation 5) The principle of magic medicines and liquids.

1) The principle of destruction and reduction: This principle has sometimes failed to overcome conflicts with the father and mother figures or their archetypical representation. On the other hand, it is usually successful in handling acute conflicts at the time of therapy. Leuner gives as an example a minor employe who had often been bypassed by his foreman in the matter of promotions. After a specially humiliating instance of this kind he consulted the therapist with symptoms of acute anxiety, tension and some depression. In the course of symbolic visualization the patient had to meet his foreman at the edge of the forest, and he appeared with his typical disdainful demeanor. The therapist summoned a lion to the spot, and the patient had him promptly devour the foreman, leaving only the bones of the foreman's feet and ankles. Therapeutic experience requires to destroy these remnants to avoid a reincarnation of a more threatening and powerful symbol from them. The therapist therefore asked the patient to visualize a stove filled with glowing coals, and throw the bones in there, after which these remnants were then actually destroyed, too. The entire session took about twenty minutes. The patient walked out relieved of his anxiety state and passed a pleasant weekend with his family.

Let me remind the readers here with regard to Leuner's use of the lion in the above example, that in the Initiated Symbol Projection Test, Leuner uses the lion as a symbol of the patient's aggressivity or hostility. As so many other people, this patient identified his own hostility with the aggressivity of the lion, in this case used to destroy his foreman. Again, as so many other people would do in a similar situation, the lion is sufficiently removed from the patient to allow the patient not to experience guilt feelings about the foreman's death.

Another result of this symbolic destruction is sometimes what Leuner calls a "synchronous change." This consists in the patient's visualization of a friendlier environment in which he finds the satisfaction of his wishes. This change in scenery is spontaneously produced by the patient after a successful symbolic destruction.

An example of a symbolic reduction is Leuner's patient with psychosomatic complaints of an incurable disease following a recent car accident. During visualization, a skeleton bursts out of a tree against which her car was crashing. This symbol of death threatened the patient, who energetically stimulated by the therapist pursued it endlessly through the plains. It was not allowed to hide in a cornfield. Later it was found under a couch in the patient's apartment as a symbolic demonstration of resistance. Again the therapist urged the patient to chase it until it finally broke down at a river bank and the river carried its bones away. The patient improved decisively after this dramatic session.

Commentary: In Psychodrama we use this principle often by means of role reversals with the threatening figure, or by reducing it in relative size, letting a patient, for instance, talk back to his father from an elevation on stage or standing on a chair or the balcony.

2) The principle of nutrition and enrichment is demonstrated by Leuner with two case histories in one of which earth opened itself like during an earthquake, and the patient was encouraged to "overfeed" mother earth by pushing her sister gently into the abyss. A dramatic reduction of symbolic threat was the consequence followed by better relationships with mother. In the other case, a failing student with a father complex had to visualize meeting his teacher, talk to him, then feed him and dine him at a picnic. He then received a home task consisting in further symbolic feedings during visualization of additional picnics, and was able to face this teacher in a following examination at school with poise and efficiency.

Let me here familiarize the reader with Jung's symbolic interpretation of the EARTH as the breast mother, to whom so many primitive people sacrifice yearly to reap rich harvests, and into which we return our dead ("Thou wast born from dust, and into dust shallst thou return"). When the earth in Leuner's case opened its hungry mouth like a "devouring mother," a therapeutic intervention of protecting the patient or attacking the mother might have been chosen by some therapists. Leuner chose the opposite tack of sacrificing to the mother, appeasing her, and by this act achieved the result of clinical improvement of the patient-mother relationship. May I remind our astonished readers, that our Bible discusses human sacrifice and its effects at least twice, namely, with Abraham and with Isaac, and with Jonah and the fisherman, respectively the whale. Also in these examples, the intended sacrifices appeased God, the results were rewarding, and the humans concerned were relieved from inner conflict.

Commentary: In psychodrama, we often use this technique similar to symbolic realization by actually feeding psychotic patients with a milk bottle.

3) The principle of reconciliation and tender embrace is followed by letting the patient pet the feared or hated animal or human figure, as described with earlier examples in this paper. This technique is especially useful in ambivalent attitudes, practically urging the patient to synthesize his conflicting ambivalent urges in a positive manner.

Leuner gives an example of a patient riding on an elephant through a dense forest in his visualization, finding great obstacles in his journey, and being threatened by snakes. The therapist urged the patient to first feed the snakes, then try to pet the biggest one. The patient agreed to caress the snake only after a lot of hesitation, but finally they became friends, and he put the snake around his neck. At this moment the snake changed spontaneously into a native girl "of divine beauty", and they both were able to continue the journey much faster, while all the wild beasts of the forest helped them during the trip. Leuner saw in the snakes a symbol of negative impulses within the patient, with which he urged him to reconciliate himself with favorable clinical results.

Commentary: We use also this technique in psychodrama, when we let patients reconcile themselves with their parents, whom they had so far only pictured as hateful and despicable. In psychodramatic action, the surprising sudden display of positive feelings by the co-protagonist (parent figure, e.g.) elicits emotional abreaction in the patients.

As an example, in one of our psychodrama groups a male patient seemed to be quite comfortable in picturing his father as a hostile dominating person, whom the patient despised. When we suddenly instructed the auxiliary ego representing the father to become tender and loving to the patient, our patient broke down in tears and admitted to having longed for such a relationship with his parent. The result was also here clinical improvement.

4) The principle of conjunction and incorporation is closely related to the principle of nutrition and enrichment, equally to Jung's demand of individuation stemming from the synthesis of opposite tendencies,

and to the mechanism of introjection of Freud and Ferenczi. Leuner demostrates this principle in a compulsive male patient, who often visualizes a young beautiful girl. In this instance she eats spontaneously the bones of the deceased mother of the patient, becomes pregnant through this act and gives birth to a baby boy who grows up fast to an attractive youngster.

The same patient experiences in visualization a change from his present size to an infant, who soon enters mother's uterus through an abdominal opening, which closes around him. He feels mother's pressing intestines and heartbeat, then pressures all around him, and finally is reborn through mother's vagina.

Commentary: In Psychodrama the very combination of protagonist and his doubles into one single person may be interpreted by this principle of conjunction. We often have the patient either assume his Mother's role in a role reversal, or have Mother's voice talk to him during a soliloquy, coming out of himself, as it were the voice of the incorporated parent. Only here I feel psychodrama to be distinctly in an advantageous position, since it manages to achieve all those effects in a much more elegant and less "phantastic" or symbolic way, a way which patients might accept easier than the florid symbols mentioned.

5) The principle of magic potions and liquids is demonstrated by Leuner in a patient who visualizes "an archetypal woman squirting from her full breasts a milk stream upon earth. On the so fertilized spots a boy is born and grows up into a youngster."

Leuner reports of the magic symbolic qualities of Mother milk in visualizations. Indeed, even so convinced psychoanalysts as S. Margolin use milk in their "analytic regression" with psychosomatic patients with equal effects but based on different theories.

Leuner scores another important point in mentioning his experience that many male patients picture negatively loaded mother figures, the "devouring mothers." They also can easily visualize young buxom females in a stereotyped fashion, which led Leuner to suspect in these latter figures the representation of Jung's "anima" in opposition to the "devouring mothers." The situation would about equal that of a dominating mother and her energetic daughter-in-law fighting for the patient in a real life situation.

Leuner uses these symbolic opponents when needed in directing a visualization, and lets the young women fight the dominating mother figures with streams of milk expressed from their breasts. He has found this milk to be a potent weapon.

Commentary: This is a use of symbol which has found application in Psychodrama only with psychotic patients to my knowledge, which by means of symbolic realization were allowed to suck milk at St.

Louis State Hospital. It is obvious that psychodrama itself does not find it easy to apply these symbolic situations in the waking state. On the other hand, this principle finds an open field of application in hypnodrama, dealing with dreams and the training of the subconscious.

DISCUSSION

In comparing the trend of many here cited authors with my views as expressed in former papers, I find that while therapists may want to analyze the patient's symbols and his manipulations of these symbols, such an analysis is not a prerequisite for skillful therapy. I insist, however, that a thorough knowledge of psychodynamics and keen understanding of the patient are necessary to help one's charges in psychosynthesis, basic knowledge of all schools is desirable since it gives the therapist the necessary flexibility in his views.

In lieu of psychoanalytic interpretation during symbolic work in psychodrama and hypnodrama, I propose training the subconscious of one's patients to overcome symbolic conflicts and fears by the successful solution of such conflicts on stage or during trance rehearsal. The therapist introduces the necessary correctives as outlined in this paper to guide the patient towards a successful ending of the session, a solution of the conflicts within the symbolic context of it. While I consider work with interpersonal problems in the patient's daily life very important, I believe this should be supplemented by work with intrapersonal problems of the patient as outlined here or, e.g., on psychoanalytic lines to achieve lasting success. Insight and interpretation on a conscious level are useful, but are not a prerequisite for improvement, since the corrective experience may be acquired also through symbolic channels with subconscious training, or at least subconscious involvement. The training of the subconscious contributes toward increased confidence, in successful role performance, and consequently toward increased spontaneity in the patient's life. It is also available to a group of patients who are ill-suited for insight therapies and who otherwise would have to rely exclusively on supportive therapies.

SUMMARY

This paper contains a description of some new techniques used by the author in psychodrama and group psychotherapy, as well as a report on some techniques used by various European and North American psychotherapists which belong to the school of psychosynthesis. Since this is not a firmly defined group, it is here presented as the "movement of psychosynthesis." The author proposes that many of their noteworthy techniques of individual psychotherapy, such as those used in "guided dreams," "waking dreams," "symboldrama," etc., may be enhanced therapeutically by providing them with psychodramatic action and skills. Some of these techniques have already been tested out successfully with psychodrama groups.

Specifically speaking, the following techniques are presented: 1) The use of minutes recorded by the patients, to enhance the active cooperation of the patient in the healing process, train his capacity for critical self-evaluation and evaluation of others in group situations. 2) The written-up dreams, serving the same purpose, but also elevate subconscious production to the rank of a communicable contribution and a means of communication within a group. 3) The initiated Symbol Projection test of Hanscarl Leuner as a means to test the psychodrama group and its members diagnostically, dynamically and provide a vehicle for symbolic correctives. 4) A summary suggestion of a similar nature is offered for the use of T.A.T. and Rorschach, as well as Make-A-Picture-Story-Test. 5) The "door" and the "heart" techniques, both as described by Assagioli & Gerard, to further the patient's skills with symbolic material, are explained as applicable in psychodrama, and some added suggestions, such as a technique of a "train" with symbolic destinations on it, are added. 6) The technique of the "inner dialogue," as refined by various authors based mainly on Jung's findings, is also proposed for use in psychodrama. 7) Finally, a paper of Leuner on "Symboldrama" is summarized in detail and its possible contributions to the theory and techniques of psychodrama are evaluated. His principles of destruction and reduction, of nutrition and enrichment, of conjunction and incorporation, of magic medicines and liquids, are explained. His use of symbolic opponents, and of archetypes in the service of the therapist, is laid open as a tool for the psychodrama director.

In the foregoing discussion the author restates his thoughts about the effectiveness of symbolic correction of conflicts in the light of the recent contributions elaborated on in this paper and calls for more inclusive goals in psychotherapy beyond the traditional acquisition of "insight."

REFERENCES

DESOILLE, ROBERT. Le Reve Eveillé en Psychotherapie, Essai sur la fonction de regulation de L'inconscient collectif, Paris P.U.F. 1945.

——— Psychoanalyse et Reve Eveillé Dirigé; Paris Chez le François, 1950.

HAPPICH, CARL. Das Bildbewusstsein als Ansatzstelle Psychischer Behandlung, Zbl. Psychother, 1932, 5, 663-77.

GERARD, R. Symbolic Visualization, A Method of Psychosynthesis, Psychosynthesis Research Foundation, Greenville, Del.

FREUD, S. The Interpretation of Dreams, Basic Books.

JUNG, C.G. Collected Works, Bollingen Series XX Pantheon Books, N.Y., 1953-61.

KROJANKER, ROLF. Training of the Unconscious by Hypnodramatic Re-enactment of Dreams, Group Psychotherapy, Vol. XV, No 2, 1962, Beacon House, Inc.

———— Narcoanalysis by I.V. Drip Surytal Sodium (Span.) Archivos de Neuropsiquiatría 1955, Quito, Ecuador, Casa Cultura Ecuatoriana.

———— El hipnodrama al servicio del entrenamiento de procesos subconscientes, Archivos de Neuropsiquiatría Vol. IX, No 36, Oct. 1961.

KRETSCHMER, W. Meditative Techniques in Psychotherapy, Psychosynthesis, R.F. Desoille, Del.

LEUNER, HANSCARL. Symbolkonfrontation, ein nicht-interpretierendes. Vorgehen in der Psychotherapie, Schweiz. Arch. Neurol. & Psychiat., 1955, 76, 23-49.

———— Symboldrama, ein aktives, nicht-analysierendes Vorgehen in der Psychotherapie, Z. Psychother. Und med. Psychol. 1957, 7, 221-38.

MORENO, J.L. Interpersonal Therapy and the Psychopathology of Interpersonal Relations, 1937, Beacon House, N.Y.

———— Psychodrama of a Dream in Psychodrama, Vol. II, Beacon House, 1958.

———— & ENNEIS, JAMES. Hypnodrama & Psychodrama, Beacon House, Beacon, N.Y., 1948.

SCHULTZ, J. H. Das autogene Training 9th ed. Stuttgart Thieme, 1932-56.

SWARTLEY, W. Initiated Symbol Projection, Psychosynthesis Research Foundation, Greenville, Del., 1958.

23
Hypnodramatics for Organizational Analysis

Ira A. Greenberg

Just as group hypnosis may be employed for creative problem solving (see Chapter 9), so may hypnodramatic techniques be used by management or command groups to learn more about the other side. Hypnodrama, the modality in which a person acts out a problem under hypnosis and uses others in the group to play involved people, includes the techniques of role playing and role training among others (see Chapter 18). These facilitate one's personal exploration and the techniques are also useful in obtaining knowledge of others and information on their thinking. For, in the achievement of special objectives, good planning is essential, and decisions that are made in the planning must be based on all available information in order to be sound. Factual information on the activities of the "other side" is obtained through many channels, which need not be of concern here. What is of possible interest is the way in which these facts may be interpreted so that the results can be appropriately incorporated in the planning for a particular operation or for an investment strategy, or for an advertising campaign or for other such endeavors.

A well-known approach to understanding or guessing what a competitor may be thinking or planning is through learning as much as possible about the individuals concerned and on the basis of this information adding a subjective dimension to the planning. This is what is involved in the Order of Battle that most military commanders seek to establish before planning to engage the enemy. An Order of Battle is nothing more than a military command's intelligence—devised table of organization of the other side, often in book form, with all available information on the personalities, histories, known strengths and weaknesses of each individual holding important line or staff positions. The information is then added to that of troop strength and deployment and used in the decision-making process of military leaders prior to a specific battle. This all boils down to seeking to know as much about the opponent as possible.

The knowledge of the other side's key individuals has in recent years been incorporated in role-playing situations in *kriegspiel* or war-game-type settings as a means of getting into the thinking of or establishing some sort of pseudo-*telic bonds* (a psychodramatic term) with members of the opposition, and this has proved useful in gaining insights into the possible thinking and planning of one's antagonists. It is contended here that the role-playing approach can be carried a step further through the use of hypnodramatic techniques, and some attempts already have been made to test this assumption. The idea explored was not so much to get into the thinking of one's opponents as to get into their very beings, and as much as possible for the role players who are to be in states of deep hypnosis to actually *be* or rather to experience themselves as *being* the people they are trying to understand better. This was done on three occasions in short demonstrations at professional gatherings that dealt with the matter somewhat simplistically.

GENERAL MOTORS BOARD

The first attempt was made on March 8, 1975, at the annual convention of the California State Psychological Association in Anaheim during a ninety-minute presentation entitled "Group Hypnosis and Hypnodrama for Personal Growth and Organizational Development."[1] The demonstration included a group hypnotic induction, plus a guided fantasy experience for personal growth for some fifty people who chose to go into hypnosis as a prelude to the hypnodramatic-type experience. After the group members had come out of hypnosis and had discussed the guided fantasy and personal growth experiences among themselves and then shared with the group as a whole, the presenter

---

[1] The idea of employing hypnodramatics for organizational analysis came to the author in early 1975, after the programs for the three conventions had been submitted; those who attended the programs were told of the change in orientation and given the opportunity to leave early, should they wish, so as to be able to attend some other convention presentation.

described what he hoped to explore in the organizational analysis approach to organizational development. At his request, eight persons who had been in at least medium states of hypnosis volunteered to participate in the exercise, and he explained to them and the others the situation they were to become involved in. Since those who had volunteered were presumed to have merely a minimum of role-playing training—and time did not permit determining how adequate they were before beginning the exercise—the presenter set up what he considered a fairly simple simulation type situation from among the number of possibilities he mentioned. These possibilities included exploring such organizations as a City Council, a Board of Education, the FBI, CIA, KGB, PLO, one's own organization (professional or where employed), a competing organization, or an organization the group could create. These were offered as possibilities, but the presenter explained that he chose General Motors as the organization to explore because most people could be expected to know something about it and to have a grasp of some of the problems it might be having at the time.

The presenter explained that the eight-member group would, while in hypnosis, be members of the Board of Directors of General Motors Corporation and would be holding a board meeting during which they would discuss their corporation's current operations and future goals in terms of such problems as the recession, the energy shortage, and competition from the Ford Motor Company. He then made up a simplified board for the purpose of the exercise and had the volunteers select their roles. These roles were board chairman (and president) and seven vice presidents in charge of finance, marketing, engineering, the Chevrolet Division, the Cadillac Division, defense production, and a conglomeration of the corporation's other divisions. The group then went back into hypnosis, and the presenter again explained the situation, stipulating that the GM board would deal with the future of the Cadillac cars and then stepped back as the meeting of the board got under way. The discussion was somewhat desultory at first, both because of the hypnotic state the participants were in and because this was a new experience for them. So the presenter periodically interjected remarks to spur the board members to deal more quickly (because of the limited time) with some of the problems they could be expected to be concerned with. Toward the end of the remaining time, before the room had to be vacated for the next scheduled presentation, the board members became more committed to the matter at hand, and they came up with several interesting proposals, among which was that the standard-size Cadillac would continue to be produced, but the division also would produce a miniature car that could fit into the trunk of the larger car so that short trips could be made from the larger car at a savings in gasoline. The obvious impracticality of such an idea should not blind one to the role involvement and the creativity that brought it forth and to the possibility that more sound ideas might be generated through this approach at other times and in other situations. However, it should be noted, the purpose here is not creative problem solving, although this may be a by-product of the process, but to attempt to get into the thinking and feeling of key members of this "other organization," which in the first presentation happened to be General Motors.

DEATH PENALTY ADVOCATES

One such opportunity at another time and in another situation occurred two weeks later on March 21 in a presentation entitled "Hypnodrama and Problem Solving" at the annual convention of the American Society of Group Psychotherapy and Psychodrama in New York City. The same initial procedure for the ninety-minute presentation was gone through as at the earlier convention, but with the previous experience gained by the presenter and with the presumption of greater role-playing training by those at the latter event, the presenter gave the participants greater latitude in selecting the organization for analysis. He again named some possibilities and then asked for suggestions from the group. The response from most of the one hundred people present was enthusiastic, although a number of people who had come to witness the excitement of classical or group hypnodrama left soon after the program was outlined. But from among the some seventy people who remained came suggestions of such organizations to be explored as the Board of Education, the top echelon of the Department of Public Welfare, and the top administration of a mental hospital, which organizations reflected the places of employment of a large number of those present. Other groups representing authority which were suggested for exploration included a mayor and city council, a state governor and his staff, and a police department administration. All were suitable organizations for exploration, so far as the needs involved in developing the process were concerned, but the presenter felt the issues concerned were somewhat muddled, at least from his viewpoint, and he was not able to find a point of focus. At last a black graduate student from Pittsburgh, a man in his early twenties, suggested, "What about a group of people who are strongly for the death penalty?" And this the presenter immediately took to.

The presenter thereupon selected ten men and women who had been in at least the medium state of hypnosis and asked them to select their roles. The man who had suggested the subject took the role of a "hanging judge," while another young black man took that of a police officer whose partner had just been killed in the line of duty. The remaining men and women chose such roles as an ambitious prosecutor, a fundamentalist minister, a conservative legislator, the brother of a guard killed in the Attica, N. Y., prison riot, the widow of a man slain in a robbery, a military leader who had seen "good men" killed in Vietnam combat, an archconservative community leader, and a police chief concerned with increased crime in the streets. The group members quickly went back into medium or deep states of hypnosis, and the presenter named the "Hanging Judge" to be chairman of a meeting of those seeking to bring back the death penalty for murder and other serious offenses. The participants formed a semicircle facing the audience, with the chairman at the apex and immediately and enthusiastically got into their roles and into the situation.

They talked about the sad state of affairs throughout the country, the deplorable conditions of danger in urban areas, the terrible leniency of the courts, the need for bigger and tougher prisons, the shame of known murderers stalking the streets, the frustration of the police, who solve crimes and made arrests and see the criminals freed by lawyers' plea-bargaining. They talked of many other things that people in their positions might be expected to be concerned about. Then at the suggestion of the presenter, they got down to the business at hand and came up with the proposals that would advance the cause of the death-penalty advocates. Many of the proposals were considered good, as judged by the presenter, and an equal number were impractical or otherwise unsuitable. However, it should be acknowledged that many of these proposals might have come forth in an ordinary brainstorming or role-playing situation where hypnosis was not an included factor. On the other hand, it is felt that the hypnosis intensified the experience for the participants, enabling them to feel and to be their roles much more effectively than might have been the case otherwise.

As all the participants were presumed to be strongly against the death penalty—on the basis of remarks they made prior to returning to the hypnotic state—their involvement in this form of role-situation experience[2] may be considered to have been much more real for them and

---

[2]Role-Situation Experiencing (R-S E) was created in 1970 by Ira A. Greenberg and is based on the contributions of J.L. Moreno, M.D., and specific works of Henry A. Murray, M.D., Ph.D. (1948) and George Kelly, Ph.D. (1955). In R-S E individuals assume new identities and adopt cover stories, which others seek to break as they interact in new roles and new situations as a means of spontaneity training and to learn more about themselves.

may have facilitated their proposing much more meaningful solutions to the problem than might have occurred if hypnosis had not been employed. One proposal that the presenter thought brilliant in regard to the problem and the way it emerged from the spontaneous interaction was put forth by a young woman who earlier had indicated she was strongly opposed to the death penalty. This called for an advertising campaign showing large photographs of physically ugly men convicted of murder, under which would be such gloating captions as this one: "They sentenced me to life just for killing some jerk, but you and I know I'll be back on the streets again soon—through good behavior, parole, and my lawyer's stringpulling. I'll be seeing you." Actually, the proposal is merely clever, but it was initially seen as brilliant because of the spontaneity of its creation and the total involvement of its creator. Nevertheless, these ideas and insights could be very useful if the group had actually been working to actively oppose those seeking to bring back the death penalty.

PENTAGON WAR ROOM

An equally successful employment of this organizational analysis procedure took place on May 25, 1975, at the Association for Humanistic Psychology's annual Western Regional Conference, held near Santa Barbara, California. In a ninety-minute session entitled, "Hypnodrama and Group Hypnosis for Creative Problem-Solving," the presenter first specified that he had changed the presentation in order to demonstrate and further explore a new procedure and then explained the purpose and the process of this approach in the manner described earlier. As on the two previous occasions, participants suggested a number of organizations and institutions they were familiar with, including those involving the top administrations of educational, social service, mental health, and police organizations, as well as various governing bodies of elected officials. The presenter kept calling for additional ideas, seeking the types of groups or organizations that might be expected to stir strong or deep feelings among the participants. They finally agreed that the three groups most worthy then of study by means of hypnodramatic techniques were the Central Intelligence Agency, the War Room of the Pentagon, and the oil interest decision makers. A plurality among the some one hundred persons attending the session chose for exploration and analysis the War Room of the Pentagon, but with the stipulation that the CIA be well represented there.

Nine persons who had been in medium to deep states of hypnosis volunteered to take part in the exercise, and the roles they chose to assume were as follows: Chairman of the Joint Chiefs of Staff, Air Force Chief of Staff, Chief of Naval Operations, commander of military forces in the Far East, a representative from the General Accounting Office, the CIA member of the War Room staff, the head of the CIA "Dirty Tricks" Department, the counterinsurgency commander, "who teaches foreign police torture methods," and President Nixon's personal and political representative. The presenter then had the nine arrange their chairs in a small oval (because of limited space) before the larger group that would be the audience, and then led them back into hypnosis, telling them that when they next opened their eyes they would be in medium or deep states of hypnosis and would be attending a very important meeting in the Pentagon War Room.

This they proceeded to do, with the Chairman of the Joint Chiefs of Staff, a woman, chairing the session, but at appropriate times deferring to the president's representative; he in turn insisted he was there simply as a passive observer, but throughout the proceedings he interjected in a mock-serious manner remarks reflecting his perception of how President Nixon's man would view the various matters at hand, together with whatever political implications they might have. After a short period of discussion involving the Mayaguez incident, as seen by the War Room members, the presenter told the group that because of the world energy crisis and this country's need to undercut the foreign oil producers' cartel, the mission of the War Room meeting was to plan the invasion of Indonesia to take over that country's rich oil fields, but the planners must also make the action as acceptable as possible to the American people and to the world at large.

The group quickly got caught up in the task, with the CIA War Room member, himself a former security officer turned humanist, becoming the dominant person, and with President Nixon's representative,[3] in his mock-passive role, becoming the second most active person. However, all participants were fully involved in what was being planned, and from these sincere and committed idealistic humanists— most if not all of whom were strongly opposed to what the War Room represented—came suggestions for assassinations, cover-ups, heavy aerial and naval bombardments and sabotage of the peaceful Far East nation, as well as the employment of diplomatic strong-arm tactics and the gearing up of propaganda efforts to make the invasion and takeover as palatable as possible to those initially against the action. The exercise went well during the half-hour of the life of the Pentagon War Room,[4]

---

[3]Although all were aware that Gerald Ford was president during the War Room meeting, the group seemed more comfortable with Richard Nixon as its *bete noire.*

[4]Much of the time was employed in arranging chairs, in explaining the process, as opposed to classical hypnodrama, in having to move to another room and again arranging chairs, and in the initial hypnotic induction.

and despite the lack of sophistication of many of the participants in military matters or in diplomatic power-play concepts, the enthusiasm shown for this form of hypnodramatic simulation and the commitment of the group members to dealing effectively with the mission at hand seems to validate the inherent effectiveness of this approach to the exploration and study of one group by that of a rival group.

For if one group of people completely opposed to what another group stands for can, with little training and on very short notice in a crowded convention room with numerous interruptions, quickly get into the spirit of the task, it seems logical to assume that under conditions more conducive to the utilization of hypnodramatics for organizational analysis, much more in the way of productive activities might be undertaken and with greater payoffs for those setting up the situation. For example, if under ideal conditions, the project were to explore the actions of the Pentagon War Room and seek to analyze the thinking of its personnel or get a subjective understanding of it, the approach would contain a number of factors missing from the exercise described. These would include more time to prepare the participants so that they would know both the mechanics of their respective roles (i.e., what would be the functions of the Chief of Naval Operations in planning an international undertaking and what kind of special knowledge of basic navy procedures and lore would a man of his rank have or what kind of information would any or all of the War Room members be expected to have at their fingertips), as well as some of the feelings and attitudes they might be expected to have. A more suitable hypnodramatic staging area with enough time available to deal with the task fully and effectively also would help, as would having specific purposes for wanting to better understand the organization and so have specific areas for exploration. The results of the exercise at the AHP conference were satisfactory, so far as the study of this technique is concerned, but it must be remembered that what was experienced at the three professional gatherings was no more than mere prelinimary efforts in an attempt to determine the feasibility of such an endeavor.

Conclusion

Obviously, more exercises involving the use of hypnodramatic techniques for organizational analysis must be undertaken before an adequate evaluation of this methodology can be made; nevertheless, the potential seems interesting. This approach could be more appropriately studied if it were employed in a setting where participants would be selected on the basis of specific skills they would bring to the project. These skills would include 1) ability to go into deep hypnosis easily, 2) training and experience in psychodrama, 3) detailed knowledge of the individual each person would portray, and 4) specific other knowledge or abilities that might be called for to add depth to particular roles. There would of course be adequate time to prepare for each organizational analysis enactment, as well as sufficient time to critique the enactment and to repeat it or do new enactments involving the same characters, should such be required. An approach to the employment of this procedure might be that of the Behavioral Studies Institute's group hypnosis for creative problem solving, in which an organization's key people involved in a particular problem, plus selected BSI personnel, work at the problem while under hypnosis, with one of the organization's principal people monitoring what occurs (see chapter 9). One difference would be: that in organizational analysis it would be better if the enactments were conducted before a group of observers responsible for proposing specific courses of action or for direct decision making, and whatever insights emerged from the enactments would be added to facts and concepts already at hand. At the present time, however, hypnodramatics for organizational analysis is merely a concept being studied—and enacted—with its worth still to be determined.

REFERENCES

1. GREENBERG, IRA A. *Psychodrama and Audience Attitude Change.* Beverly Hills, Ca.: Behavioral Studies Press. 1968.

2. _____ (Ed.) *Psychodrama: Theory and Therapy.* New York: Behavioral Publications. 1974.

3. _____ "Psychodrama, Hypnosis, and Hypnodrama Workshops." Chapter in *Workshops of the Mind,* edited by Bernard S. Aaronson. New York: Doubleday Anchor Press, 1975.

4. KELLY, GEORGE A. *The Psychology of Personal Constructs.* (2 Vols.) New York: W.W. Norton & Company, Inc. 1955.

5. MORENO, J.L. *Who Shall Survive?* (first published in 1934.) Beacon, N.Y.: Beacon House, Inc. 1953.

6. _____ *Psychodrama, Vols. I, II, III.* Beacon, N.Y.: Beacon House, Inc. 1946 & 1964, 1959, and 1970, respectively.

7. _____ (Ed.) *Sociometry and the Science of Man.* Beacon, N.Y.: Beacon House, Inc. 1956.

8. _____, *et al.* (Eds.) *The Sociometry Reader.* Glencoe, Ill.: The Free Press of Glencoe. 1960.

9. MURRAY, HENRY A., et al. O.S.S. ASSESSMENT STAFF. *The Assessment of Men.* New York: Rinehart & Co., Inc. 1948.

24
Imaginary Hypnodrama

Ira A. Greenberg

Imaginary hypnodramas are what this writer terms the fantasy technique in individual hypnotherapy during which the patient or client, while in the light to deep state of hypnosis, visualizes himself in a particular scene or actually experiences himself in the scene and in this imaginary hypnodramatic situation interacts with the people he either cognitively places there or whom he simply finds there. This can be accomplished either in a stipulated period of time in which the therapist utilizes time-distortion to facilitate the process or in an open period of time, in which the patient indicates when he has completed the task decided upon. The task might be to return to the period when the patient was falsely accused of cheating and to direct his anger to the teacher or vice-principal who had accused him or it might be to set up a scene on the job and to try various ways of dealing with the fellow employee who has been giving him trouble. The patient is informed that he can role-reverse whenever he needs to during the imaginary hypnodrama and to utilize these opportunities to get whatever insights he is ready for. At the conclusion of the imaginary enactment, the patient and therapist discuss what has occurred. Another way of doing this is to have the patient place himself in a particular situation while under hypnosis, the situation being selected by the patient or the therapist, and to interact aloud with the people in this situation; in this type of enactment, the therapist becomes an active director in the hypnodrama and will call for verbal exchanges with specific important others in the patient's life, often playing the roles himself, and he will call for role reversals, scene changes, the escalation of anger and the hitting of a cushion, just as in an actual hypnodrama or psychodrama. The imaginary hypnodramas are usually of short duration, but the catharsis that invariably occurs and the insight that often occurs support the feasibility of this approach. A couple of recent enactments will be described briefly, and a few others listed.

THE KID WHO WAS PICKED ON

Martin Bradford, a forty-year-old mechanical engineer who was in therapy because of insomnia and depression, was slow in learning to become a good hypnotic subject. But he had quickly learned the Cheek-LeCron ideomotor response technique (1968), and so we were able to pinpoint areas in his past that he was ready to deal with. In a light state of hypnosis, he returned to the period when he was in the sixth grade and was being picked on by some of the boys in his class. Although this was not a complete age-regression, he was able to name the boys who in this particular scene were picking on him, and he demanded to know why they were doing this. Through a simple role-reversal in which Martin became the chief tormentor, he told the therapist, in the role of Martin, "Because you're such a dumb, snotty kid; you're always sticking your nose in where it's not wanted; you just stink." Reversing roles, Martin, as himself, replied to this accusation with the anger and frustration of a youngster unable to cope. When told to tell the other kids why he acted the way he did, Martin told them how lonely he was, how unhappy he was at home, how he wanted to make friends but did not know how to and so did what he could to gain attention. On coming out of hypnosis, he remarked, "Well, *that's* something to think about."

THE ODIOUS ONE IN HER LIFE

Katherine Henderson, a shy, attractive, and very bright twenty-year-old file clerk who has never had a boyfriend, was in therapy because of a chronic stomach upset that would manifest itself during times she might have dinner with an eligible man, so she simply did not date. A very conscientious person who enjoyed her work, liked her place of employment, and got along well with her coworkers, Katherine had difficulties with her superiors. She liked and admired the two partners heading the small firm, and they in turn liked her, but she could not relate to them, felt very inadequate in their presence, and often could not think of anything to say when either talked to her, especially the more senior partner. But her main problem at work was her immediate superior, a

married man a few years older than Katherine who teased her occasionally and made sexual advances toward her and toward the other young
woman she worked with. On occasion she would fly into a murderous
rage that often caused her to think of suicide when he angered her with
his teasing or pass-making, whereas the other young women would
reject his advances with a casual joke or flippant remark and would
think nothing more of the matter.

Katherine had been a happy and outgoing child until the age of ten
when she went to live with her newly remarried father and found herself
in the Cinderella situation, where her stepmother mistreated her to the
advantage of her own children. Two years later, the chronic stomach
upset made its first appearance. During her fifth therapy session, the
hypnotherapist suggested that she return to the period between her tenth
and sixteenth year when she was an unwanted resident in her father's
new household, the intent being to help Katherine explore some of her
feelings toward her stepmother, the obvious cause of her problems.
Katherine quickly and easily went into a medium-deep state of hypnosis
with the idea being to get at one of the major causes of her problems.
Soon she began getting angry, muttering to herself, and then in a small
voice shouting in quiet desperation, "I told you to stay away, keep away
from me, stay out of my business, just leave me alone!" The therapist
thought she was involved with her stepmother, and replied, "No, I won't
leave you alone, I don't like you." "Well, I don't like you either, Larry,"
she shouted back. "You're selfish, and you tell lies about me, and you
just want me to get in trouble with her. You're no brother of mine." The
therapist quickly switched into the hated brother who was four years her
senior and whose name had not been mentioned in previous sessions
although she had included it on the background information form she
had filled out on entering therapy. "Yes, I am your brother, and you're
supposed to like and appreciate me for all the things I've done to help
you." Katherine screamed at this point, "You've done nothing but try to
hurt me; you're no good; you should be dead; I could kill you with my
bare hands!" The therapist thereupon presented a soft pillow to her that
she could crush. "Here he is," the therapist said. "Here is your brother,
Larry, and you can kill him." She cringed, and with her eyes closed
huddled deep into the chair trying to get away from the approaching
brother. "Here he is, hit him if you want, kill him if you want to," but
she cringed further. "Get him away," she shouted flailing her arms
about, hitting the pillow accidently and again cringing from it. She then
pushed at it with her feet, pushing it away and crying, "Keep him away,
stay away from me, stay out of my life," her body wracked with sobs.

The therapist threw the pillow at the door so that Katherine could hear it and said, "There he's gone; he's no longer a part of your life; you can relax now," and this she immediately did. He brought her out of hypnosis, and they discussed what had occurred, with no interpretation whatsoever offered by the therapist and with no great leaps of insight made by the patient. She did feel much better, however, as a result of the catharsis experienced, and the therapist let it rest there, intending at the proper time to again provide the opportunity for her to experience these strong feelings in hypnosis with the hope that on this occasion some insights might be achieved. As of this date, April 21, 1975, five sessions following the imaginary hypnodrama, the patient was not ready to again undergo this experience, but the therapist is confident that at the appropriate time Katherine will be ready to gain some important insights into her situation and respond to these gains with positive changes in her manner of functioning in the various aspects of her life.

OTHER TRAUMAS REVISITED

Imaginary hypnodramas employed on a one-to-one therapeutic interaction basis in an office setting have occurred quickly and too frequently to list fully here, but a few will be mentioned to give some idea of traumatic experiences dealt with through this modality. They include: a twenty-five-year-old emotionally constricted electronics technician who lives a lonely and somewhat ritualistic life interacting with the father who had beaten him capriciously and maliciously when he was a child; a fifty-five-year-old self-defeating businessman—he had caused himself to be kicked out of a posh medical school as a young man and periodically overextended himself so as to come close to financial catastrophe—whose mother had caught him "playing doctor" with the neighbor girl when they were six and who told him he was dirty and would never amount to anything; a very refined sixty-eight-year-old woman whose minister-father had threatened her about the evils of sexuality and who unconsciously feared that her mother would choke her while she was an infant; a 31-year-old poised and sophisticated woman artist who often found herself the victim of others and who relived an experience when as a four-year-old she found herself "abandoned" in a hospital where she was to have her tonsils out and where she was frightened by an angry nurse; a thirty-year-old bright and personable housewife with great literary, artistic, and scientific potential, who had already made exceptional progress in hypnotherapy and who, in the imaginary hypnodramatic exploration of a dream, discovered that a principal reason she as a girl had never been able to establish a close relationship with her father was that every time this seemed about to happen her mother would intrude and do something to spoil the moment; she became so enraged on discovering this that she grabbed the pillow (the same symbol that Katherine had been afraid of) and supported by the power of her anger tore it apart. Many other instances, just as diverse as the above, could be cited to illustrate the effectiveness of the quick and simple method of imaginary hypnodrama, but it would be without point. The principal point to be made is that the insight often occurs, but even when it does not the therapeutic gains during the intense few minutes of the session are usually of great import.

25
When Psychodrama Can Slip into Hypnosis

Edward M. Scott

The present author is unaware of material reaching the literature which indicates that hypnosis is, at times, the end result or the natural consequence of psychodrama. There are reports which suggest that hypnosis does occur without conscious intent; both ·Orne (1964) and Scott (1968) mentioned this phenomenon. Although psychodrama and hypnosis have been utilized—even hypnosis in group therapy (Scott, 1966)—I was not alerted to the "connection'" between two therapeutic modalities.

Some time ago during a group therapy session, a thirty-five-year-old female alcoholic patient related guilt feelings associated with an attempt of choking one of her children fifteen years earlier. Since it seemed apparent that there was a residue after the verbalization, it was felt that a psychodramatic reenactment would be of further help. The psychodrama was set-up and at the climax—when the patient was reenacting the choking of her child—she suddenly (and naturally?) went into a state of altered consciousness in a hypnotic reaction. The term *hypnotic reaction* means a loss of the present time, an altered awareness. When the patient *came out of it* (returned to the present time), she inquired, "What happened?" adding, "Wow! That was awful." She appeared confused and a bit stunned. As a kind of confirmatory note some of the patients in the group asked, "Did you hypnotize her?" I replied that I hadn't—at least I was not aware of this intent.

In a second example, a woman patient had experienced bitter rejection by her husband and had thought of suicide (went to a bridge to jump off). As she continued to relate events of the past week, it was decided that she needed to experience acceptance and love. The patient was asked to choose a member of the group to play her mother. Following her choice of a "mother" the patient followed directions of putting her head on her "mother's" lap to experience being accepted. In a short time the patient began to cry; then suddenly started to talk in a foreign tongue—the language of her childhood! Without any attempt to hypnotize her, the psychodramatic technique alone was sufficient— carried along by her own inner mind to an altered state of awareness, to hypnosis.

Another illustration might be more convincing. I have group therapy for convicts on work release. Jim (let's call him that) was quiet during the first hour of his initial group therapy session. He was asked to tell the group about himself, and he related that he had spent eleven years in the state penitentiary for murder. As I questioned him more (although he initially resisted) he began to relate further details. He and another fellow got drunk, eventually got into a fist fight, and "I shot him." When asked if he could tell a little more, Jim said, " . . . he was my brother." I asked him to set the scene, stating that we would play act it. As the climax approached—his brother was dying from the bullet wound (I was lying on the floor as his "dying brother")—Jim leaned over and I took his hand as his brother had done. Suddenly Jim said, "What's happening? What's going on? What did you do to me?" He found himself crying, much to his surprise, since he later mentioned he had not cried about this during his eleven years in prison. He had kept a mask on. "They couldn't get me—I'm not weak," he declared. "Why am I crying? What did you do to me?" He held his head in his hands, then bolted back in his chair, stared at the ceiling, leaned forward, head in his hands, asking, "What did you do?" I replied, "I just helped you along a little." For the next half-hour, Jim alternately cried and ceased crying, much to his surprise. He related his thoughts, his fears, his feelings of anger, of disgust, and of worry. Here is an illustration of a patient who at his very first group session, without previous experience of hypnosis or without witnessing it in group and without knowing my interest in hypnosis, just let go with the help of a psychodramatic technique.

For a fourth example, I will allow a cotherapist to describe what he saw, what he felt, and what kind of interpretation we gave. At this particular time, I was conducting group therapy at the Department of Psychiatry, University of Oregon Medical School. The cotherapist, James W. Eastman, M.D., recounts it thus:

Early in the group therapy session, Art revealed that he had a hang-up about an incident that occurred during his tour of duty in Vietnam. Although he was reluctant, he was encouraged to describe the incident to the other members of the group. As he did so, he was encouraged by the group leader (yourself) to try to visualize the actual situation and to put himself into that situation. At this point, there were no other participants in the conversation except Art and you. The remainder of the group was silent.

As Art began to describe the details of the setting, he was sitting back in his chair and either looking straight ahead at nobody in particular or sitting with his eyes closed. His hands were tightly gripping the arms of the chair and he had a somewhat pained look on his face. He then went on to describe the incident in which he accidently shot and killed his best friend. As he described this, he was encouraged to reenact the situation with him playing his own role and you playing the role of the felled buddy. Although he verbally resisted doing this, he did respond to your playing the role of his friend. By this time, it was fairly obvious to this observer that he was undergoing a great deal of anxiety and seemed to be fully occupied with thoughts and feelings regarding the incident. There was no indication that he was responding to anything but reliving the situation. At the point that you in your role as the friend actually were shot and killed, Art became very agitated, making utterances of apparent anxiety and struggling to get up from his chair. Then other members of the group gathered around to hold him down and to give him physical evidence of reassurance. At this point, he was sweating heavily, crying, but making no understandable utterances.

After some several minutes of giving Art verbal and nonverbal support, we then returned to our seats and began to discuss the experience that he had gone through. What he described was the experience of being back in the situation in which the incident occurred. He also described feeling a great sense of relief for having shared his experience with the group. In general terms, I would describe his condition at the time of the reenactment of the scene as that of a trance that from my viewpoint is indistinguishable from a hypnotic trance. I say this because he seemed to be in an altered state of consciousness and because he was responsive to suggestions made by you and to his own internal cues. No matter what it is called, it was a very useful technique for Art with his particular problem. (James W. Eastman, M.D., January 21, 1971)

To conclude, what this brief chapter hopes to convey is: (1.) Psychodrama can in some cases lead into hypnosis. (2.) Psychodrama can be seen as a prelude to hypnosis (3.) In either case professional therapists should be alerted to this potential. (See, Sacerdote, 1970) (4.) Ludwig and Associates (1970) write, "In almost all brief "healing" practices, the production of an altered state of consciousness is a crucial prerequisite for therapeutic change to occur." (5.) Lastly, psychodramatists should be cognizant of this phenomenon, and as a result some understanding of hypnosis would seem appropriate in the training of a psychodramatist.

REFERENCES

1. LUDWIG, A., LEVINE, D. and STARK, S. *LSD and Alcoholism.* Springfield, Ill.: Charles C. Thomas, Publishers, 1970.
2. ORNE, MARTIN T. "A Note on the Occurrence of Hypnosis Without Conscious Intent". *International Journal of Clinical Experimental Hypnosis,* 1964, *12,* 75-77.
3. SACERDOTE, PAUL. "An Analysis of Induction Procedures in Hypnosis" *American Journal of Clinical Hypnosis,* 1970, *12,* 236-53.
4. SCOTT, E.M. "Group Therapy for Schizophrenic Alcoholics in a State Operated Out-patient Clinic: With Hypnosis as an Integrated Adjunct". *International Journal of Clinical and Experimental Hypnosis,* 1966, *14,* 232-42.
5. _____ "Hypnosis without Conscious Intent in an Alcoholic." *Quarterly Journal of Studies on Alcohol,* 1968, *29,* 709-711.

Part VI

THERAPEUTICS:
Habit Change and
Intensive Intervention

26
The Treatment of Obesity by Individual and Group Hypnosis*

Frederick W. Hanley

Obesity is a disfiguring psychosomatic disorder with many causes. Regardless of etiology, any individual patient, with his specific genetic, metabolic, and emotional make-up, gains weight because, in the last analysis, he is taking in more food than he actually needs for energy and maintenance. For the obese, overeating is not simply an occasional practice but has become a habit, a learned pattern of behavior involving longstanding attitudes to food and eating. Added to this are self-dislike generated by the disfigurement and discouragement due to the frequent failure to reverse the process of weight gain or even to control it adequately by dieting. The obese person gradually comes to build up rationalizations and other defenses about his condition but these do not resolve the underlying feelings of guilt and self-dislike, which he very often assuages by further eating. Thus the corpulent are caught in the familiar vicious circle.

The basic problem with obesity is to help the patient to learn new, more satisfactory eating habits and to have these become so firmly implanted that they will last indefinitely. It is true that in many cases eating is an emotional outlet for other problems, but psychotherapy directed solely toward these and the maturation of the personality is very

*Reprinted with permission from the author and the publisher from the *Canadian Psychiatric Association Journal* (1967), 12:549-51.

seldom successful without, in addition, direct attention to the habits themselves. The situation is similar to that of the alcoholic in whom the drinking has become a major part of the disease, causing its own repercussions and ravages to the personality. In the obese person the very acquisition of better eating habits and the loss of weight bring a feeling of encouragement and control which can lead to significant development and maturation of the personality and hence less and less need to use the primitive gratification of eating. A positive cycle is established to replace the former *impasse*.

To achieve the goal of relearning, hypnosis can be of great value as a method of communication to increase rapport, to motivate learning and to facilitate the acquisition of new eating patterns. It is not used to deprive the patient of satisfaction, i.e. to remove a symptom, but to alter the eating behavior on the basis of the patient's needs.

The first step is to define clearly the patient's goals and motivations. How much weight does the patient want to lose? What would he like to weigh and how long does he think it will require to reach his weight? Discussion of these concrete matters helps the patient to adjust to a realistic expectation and at the same time communicates the physician's understanding that he is prepared to work with him on a relatively long-term, consistent program which he expects the patient to maintain after the termination of treatment. The motivations for losing weight are brought out and explored and all positive aspects are strongly supported. The eating habits are then carefully examined to learn how the patient overeats and his lifelong as well as his present attitudes to food are looked into. At this point some tentative agreements are reached, e.g. that it would be best to eliminate eating between meals or perhaps that a mid-morning snack should replace the usual mid-day meal. Individual variations must be taken into account. In this whole process a good rapport is being established and the patient is committing himself to a definite program.

At this stage the patient is trained to enter a hypnotic trance, which usually requires only one or two sessions. Acting on the knowledge that has been gained the physician then formulates positive suggestions. The patient is told that he will derive a great deal of pleasure from eating, that he will enjoy even more the taste of his food and the satisfaction of chewing it and that when he swallows the first mouthful he will begin to feel satisfied and full. It is suggested that by the time he has eaten a very small portion of food he will feel so satisfied and full that he will have no desire to eat anything more until the time of the next meal. Increased feeling of confidence and self-esteem are suggested. He is also asked to visualize himself at the size and weight he would like to be, doing the things he cannot do now, wearing the clothes he would like to wear, enjoying additional energy and so on. As one learns more about the individual patient, one can formulate various suggestions to suit the specific case. The unconscious is reeducated so that the satisfactions of achievement come to outweigh the primitive gratifications of eating, and food loses its central place in the patient's life. Practice and repetition are essential until the new eating habits are thoroughly learned.

An important feature of the learning process which is often overlooked is the relapse and discouragement following the initial enthusiasm and accomplishment. It is at this point that the patient has often given up in the past but it is precisely at this stage in the learning process that there is a potential for basic change. The initial success is always superficial and deeper change does not occur until at least one recrudescence of the old habits. When the relapse comes it is carefully explained to the patient that this was expected and that it is part of the learning process. In fact he is congratulated on having relapsed so quickly and so well. At this juncture the patient will often bring out some of his deeper attitudes and problems and the rapport will be greatly strengthened. It is sometimes useful in the hypnosis sessions at this time to give the patient permission to fail at any time he feels he really needs to. This is not only supportive but subtly transfers the responsibility to the patient. Depending on the degree of personality problem present, a considerable amount of psychotherapy may have to be done at this time. This may be usefully combined with hypnotherapy. After passing this phase, the patient often settles down to more or less steady progress in acquiring his new eating habits, but in many cases the relapse may have to be repeated several times.

Recently the author began group treatment of six to eight females aged 21 to 44. The first forty minutes of the hour are used for group discussion, which at first centers around the problem of obesity, but later extends into areas of other personal difficulties. It has been found that this group therapy has been most valuable for the ventilation of feelings of guilt, discouragement, and hostility associated with eating and obesity. Patients express their feelings and their attitudes more freely when they find that others feel the same way. There is a great deal of mutual support and an interchange of helpful ideas. Motivation is maintained and friendly competition may develop. When a patient announces that she has lost seven pounds in the previous week, the motivation of the others is increased. On the other hand, when patients relapse others come to their support, thereby increasing their own motivation. In fact, several of the patients have worked out a procedure similar to that of Alcoholics Anonymous—if one is feeling depressed or otherwise tempted to overeat, she will call another member of the group to be "talked out of it." The group has been found to be especially useful for the withdrawn patient.

Following the group discussion, twenty or thirty minutes are spent on group hypnosis. When everyone is in a satisfactory trance state, general suggestions outlined above are given and then specific suggestions are offered to individual patients by referring to them by name and by telling other patients that they may disregard these remarks. It has been interesting to note that sometimes a specific suggestion was rejected by the patient to whom it was offered but has been picked up and used effectively by some other member of the group. The fundamental fact holds true here that patients accept those suggestions and only those suggestions which are meaningful and useful to them.

Each member of the group loses weight at her own individual rate, the average loss being around two to three lb a week. The greatest weight loss has been seventy lb in six months. Invariably, patients report that their outlook on life changes and that they find themselves improving in many ways they had not expected. This is contrasted with their previous experience in losing weight by dieting, where the effect was limited to the one specific matter of weight and there was little or no effect on other aspects of their lives. Although it is too soon yet for meaningful follow-up, most patients feel that they will be able to maintain their new weight because their attitudes to food have changed, their new eating habits are firmly established and their accomplishments and satisfactions in life preclude the necessity of using food for emotional relief. Patients with a poor prognosis are the very immature who expect hypnosis to accomplish magic with no effort on their part.

REFERENCES

1. BRODIE, EARL I.: A hypnotherapeutic approach to obesity. *Am J Clin Hypnosis,* 6: No. 3, 1964, p.211.
2. ERICKSON, MILTON H.: The utilization of patient behavior in the hypnotherapy of obesity: Three Case Reports. *Am J Clin Hypnosis,* 3:No. 2, 1960, p.112.
3. WOLLMAN, LEO: Hypnosis in weight control. *Am J Clin Hypnosis,* 4:No. 3, 1962, p.177.

27
The Use of Group Hypnosis for Weight Reduction*

F. Scott Glover

Herein are recorded my experiences with the use of group hypnosis for weight reduction. My first use of group hypnosis for weight reduction was highly successful and the results were reported in the American Journal of Clinical Hypnosis, Volume 3, No. 4, April, 1961.** Treatment of obesity by hypnosis was ordinarily on a one to one basis. However, due to a tremendous backlog of patients wanting appointments, in mid 1974, I began to employ hypnosis in groups of 3 to 5, gradually expanding to groups of 16, presently groups number up to 32 and in the near future groups will number up to 48.

Patients are seen at weekly intervals the first month, because there is an apparent attrition rate for hypnosis for weight reduction. My patients tell me they begin to notice an increase in hunger around the sixth day after a group session, therefore, it is necessary for patients to be seen more frequently the first month. Then after they have been seen about five times, if a patient so desires, the interval between visits may be extended to two weeks without an appreciable decrease in rate of weight loss. I have found, however, that few are able to go for three weeks between

*A paper presented on Oct. 19, 1975, at the 18th annual convention of the American Society of Clinical Hypnosis in Seattle, Washington, and published with the permission of the author.
**Reviewed by Perline in Chapter 5 of this volume.

visits without a marked reduction in rate of weight loss so that it is not as economical to extend the intervals between visits to three weeks. Hypnosis used for weight reduction of large groups has proved to be equally effective as hypnosis used on a one to one basis and may even be more effective because the element of competition is introduced. Additionally, when friends share the same group they tend to be mutually supporting.

The first step of the program is to establish each individual's goal for total weight loss as well as monthly weight loss based on a calorie requirement of 15 calories per pound per day for maintenance, assuming a loss of one pound per week for each 600 calories a day deficit. Patients are placed on a high protein, low fat diet. Each day carbohydrates are not to exceed forty grams and calories are not to exceed 1,000. The advantages of this diet are many. Patients will feel better and remain full longer because their stomach will still have food in it at the end of a four hour period as the stomach empties very slowly on a low carbohydrate diet. Because they are consuming less than 40 gms of carbohydrates a day, patients will develop a mild ketosis which will reduce their appetite without causing them to feel weak. Patients may substantiate their ketosis by using Ketosticks to test their urine; they will recognize it when they notice a bad taste in their mouth or bad breath. I tell them, however, this is a good thing as it indicates they are spilling out unburned energy and are losing weight rapidly. I inform them that if they eat three meals a day rather than one they will not get as hungry; they will feel better as they will maintain an average higher level of blood sugar; they will lose weight faster because they are bringing into play the specific dynamic action of protein three times as often.

I ask what knowledge the patients have of hypnosis. As a general rule they either have none or are grossly misinformed. I explain that they will not "go to sleep", they will still be aware of their senses and will be able to see, feel and hear. I assure them they will not develop any amnesia and explain that there is no dominance of one mind over another and that actually I do not hypnotize anyone, that patients hypnotize themselves and that I act as their guide or teacher helping them to attain a hypnotic state during which time they will be more receptive to suggestions regarding their attitude toward food and their environment. I explain they are going to develop a philosophy where they will not allow minor things to be stressful to them which have been so in the past and they will learn to put people, events and circumstances in proper perspective and not respond to stresses by eating and overeating.

I explain that most obesity is of two types: the childhood onset type which is generally due to a mother overfeeding her infant because she equates a fat baby with a healthy one. This results in a fat infant, a fat child and a fat adult. The second type is adult onset obesity which occurs in the female around the age twenty or twenty-one after she acquires a spouse or after she has a child. These two situations subject her to more stress than usual and she responds to it by eating and overeating. In the male, obesity occurs slightly later when he acquires a new job, wife and child with increased responsibilities and decreased physical activity. He then is subjected to more stress to which he responds by overeating. I explain that eating is an infantile response to stress. The infant is happiest and most secure when it has something in its mouth or a full stomach. When the infant grows up and is subjected to stress, instead of exercising, which is the proper response, it evokes an unrecognized memory of security which tells that person to go eat something. He does and feels more secure until he walks past a mirror and sees himself. This increases his stress so he goes back to the refrigerator for more security. The adult under stress is prepared, as was the caveman, to fight or run away when his security is threatened, but in modern society it is no longer necessary or appropriate for him to use physical force; therefore, to relieve stressful tension it is suggested that patients get a sufficient amount of exercise daily.

I emphasize the advantages of developing a philosophy where events and people are put in proper perspective and explain when patients can do this they will lose their compulsion to overeat. I ask how many can remember specifically what happened three months, or one month ago that was so important to make them so nervous and upset they had to eat something. I point out if they can't remember what happened one or two months ago, it was not important enough to justify their overeating to feel more secure. I emphasize the importance of attitude by asking how many would be willing to make a speech before a thousand people without being nervous; very few would do so. I suggest the reason they would not is because they would be afraid of making a mistake and looking or feeling ridiculous in front of others. I explain that excellent speakers frequently poke fun at themselves as it establishes an empathy with their audience which then identifies with the speaker. I point out most people are their own worst enemies, underestimating their own ability and overestimating either the difficulty or the importance of whatever it is they need or desire to do. Consequently, they do not even attempt to achieve what they are perfectly capable of accomplishing; they deprive themselves of the rewards, monetary and otherwise, they are capable of receiving. I also state categorically that I believe anyone is capable of having anything they desire; that only three elements are necessary for this: 1. they must want it, 2. they must believe they can get it, 3. they must be willing to pay the price for it, as no one in this tough world is going to give them anything except the opportunity.

I use the young man, Mark Spitz, as a perfect example of this belief. First, he wanted to be the world's greatest swimmer; second, he believed he could be; third, he paid the price. Month after month of torturing, vigorous exercise, he trained until he was physically and emotionally prepared for the Olympics. When he was awarded the seven gold medals in Munich he received the admiration and respect of the world, a million dollars in contracts, and he married the girl of his choice. He will continue to have a happy, successful life because he believes in himself and is a disciplined man.

I continue to express the importance of belief in one's self, pointing out that all great men have had one thing in common: complete confidence they could achieve their goals. Civilization has advanced because men and women did not listen when they were told it could not be done. I continually remind patients each time they come in for a group hypnosis session that good things will begin to happen to them completely unexpectedly. This is because they are going to undergo a personality change. They first came in because they did not like themselves, or if they did they would not be here. Over a period of time as they lose weight, their personality will undergo tremendous changes; they will begin to believe in themselves; they will like themselves. As they approach their goal and look at themselves in a mirror they will no longer be depressed by their image, instead they will say to themselves confidently, "Doll, you've got it made."

I also stress the importance of exercise as I have observed the obese person usually gets little if any exercise. While one cannot lose weight by exercise alone, exercise coupled with a low carbohydrate, low calorie diet has an anorexogenic effect, probably because it increases the amount of ketone bodies produced. Additionally, the person feels better, his circulation and physical condition improves, muscle mass increases with a concomitant decrease in fatty tissue, and over a period of time the extra calories burned will increase weight loss. Moreover, exercise is the proper response to stress.

I point out that it is possible for a woman to maintain an excellent figure throughout life as demonstrated by so many movie stars; however, to do so they must exercise daily.

The hypnosis session follows. The induction of hypnosis uses various techniques so as not to permit sessions to become stereotyped or boring. Suggestions for better eating habits, proper choice of food, early satiety are offered. It is also suggested the person will not permit others to tempt him off his diet. Most of the time during a hypnosis session is spent in instilling in the subject an adequate philosophy together with the expectation of a far better life as fat is lost. I try to let patients see themselves as they will be after they have completed their weight loss. I assure them they will have no difficulty in maintaining their normal weight once it is reached. The hypnosis is then terminated and a question and answer period follows. A calorie and gram counter booklet is passed out together with a diet sheet and weekly diet form. The diet is discussed with the group. I stress the importance of keeping a written account of everything consumed. Patients must write down each day what and how much they eat; they must also count both calories and grams of carbohydrates and list them on the forms provided to be returned the following visit. I want my patients to really learn calorie and carbohydrate values. I tell each one how much he or she is expected to lose the following week. It is amazing that patients usually lose more than their weekly goal. For the purpose of this paper, we took 100 consecutive patients and followed them for a two month period. Two dropped out after one visit, reason unknown.

1. The total original weight of the other
   98 patients   18,192 lbs.
   At 2 months total weight of the 98 patients   16,123 lbs.
   Total weight loss in 2 months   2,069 lbs.
   Average weight loss per person   21.11 lbs.
   Average % weight loss per person in
   2 months   11.38 %
   Most % weight loss per person in 2 months   17.18 %
   Predicted weight loss for the group was: 2,213 lbs.
   Actual weight loss for the group was: 2,069 lbs.
   (This means each person lost only 1.5 lbs.
   less than predicted in a 2 month period.)
   Maximum weight loss was 42 lbs. in 6 weeks.
2. TRIGLYCERIDES
   Original total triglyceride level of
   98 patients   17,920 mg.%
   1 month total triglyceride level of
   98 patients   8,490 mg.%
   Difference total triglyceride level
   of 98 patients   9,430 mg.%
   Original triglyceride level per person   178.78 mg.%
   1 month triglyceride level per person   86.63 mg.%
   Decline in triglycerides   92.24 mg.%
   Maximum decline in triglycerides in a person   540 mg.%
   (800 - 260 = 540)

In 2 cases there was no change in
   triglyceride level
(One was 80 and one was 50)

3. T-4

Number declined	54%
Number increased	41%
Number same	3%

4. CHOLESTEROL

Total original cholesterol of 98 patients	20,510 mg %
Total cholesterol of 98 patients 1 month	18,520 mg %
Total cholesterol of 98 patients 2 months	19,730 mg %
Total cholesterol drop in 2 months	1,990 mg %
Cholesterol drop per person in 2 months	20.31 mg %
Largest cholesterol drop in an individual	110 mg %
Average original cholesterol of 98 patients	209.20 mg %
1 month cholesterol average of 98 patients	188.98 mg %
2 month cholesterol average of 98 patients	201.32 mg %

5. BLOOD SUGAR

Original blood sugar of 98 patients - total	9,931 mg %
1 month blood sugar of 98 patients - total	10,021 mg %
Total difference increased 98 patients	90 mg %
Original average blood sugar 98 patients	101.33 mg %
Average blood sugar per person after 1 month	102.25 mg %
Average increase in 2 months per person	6.64 mg %
Largest increase blood sugar in person 1 month	40 mg %
Total blood sugar 98 patients in 2 months	105.82 mg %

Difference in original and 2 months	651 mg %
Average blood sugar per person 2 months	107.97 mg %
Note: Average number of visits in 2 mos. per person	6½

6. URIC ACID

Number increased = 66 =	67%
Number decreased = 29 =	30%
Number same = 3	

On my diet of less than 1,000 calories, high protein, low fat, and 40 grams carbohydrate, the following changes are noted in the patient's blood chemistry: (1.) A marked drop in triglycerides   (2.) T4 changes unpredictable and should be checked   (3.) There will be a drop in cholesterol even though a patient may be eating four eggs a day   (4.) Uric acid levels tend to increase, so symptoms of gout should be watched for   (5.) There will be an increase in four-hour blood sugar levels, so patients do not get as hungry or weak and no hypoglycemic reaction is noted.

Conclusion:

The use of group hypnosis for weight reduction is extremely effective and when total weight loss is achieved patients experience little difficulty in maintaining their weights at a normal level.

In the past six months, I have seen 1,243 new patients and 5,278 return weight patients. The most dramatic change was the improvement in personality and health. Further papers on this subject will be presented.

28
Post-Hypnotic Suggestion in Group Therapy: A Note*

William B. Singer

In Veterans Administration general, medical and surgical hospitals which have a neuropsychiatric service, the admission rate is high, and the average period of hospitalization is limited by consideration of bed space. In this setting there is a distinct need for abbreviated types of psychotherapy. At this hospital this need is met to some extent by an intensive program in which individual therapy, group therapy (discussion) and psychodrama are integrated so that each supplements the other. An additional technique has been developed which involves the use of hypnotherapy with the two forms of group therapy.

Hypnotherapy has been found useful at this hospital for expediting the penetration of resistance, the elicitation of significant repressed material and the integration of this dynamic material with the conscious mind. Although the efficacy of direct post-hypnotic suggestions directed toward the development of salutary changes in the patient is very transitory, it is nevertheless possible to exploit this short-term effectiveness to prepare patients for maximal participation in group forms of therapy. A number of the patients having hypnotherapy also participate in the group therapy and psychodrama programs. The following procedure is used with the patients of this group who are capable of

*Reprinted with permission. *Journal of Clinical Psychology* (April 1952), Vol. 8, No. 4, p.205

322 / Group Hypnotherapy and Hypnodrama

attaining deep or somnambulistic trance depth and can reliably execute post-hypnotic suggestions.

When certain problems which are valuable and feasible for group discussion emerge under hypnosis, the patient is given a post-hypnotic suggestion that he will discuss this problem in the next group therapy session. He is instructed that he will become acutely aware of this problem at the next group meeting, will discuss it freely and will express all of the significant feelings associated with it. He will be alert to and ready to accept any feelings and insights generated in the group discussion. When the patient subsequently discusses these problems in the group session, he receives the therapeutic benefits which are intrinsic to the group situation, such as reality testing, group acceptance, etc. In addition, his high level of motivation and emotional participation acts as a ferment or catalyst to elicit a high degree of emotional participation in the members of the group.

The same technique has been applied to prepare patients for maximal participation in psychodrama. It is suggested to the patient that before the next psychodrama meeting, he will become very interested in dramatizing a certain problem and will develop an appropriate plot. He will react to the other participants as if he is in a lifelike situation, will throw himself into his role with intense emotion, and will be keenly receptive to significant feelings and insights occurring during the performance.

29
The Use of Extended Group Hypnotherapy Sessions in Controlling Cigarette Habituation*

Milton V. Kline

A variety of approaches and methods have been employed in dealing with the problem of smoking habituation. Many individuals are capable of eliminating smoking voluntarily with little apparent difficulty and without withdrawal behavior of any significance. Others require psychological help; this type of help has ranged from educational approaches in smoking clinics to more formalized psychotherapeutic procedures, including the use of hypnosis, either as a motivational or aversive technique. Individual hypnotherapy, ranging from one to four or five sessions, has generally indicated whether this modality would be effective for a patient with this problem. Crasilneck and Hall (1968) have presented the best documented and controlled investigation of the use of hypnosis in the treatment of smoking habituation, and their statistical results generally coincide with those that have been clinically observed and reported. Follow-up studies after a period of one year indicated that 64 percent of the individuals acceptable for hypnotherapy in connection with smoking habituation were still not smoking.

On the other hand, the drop-outs, the recidivists, those who are unable to profit from any educational or therapeutic approach, have

*Reprinted with permission from the author and publisher. Originally published in *The International Journal of Clinical and Experimental Hypnosis* (1970), Vol. 18, No. 2, 270-82.

continued to constitute a significant hard-core group of smokers. For this group, smoking may frequently be not only undesirable in terms of its general implications, but also actually contraindicated in terms of presenting psysiological evidence of emergent pathological medical conditions.

The patient population described in this paper consisted of a group of individuals who had made serious attempts to stop smoking, first on their own, and then with professional help. Many had attended smoking clinics, psychotherapy sessions, and a significant number had received hypnotherapy in an attempt to deal with this problem. All had failed. The construct for this experimental therapeutic approach was an extended group hypnotherapy session, emphasizing the role of hypnosis as a desensitization technique, within a therapeutic framework consistent with the concept of cognitive dissonance (Zimbardo, 1969). Earlier observations,[1] as well as data collected in this therapeutic setting, have indicated that a reasonably large number of habitual smokers who have difficulty in giving up smoking reflect deprivation reactions on polygraphic examination characterized by irregular patterns of respiratory activity and galvanic skin responses (GSR). The general psychophysiological state of these individuals can best be described as dysphoria with noticeable irritability, depressive reactions, and signs of greatly increased stress. Laboratory studies reported by other investigators have indicated that alterations in electrocortical activity as evaluated by EEG studies and distinct changes in blood pressure accompany a state of dysphoria (Ulett & Itil, 1969).

Since Festinger's (1957) theory of cognitive dissonance emphasizes the issues of commitment, choice, and clarification as central in human decision-making, it has particular relevance to psychotherapeutic approaches dealing with habituation disturbances. As articulated by Zimbardo (1969), a state of cognitive dissonance is created when a person has the cognition that he has voluntarily chosen to commit himself to a behavior which has negative consequences in order to satisfy some immediate motive. The awareness of discomfort caused by the tension associated with a given motive is inconsistent with the knowledge that one has agreed to accept this tension, to endure more of it, and to alter or postpone behavior directed toward available goals which would reduce the drive or habit. Dissonance, thus, can be defined as a general tension state which motivates behavior, the terminal response of which results in the reduction of the level of tension. Therapeutic efforts to reduce

[1]Unpublished study entitled "Polygraphic Patterns of Deprivation Behavior in the Treatment of Smoking Habituation and Obesity," 1969.

dissonance must attempt to redefine the situation by adding new cognitions or modifying existing ones, thereby decreasing the ratio of inconsistent over consonant cognitions.

Thus, a therapeutic approach emphasizing reduction of tension, the gaining of voluntary control over tension states, and the ability to anticipate the onset of tension, is consistent with the concept of cognitive dissonance. It permits the structuring of a therapeutic approach which is both specific and, in this instance, symptomatically oriented.

All participants in the 12 hour group hypnotherapy session, beginning at 10 A.M. and terminating at 10 P.M., were required to refrain from smoking for 24 hours prior to appearing in the group. The effectiveness of hypnosis in altering the characteristics of dysphoria was noted almost immediately in a large number of participants. Polygraph recordings, taken during an initial interview prior to the group session while the participants were still smoking were compared with recordings, taken upon first entering the group situation and then again some time later, following the use of hypnosis as a prolonged relaxation and desensitizing procedure.

An Arther polygraph was utilized to record upper thoracic breathing and mid-thoracic breathing as well as GSR and blood pressure variations. For the purposes of this study, the upper thoracic respiratory tracings are presented (Figures 1 and 2). Previous studies have shown that tension states are readily recognized through breathing patterns and that the influence of hypnosis on respiratory patterning is both distinct and reliable (Kline, 1967). The tracings reported here are

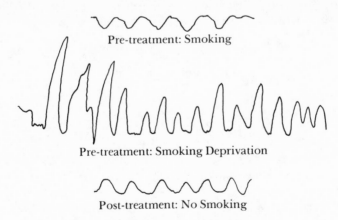

Pre-treatment: Smoking

Pre-treatment: Smoking Deprivation

Post-treatment: No Smoking

Fig. 1. Upper thoracic respiratory tracing segments typical of an individual patient's response prior to, during, and after treatment.

typical and representative of most of the patients in this treatment group. Although the recording for each patient represents approximately a 2-minute interval, in each instance the segments reported were of the same pattern consistency for as long as 15 to 20 minutes in tension states, and for as long as 40 to 50 minutes in relaxed states. Although in a therapeutic situation, subjective reports do have clinical validity, utilization of respiratory tracings gives a more objective indication of the presence of tension, regardless of verbal reports by the patient, and of the effectiveness of hypnosis in establishing relaxation and homeostasis. Showing patients their respiratory tracings recorded during tension states and during hypnotically induced relaxation states has also proven valuable as a feedback device.

During the 12-hour period, patients were required to have visual, tactile, and olfactory contact with cigarettes of their own choosing, but no oral involvement. Periods of hypnosis were used to intensify the need to smoke, and these were followed by relaxation and hypnotically induced sensory gratification of a tactile, oral, and olfactory nature.

While in the group situation hypnotic desensitization might be directed in a rotational manner toward one member of the group at a time, our findings indicate that the effects rapidly become somewhat generalized and are often transmitted to the others. Some members of the group also observed that although they had experienced hypnosis previously (usually with minimal response to induction and certainly with minimal response to alterations in their smoking behavior), the hypnotic experience within the group significantly potentiated their own involvement in hypnosis and the degree to which they could experience a reduction in smoking deprivation behavior.

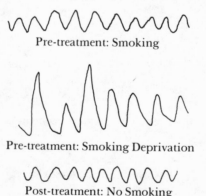

Pre-treatment: Smoking

Pre-treatment: Smoking Deprivation

Post-treatment: No Smoking

Fig. 2. Upper thoracic respiratory tracing segments typical of an individual patient's response prior to, during, and after treatment.

The rationale for both the intensification of tension associated with deprivation and the capability of reducing this tension, initially through therapeutic approaches and eventually through self-hypnosis, is consistent with the concept of desensitization. Desensitization permits the individual to experience, within a therapeutic framework, variables in his own behavior which are discomforting. This process allows for an increasing reduction in discomfort and an allaying of the anxiety associated with its uncontrollable characteristics. Although the concept of reciprocal inhibition may be applied in this context in a broader approach, the use of a desensitizing hypnotherapeutic approach enables the patient to gain a sense of self-mastery in being able to anticipate tension states without the anxiety that is associated with an uncontrollable experience, and to acquire a readiness to manage his own tension in an effective and readily available manner. Within this framework, the earlier emphasis on the ability to create and maintain a state of psychophysiological homeostasis had been reflective and indicative of positive and lasting therapeutic gains with the use of hypnotherapy (Kline, 1969).

Six extended group hypnotherapy sessions, with a total of 60 patients, were included in this study. At the end of one year, 88% of those involved had not resumed smoking (Table 1). The results from this study reflect the meaningfulness of a therapeutic approach within which hypnosis becomes an effective modality for maintaining psychophysiological homeostasis, and for producing marked diminution in dysphoria and in the psychophysiological instability associated with deprivation behavior (Kline, 1968; Kline, Wick & Sigman, in press). Further work with this approach would certainly seem to be indicated, and the possibility of developing a means of controlling smoking habituation more rapidly and effectively is strongly suggested.

TABLE I

One Year Follow-Up of Smokers Treated by a 12-Hour Group Hypno-Therapy Process

	Male	Female	Percentage of Group
Smoking Controlled............................	43	10	88
Continued Smoking..........................	7	0	12

TREATMENT PROCEDURE

Each hypnotherapy group consisted of a maximum of 10 individuals previously referred for the use of hypnotherapy in connection with eliminating smoking habituation. In the entire series of patients reported on in this study, 15 had made previous attempts to stop smoking by attending smoking clinics, utilizing adjunctive techniques such as Nikoban, and, in 12 instances, undergoing hypnotherapy. None of these techniques had proven effective and, in all instances, attempts to eliminate smoking through self-effort had been undertaken.

Each patient was seen for a brief initial interview of 30 minutes. During discussion with the patient, an assessment of motivating factors for eliminating smoking was made. Hypnotic productivity was evaluated clinically (Kline, Wick, & Coleman, in press), and a polygraph record of respiration and GSR patterns was obtained. A brief orientation was given to each patient, describing the nature of the treatment process: A group of 10 patients would meet together at 10 A.M. and remain together until 10 P.M. During this time, all patients would follow the group procedure. There would be minimal amounts of food and beverages available, and the patients would be allowed to leave the group situation only to attend to matters of personal comfort.

In addition, patients were instructed that, for 24 hours before the group session, they were to eliminate all smoking. All patients agreed to this condition, and it was further understood that if they could not follow the request, they would notify the therapist, and a date for another group session would be set when they could comply with this requirement. The importance of this criterion was stressed as an essential ingredient of the therapeutic process.

Of the 60 patients seen in group settings, only one failed to meet this requirement, and she subsequently attended another group session, having met the requirement the second time. Drop-outs from group situations were balanced by available extra patients who had been seen and requested to go through the same procedure with the idea that if they could not be admitted to the current group situation, they would be able to attend the following one.

Each patient was instructed to bring an unopened pack of his favorite cigarettes. When the group assembled, the general orientation which had been presented in the initial individual sessions was amplified. The group was told that during the 12 hours they would be together, the focal topic of discussion would be the desire to eliminate smoking and the recognition of those feelings which made the elimination of smoking difficult. Each member of the group was then instructed to open his pack of cigarettes and place them on a small table near his chair. Hypnosis, which had been induced individually in the initial sessions, was again induced individually in a rotational manner, and when the entire group was in a state of hypnosis, relaxation was produced for the entire group for a period of 15 minutes. Following this period, there was no formal termination of hypnosis, but simply instructions to open the eyes. There was no indication that there would be an alteration of the hypnotic state, but the suggestion was given that increased relaxation would be available when needed. Patients were instructed to recognize the onset of tension throughout the entire course of the therapy session and to bring it to the attention of both the group and the therapist as soon as recognized. At this time additional direct use of hypnosis or self-hypnosis was used to reestablish relaxation and, at times, if indicated, to permit discussion for clarification of the nature of the tension; this discussion, in itself, would frequently have a relaxing effect without further recourse to hypnosis.

Discussion was initiated about how the group members were reacting to the period of smoking deprivation from the day before. The various expressions of this deprivation were contrasted and evaluated within the group setting. Most members indicated a strong desire to smoke, a feeling of some tension in not being able to smoke, and considerable anxiety that they would not be able to give up this habit. Deprivation behavior as experienced and expressed by the group was discussed and interpreted by the therapist. The significance of deprivation as a psychological reaction was singled out as the most important consideration in the treatment of smoking habituation.

Techniques to Intensify Smoking Deprivation

Following the period of relaxation, the group was told that it would undertake a series of procedures designed to intensify the feelings of smoking deprivation. A discussion of the various characteristics and patterns of smoking for each member of the group was undertaken in order to indicate in which context each individual experienced the strongest desire to smoke and obtained the greatest pleasure from smoking. For example, many patients indicated that they greatly enjoyed a cigarette with a cup of coffee or following eating. Others indicated they enjoyed smoking when involved in discussions with others, either on a social or business basis, and that intensive interpersonal experiences tended to make them reach for cigarettes.

An evaluation of some of the sensory factors involved in smoking gratification for the various members was presented by the therapist. Many group members liked the feel of a cigarette in their hands. They liked the sensation of holding the cigarette and frequently they held cigarettes more than they actually puffed them. Others revealed the tremendous satisfaction gained from the inhalation of smoke and the respiratory sensations that accompanied inhalation. It became clear that a variety of sensory experiences were involved for each group of smokers, with some individuals finding satisfaction closely related to sensory experiences in the throat and the respiratory apparatus, and others finding tactile and kinesthetic sensations of equal, if not greater significance.

Techniques to intensify deprivation were undertaken through the use of hypnosis. After each individual had described those characteristics which gave him the greatest pleasure, hypnosis was used to intensify the sensations of touching, holding, and inhaling, emphasizing specifically those qualities the patient himself had described as being most stimulating and satisfying. Along with this, vivid imagery of the smoking process was suggested. During this phase of therapy with each individual patient, the other members of the group were requested to pick up their cigarettes, to hold them, to smell them, but not under any conditions to place them in their mouths. They were instructed that they were free to touch, to hold, and to smell the cigarettes whenever they wished. They were also told that when they were requested to do this as part of the group process, it was mandatory that they participate in the group experience. At times, the entire group was asked to hold cigarettes, to smell them, and, along with these actions, to visualize themselves smoking through hypnotic visual imagery. At no time were they permitted to place cigarettes in their mouths.

Oral stimulation was produced in a variety of ways. The use of the tongue to lick the lips as a form of erotic stimulation was requested on a group and individual basis along with imagery of smoking. Coffee was available and was of a decaffeinated nature so that the element of caffeine, itself, would not be unduly stressed. Minimal amounts of food and other beverages were also available.

Following each intensification of smoking deprivation, hypnosis was used in a systematic manner to produce complete relaxation. Hypnotically induced gratification similar to that which had been reported following smoking was induced first by the therapist and then by each patient using self-hypnosis.

All hypnotic relaxation procedures immediately followed the intensification of deprivation behavior and visual imagery of smoking. During a typical hour, some 10 to 15 minutes would be spent in the intensification of smoking deprivation and the remaining time devoted to discussion and interpretation of these feelings along with the induction of relaxation. Approximate imagery selected and constructed by each patient was incorporated into the stress reduction phase (Kline,

1965). As part of the exposure to deprivation situations to which the patient must adapt in effective smoking control, an assistant was present who smoked cigarettes frequently. The therapist himself did not smoke.

Patients were encouraged to report their continuous subjective feelings and, in addition, certain objective evaluations and observations were made. These included periodic recordings of polygraph responses measuring respiration and GSR. Blood pressure and pulse rates were also obtained for each member of the group at various times throughout the sessions. Measurements were taken during intensification of deprivation and following periods of stress reduction and hypnotic relaxation. A room adjoining the group therapy room was equipped with a polygraph and apparatus for measuring blood pressure and pulse rate; these measurements were taken by the research assistant.

RESULTS

Initial follow-ups from all groups were on a 6-week basis, second stage follow-ups on a 10-week basis, followed by a 6-month and 1-year follow-up. At the 1-year follow-up, 88% of the treated group reported that they were still not smoking. Of the remaining patients, all but one reported a reduction in the number of cigarettes smoked, but no discontinuance.

Clinical observation during the therapeutic sessions indicated varying degrees of deprivation behavior. Some patients showed great anxiety and tension, with most displaying within a few hours, if not initially, a very marked and clinically observable state of dysphoria. This state was characterized by motor restlessness, fidgeting, generalized statements of discomfort, dissatisfaction with physical surroundings, and, sometimes, dissatisfaction with the entire therapeutic setting.

Compared with pretreatment recordings, polygraph measurements of respiratory patterns reflected significant irregularities during all periods of smoking deprivation, with a rapid return to predeprivation levels during periods of hypnotic relaxation. Self-hypnosis procedures noticeably altered respiratory irregularity for most of the patients within a few hours and, with additional experience, the amount of time required to achieve this level of relaxation became shorter for most group members.

Hypnotic relaxation was always followed by a period of hypnotic imagery involving self-activation. Patients were instructed to visualize themselves involved in physical activities which they liked, such as swimming, walking, skiing, or any other physical activity. Following the combined relaxation-activation periods, polygraph records, systolic blood pressure, and pulse rate tended to show relatively little variation from waking pretreatment levels (Kline & Linder, 1967; Maiolo, Porro, & Granone, 1969).

DISCUSSION

Follow-up studies indicate that the use of a group therapy situation of a time-extended nature in which hypnosis is used first to intensify deprivation behavior and then, within the same setting, to reduce psychophysiological manifestations of deprivation reactions (Kline, 1969; Kline, Wick, & Sigman, in press), has produced, for the group of patients studied here, significantly better results in the control of smoking than have been produced through individual hypnotherapy.

Previous studies have indicated that smoking withdrawal may affect brain functions. Hauser, Schwartz, Ross, and Bickford (1964), Lambiase and Serra (1957), and Brown (1968), as well as a recently reported study by Ulett and Itil (1969), have demonstrated that a significant increase in slow-wave EEG activity following smoking deprivation is a typical sign of decreased vigilance. This finding is consistent with the view of cigarette smoking as a complex psychosomatic phenomenon similar to other habituation disorders. These studies indicated that the electrocortical changes were in the direction of what is usually classified as EEG abnormality.

The effectiveness of hypnosis in altering the characteristics of dysphoria, reducing stress states, and, in general, controlling the behavioral concomitants of smoking deprivation, tends to be associated with the capacity of individual patients to eliminate cigarette smoking. This relationship is consistent with a concept of desensitization and homeostasis associated with the treatment of a wide range of emotional disorders and psychophysiological disturbances (Kline, 1968, 1969; Kline & Linder, 1967). The effectiveness of this form of hypnotherapy would seem to be related to the capacity to obtain relief from the discomfort of deprivation behavior. Although, as Bernstein (1969) pointed out, it is difficult to evaluate which factors in the total treatment of smoking habituation are responsible for change, this evaluation is not essentially different from the problem of determining which variables play the critical role in any type of therapeutic change, particularly when a number of different therapeutic contexts are involved. Nevertheless, the patients in this treatment group serve as rather adequate controls in view of the fact that each one had a personal history of being refractory to previous treatment for smoking habituation. The findings based upon the 1-year follow-up suggest that the treatment procedures used in a prolonged group therapy plan, within which hypnosis and the direct management of deprivation behavior are emphasized, appear to play a significant role in therapeutic outcome. Further studies of the variables involved would certainly seem to be necessary and of interest not only in the evaluation of the treatment of smoking habituation, but in the more generalized problem of evaluating the role of hypnosis in many of the more direct psychotherapies.

The specific influence of hypnosis in creating freedom from deprivation behavior and from the psychophysiological mechanisms which are associated with dysphoria is consistent with the work recently reported by Kline and Linder (1967), indicating that in the face of intensified emotional stress, particularly involving abreactive components, the hypnotic experience tends to create a state of homeostasis. The maintenance or the reinduction and reinforcement of homeostasis would seem to be essential ingredients for increasing the degree of voluntary behavior which individuals are capable of exercising in conflict situations; they constitute important factors in the therapeutic results obtained through hypnotherapy. Relaxation of the sort that is obtained within the hypnotherapeutic context would seem to be a significantly more complex phenomenon than simple muscular or skeletal relaxation (Kline, 1969; Kline & Linder, 1967).

REFERENCES

BERNSTEIN, D.A.   Modification of smoking behavior: An evaluative review.*Psychol. Bull.*, 1969, 71, 418-40.

BROWN, BARBARA B.   Some characteristic EEG differences between heavy smoker and non-smoker subjects. *Neuropsychol.*, 1968, *6*, 381-88.

CRASILNECK, J.F., & HALL, J.A. The use of hypnosis in controlling cigarette smoking. *Sth. med. J.*, 1968, *61*, 999-1002.

FESTINGER, L.   *A theory of cognitive dissonance.* Stanford, Calif.: Stanford University Press, 1957.

HAUSER, H., SCHWARTZ, B. E., ROSS, G., & BICKFORD, R.G Electroencephology. *Clin. Neurophysiol.*, 1964 *17*, 454. Cited by Judith A. Ulett and T. M. Itil, Quantitative electroencephalogram in smoking and smoking deprivation. *Science,* 1969, *164*, 969-70.

KLINE, M. V.   Hypnotherapy. In B. B. WOLMAN (Ed.), *Handbook of clinical psychology*. New York: McGraw-Hill, 1965. Pp. 1275-95.

KLINE, M. V. (Ed.)   *Psychodynamics and hypnosis: New contributions to the practice and theory of hypnotherapy.* Springfield, Ill.: Charles C Thomas, 1967.

KLINE, M. V.   Sensory hypnoanalysis. *Int. J. clin. exp. Hypnosis,* 1968, *16*, 85-100.

KLINE, M. V.   The role of desensitization and homeostasis in relation to the therapeutic gain derived from hypnotherapy. Paper read at Amer. Psychol. Ass., Washington, D.C., August 1, 1969.

KLINE, M. V.   Research in hypnotherapy: Studies in behavior organization. In N. Petrilowitsch (Ed.), *Beitrage zur Verhaltensforschung.* New York: Karger, 1970.

KLINE, M. V., & LINDER, M.   Psychodynamic factors in the experimental investigation of hypnotically induced emotions with particular reference to blood glucose measurements. *Proc. 7th European Conf. psychosom. Res.,* Rome, September, 1967.

KLINE, M. V., WICK, E., & COLEMAN, L. L. (Eds.) *The etiology, evaluation and management of obesity.* Springfield, Ill.: Charles C Thomas, in press.

KLINE, M. V., WICK, E., & SIGMAN, R. Hypnotherapy and therapeutic education in the treatment of obesity. *Psychiat. Quart.,* in press.

LAMBIASE, M., & SERRA, C. Fumo e sistema nervoso: 1-Modificazioni dell'attivita elletrica corticale da fumo. *Acta Neurol. (Napoli),* 1957, *12,* 475-93.

MAIOLO, A.T., PORRO, G.B., & GRANONE, F.   Cerebral haemodynamics and metabolism in hypnosis. *Brit. med. J.,* 1969, 1, 314.

ULETT, JUDITH A., & ITIL, T. M.   Quantitative electroencephalogram in smoking and smoking deprivation. *Science, 1969, 164,* 969-70.

ZIMBARDO, P.G.   *The cognitive control of motivation.* Glenview, Ill.: Scott, Foresman & Co., 1969.

30
Group Therapy for Schizophrenic Alcoholics in a State-operated Out-patient Clinic: With Hypnosis as an Integrated Adjunct*

Edward M. Scott

All authorities in the field of alcoholism agree there is no such entity as the alcoholic personality. Alcoholism can and does appear in a variety of personalities. It is a major mistake to group all alcoholics together simply because of their alcoholism, and hope for therapy. The variations in intelligence, inner resources, and emotional disturbances strongly indicate that these patients should be placed in therapy situations which will tap their resources and meet their basic needs.

There are some beginnings on special techniques for alcoholics in group therapy, for example Scott (1956). In addition, there is evidence which indicates the advisability of utilizing diagnostic criteria when planning group therapy for some alcoholics (Scott, 1963).

Parker, Meiller, and Andrews (1960) found that alcoholism can mask major psychiatric disorders. In their study of 70 manic-depressives, for example, 32.8% had been "considered at one time or another by relatives or physicians to be alcoholic" (p.562), while in 150 schizophrenics, 22% were thought at one time to be alcoholic. This finding in itself might not be startling or new. The implication is important: "Of the manic-depressive group who were alcoholic, not one has been

*Reprinted with permission from the author and the publisher. Originally published in *The International Journal of Clinical and Experimental Hypnosis* (1966), Vol 14, No. 2, pp. 232-42.

successful with [Alcoholics Anonymous] A.A." (p. 563), whereas, "although the schizophrenic patients usually passively and irregularly attended meetings (A.A.) held at the hospital when it was suggested to them, they did not continue to attend on their own initiative once they were no longer hospitalized" (p. 563). These authors add that the schizophrenics who "use alcohol excessively generally seemed non-responsive to therapeutic measures" (p.563).

At the Oregon Alcoholism Treatment Clinic in Portland, a schizophrenic alcoholic would be placed in a "typical" group—without benefit. The schizophrenic simply could not function in that he felt he was not understood, or assumed a passive role and would leave the group. In view of the above considerations, group therapy exclusively for schizophrenic alcoholics was begun.

In the structuring of this new group, the fundamental nature of schizophrenia, as delineated in standard texts, was accepted. Typical therapeutic techniques, orientations, and modalities were carefully considered. The work of Forer (1961), Frank (1952), Fromm-Reichmann (1950), Gendlin[1], and Slavson (1964), for example, was pursued and accepted in basic form. Yet, certain features of the schizophrenic alcoholic had to be acknowledged.

In the past three years, 24 patients (10 female, 14 male) have been referred, through the clinic staff, to this group. All have been diagnosed as schizophrenic with alcoholism. The age range of the patients was from 21 to 48 with the average age being 38. All patients were white and of at least average intelligence.

In an effort to describe the kinds (or types) of schizophrenics in the present study, the types which were not present will be indicated first. There were no catatonic, hebephrenic, or senile schizophrenics. Two paranoid schizophrenics were included. One was a male who remained in the group two months, then had to be returned to the state hospital; the other was a female, who had remained in the group one and one-half years. Presently, she is working and recently related to the group that she had an advance in her position as a secretary. This woman had tried A.A. and been in and out of state hospitals for an extended period of time.

The remaining patients could best be described under one of the following categories: (1) schizophrenic-reaction, chronic undifferentiated type, and (2) schizophrenic-reaction, schizo-affective type. The first category comprised the majority of the population (16 of the 24 patients).

[1]Gendlin, E. Client-centered developments in psychotherapy with schizophrenics. Unpublished report.

Presently the group consists of 10 members, 5 female and 5 male. Four patients have terminated participation. Two of these are women; both are working and from our observations they appear to be doing well. One has been reestablished as a registered nurse. The other self-terminated patients are males; both are successfully employed.

The "drop-outs" (11)—those who no longer attend the group and seemingly have not been helped—include the following: (a) one woman patient was returned to the state hospital, (b) one woman left this part of the country to live with relatives, (c) one woman was an avid A.A. member and could not tolerate the group, (d) three male patients were returned to the state hospital, (e) one male stated he couldn't tolerate the group (there was intense hostile transference to the therapist), and (f) four male patients have disappeared.

The group sessions were held twice a week. All patients were under medical supervision. The use of drugs was employed as with other schizophrenic patients for symptomatic treatment of anxiety, depression, etc. Additionally, the utilization of Antabuse was periodically instrumental in assisting two patients.

The first phase of group therapy was linked to the author's philosophy of attempting to portray the "good parent," namely, to be kind, understanding, and accepting. Furthermore, it was felt that a sense of humor could be crucially curative. The desideratum hoped for was the "playful father." In view of the bitter and traumatic experiences of the schizophrenic, plus the prevalence of anhedonia, the group experience was intended to be relaxed, warm, and sprinkled with humor. This attempt was occasionally misunderstood by some of the patients in the early life of the group. Once convinced, the patients themselves often "introduced," or explained, this aspect to new members. Eventually the patients "caught" this spirit. One of the patients, for example, said she was going to write a play called, *The Case of the Dangling Libido*.

Most of these patients entered group therapy with a feeling that they were still hospital patients. When they were confronted with disappointments and problems in the world, a regressive drive frequently appeared as exemplified by, "It is easier to return to the hospital, at least I'm taken care of there." Those group members who have made progress encourage the discouraged patient to fight it out, stressing that nothing is really gained by returning to the hospital.

In attempting to combat the struggle of living in the world, these patients experience a somewhat common phenomenon, that of abulia. An instance can be cited of a patient who did not get out of bed for two days "because I didn't know which shoe to put on first." Discussion in the group revealed the deeper problem, "Why should I get out of bed?"

This problem of abulia, which was so severe and constant in the beginning, is now, one year later, no longer present. The patient has been working regularly for the past six months. He needed the assistance of Antabuse, as did another male patient; although both resisted Antabuse for some time.

Another patient, this time a woman who had spent eight years in the state hospital, was initially principally concerned about her inability to find a girdle which would fit. In fact she spoke of going to Seattle (200 miles away) to find a girdle, since, she said, none in Portland fit her. Although on the verge of returning to the state hospital on several occasions, the ego-support she received from the group managed to tide her over. She began to see the girdle indecision was symbolic of the more significant problem of her fear of facing life in the world. Although a teacher, she no longer wanted to be a teacher (and most probably couldn't find employment in that field if she applied) and had to seek a new area of employment. As she became involved in this real problem, her concern about girdles disappeared. The group came to mean something real to her—a place to discharge feelings, frustrations, and anger; but also a place to seek encouragement, strength, and support. Hypnosis was an especially effective therapeutic modality. She particularly liked the hypnotic suggestions of growth, of relating to the healthy part of the self, etc. This patient has been working for five months, her first employment in 10 years.

The second phase of the therapy was an attempt to make it real—where one could say whatever he wanted, could observe, and verbalize his feelings about himself and others. But it was also a place where one eye was kept on reality; that is, of formulating some real goal in the world.

It would be pleasant to report complete success in all similar cases, but the problem of struggling with the self, the self hatred, and defeat is clearly etched out by a portion of a group therapy meeting:

Ken: I'm dying inch by inch by inch by not doing what I want to do. I get tough and work a week and have to reward myself with a drink—I don't even enjoy. Somehow I have to be rewarded for the persecution I'm going through—ordinary work—others wouldn't consider it persecution; the things I say don't make sense. I don't know how to change. My own image is getting in the way and I don't like what I see. Others don't realize it at first, what a lousy image it is.

Therapist: How are you accepting group therapy?

Ken: Better than anything, ever, but it implies an obligation that I don't want, I want to give a better image of myself, than what I am and yet at the same time, I don't. I gave up trying to mix with groups of kids at a very early age, as being worthwhile, that's important, not just being put up with.

Kris: You're trying, aren't you?

Ken: I gave up too early. I feel I have the potential I've never exploited. The spastic who is trying to walk is better than I. I hate to make an appearance on the street, whether anyone can see it or not, I can. I don't trust people, or myself either. I feel people are putting forth their best efforts and are therefore better than I. They accept their obligations, I've never done it.

Mary: Poor Ken!

Ken: Okay, so that's it! I feel sorry for myself, but I can't do anything.

Mary: You recognize it?

Ken: Intellectually, but the emotions don't match. I should have been a criminal. I'd like to pull a big bank job.

Wayne: What would you do with the money?

Ken: I'd like to go to another country and be a Robin Hood.

Ken still comes to the group and presently is facing a problem which he has avoided for 15 years—income tax evasion. He is taking Antabuse and is struggling with his problems.

All the implications of these statements and feelings cannot be explored in this paper, but it might be sufficient to indicate some of the essential problems; namely, "bad image," the comparison of the self with others, the separation of intellectual and emotional factors, the distrust, and the self hatred. Focusing on this latter element (self hatred) which is so typical of schizophrenics, attention is drawn to the present population by their unique "solution." As one patient explained, when he drinks he can, "go back and live as I was before I was bad." Yet the ensuing hopelessness which follows a drinking bout quickly merges into self hatred. Here there seems to be a combined self hatred, of the schizophrenic and the alcoholic. The third phase of the group therapy was aimed at the elimination of alcohol, working through of transference, eliminations of hatred, and finally the struggle to establish a more healthy, functioning personality.

We would disagree with Hill (1955) when he wrote, ". . . in a general way schizophrenics are not particularly interested in alcohol. It would seem that they already suffer from defective ego abilities and are afraid of alcohol because it might produce panic in them" (p. 64). This might be true of many schizophrenics, but, in our experience it is not true of all of them.

The following group dialogue suggests some of the reasons why alcohol is used by the schizophrenic-alcoholic. It is, also, interesting to observe the struggle among the group members—between a relatively new member (Pat) and the older members.

Pat: I used to hold up a glass of wine, look at it, and say, gosh, isn't that beautiful, wine is a beautiful color, isn't it? Even cheap wine! What it takes to make all this! Just like God reached up, puts His arms around all these grapes, lets the sun shine on them, fills them up with sugar, and through His magic, turns it into wine: there's a certain poetical quality about alcohol. It makes you feel so warm and comfortable and a-a-a nearly anyone appreciates comfort.

Jim: When you realize that you have to have this because you can't take life the way it is, or yourself the way you are—

Pat: What?

Jim: If you can learn to turn to the good part of yourself and a—whatever power you have, when the chips are down and a-a- turn to that.

Wayne: I was like cold macaroni—before I found alcohol—just a whole bunch of ends pulling every way. When I drink it seemed to make sense, a direction to things, and a- got rid of the turmoil.

Pat: I can't accept life—apply it to drinking people who could take it or leave it—don't really like it, not the way I do—

Wayne: A need for what alcohol does—

Pat: I'd say, as far as I'm concerned, not so bad, oh brother, I'm nearer to heaven, being half stiff! I think a person who doesn't experience that—can take it or leave it—they don't get their money's worth—might as well drink pop.

Kris: But it doesn't always do that for you, you keep searching, you don't always hit that level.

Therapist: Pat, you said you felt near to heaven, what does that mean?

Pat: Real close to God.

Therapist: Half drunk!

Pat: (laughs) You asked me—good conversations with God! For awhile I'm a bit closer to heaven and this world seems more normal.

Fran: That's the way you're supposed to feel, without the booze.

Pat: No, I don't think so; you're supposed to be miserable.

Wayne: No, maybe half the people enjoy themselves.

Pat: No, if you took a poll of people, they'd all have deep problems.

Wayne: You can't stop people on the street and ask if they're happy.

Pat: Take all the fear out of the world and the economic structure would collapse.

It is important to note a further statement by Hill (1955), "This leads to the statement of what has been obvious in all our approaches to the schizophrenic: schizophrenics, as compared with other people, are extremely serious and are interested in meaning. They are trying to find some unifying principle, trying to find some sort of peace, symmetry, or harmony in the world. Since it is not in the real world, they look for it elsewhere" (p. 67). Our contention, indicated by the above group dialogue, is that for the schizophrenic-alcoholic, alcohol does function as a unifying principle. No claim is made that alcohol serves this purpose for the schizophrenic who is not alcoholic.

The negative manner of relating to the self is universal with these patients as verbalized by one patient, "I'm not only an alcoholic, I'm also nuts."

In order to combat the above pathological dynamics, a theoretical orientation with accompanying specific therapeutic modalities has been utilized.

We have selected from psychosynthesis, founded by Assagoli[2] and expanded by Gerard[3], two principal elements. First, that the self is an inner citadel, the source of growth and strength. Second, a person is not entirely what he does, or how he behaves, even if his behavior is marked with consistent mistakes and defeats. He is a person facing some defeats, and some mistakes; he is not defeat itself and that only. He can learn to dis-identify himself from his mistakes and defeats. This orientation is most important for the present patient population. They are notorious for identifying themselves with their defeats, foolishness, drunkenness, etc. One patient definitely marked his beginning of recovery to this concept.

One possible explanation for the effectiveness of this therapeutic modality is that although the schizophrenic (as the term implies) begins his psychosis with a "split mind" eventually the patient becomes "all bad!" By "re-introducing" through the process of disidentification the good self, the patient can once again observe and experience himself, all of himself, or at least more than formerly.

Recall that in the previously quoted group dialogue Jim said, the "good part of yourself" should be sought as a source of strength. This theme of identification with the good self is reiterated constantly in the group and patients are quick to spot one of the members who starts out in a negative manner.

Two examples may serve to indicate the effectiveness of this concept. For instance, one patient (a 30-year-old, single male), while in a

[2]Assagoli, R. Dynamic psychology and psychosynthesis. Unpublished report.
[3]Gerard, R. Psychosynthesis: A psychotherapy for the whole man. Unpublished report.

schizophrenic episode, thought himself the leader of the universe, and while in this condition attempted to carry out many bizarre actions which finally were terminated by his hospitalization. Upon release from the hospital and the beginning of therapy at our clinic, he would say, "All I am is nuts and an alcoholic." Now, after two years of therapy, the relationship to himself is quite different, as indicated by, "I can, I can look at it and think, I'm better off than a lot of people. Am I such a bad guy or so terribly rotten? No." It should be added that he is regularly employed and attending college classes in the evening.

Another patient (26-year-old male) after a visit to his parent's home reported the following: "My father said, 'I see you have a guitar, you'll sell it and drink up the money, just like you always have. You're just a bum.' I remembered what you said and it helped." On previous occasions this patient had carried out serious murderous attacks against his father. He was able to say to himself that he was more than what his father had stated, that he wasn't just a no-good alcoholic.

Hypnosis was regularly employed. Abrams (1964), in a review of the literature regarding hypnosis with psychotics, concluded, "that little or no risk is involved when this method is employed by a professional person who has been trained in both therapeutic and hypnotic techniques. When used in this manner, it has been demonstrated to be a highly effective treatment modality with some psychotic patients" (p.92).

The theoretical orientation, and the applicability of Bowers (1961) hypnotic procedure with schizophrenics appeared to be especially suitable to our present task. Bowers stated that in the schizophrenic the "sense of self, his 'little me' is hidden in the depths of his body and cannot make contact with the outside world" (p.41). Hypnosis, Bowers suggests, is a method of reaching the "little me," so tightly guarded by the schizophrenic.

We have also assumed the concept following Slavson (1964) and Wexler (1952)—but especially the latter—of the destructive action of the schizophrenic's superego. The importance of attempting to counteract this pathological trend was made a major task of therapy.

This task has been attempted by coordinating the following orientation and techniques (1.) To reach the "little me," mentioned by Bowers, through hypnosis. (2.) To help the patient to overcome his tendency to evaluate himself only on the basis of his defeats and failures by employing a concept of psychosynthesis through hypnosis. (3.) To lessen the severity of the superego by incorporating the "good parent" image of the therapist through hypnosis. With these orientations, the following group hypnosis technique has been developed. In order to alleviate the deeply felt and constant anxiety, a relaxing method is first utilized. This is done by "draining" the tension out of the body with suggestions of growing comfort, relaxation, and peace. When in this condition, further (or deeper) hypnosis is employed, and then the patients are directed, or urged, to contact their healthy selves (Bowers' "little me," or Assagoli's "self") or what can also be termed a return to their original primary narcissism. The assumption is that at one time, in early childhood, the patient was trusting, autonomous, unhampered, "unappraised"—in short, healthy. But this has been hidden or so damaged that the patient feels there is nothing to build on. Hypnosis is an especially appropriate vehicle to "recapture" this aspect of the self.

Under hypnosis the patients are given suggestions to recall positive relationships, or at least events. For instance, they are asked to recall a happy incident of childhood. Frequently, the patient is surprised at being able to recapture a happy event of childhood, having felt that his entire childhood was bereft of any happiness. As regards their present existence, they are asked to see pleasure in things they have taken for granted—a smile, a flower, a bath, a sunset, etc. They are reminded of how much they share with everyone, with illustrations that the water they bathe in isn't any different from the water the President bathes in, or the food they eat tastes just as good to them as food eaten by anyone else, etc. In this manner, there is the growing awareness of sharing some fundamental pleasures with mankind. During this three-year period, none of the patients experienced any psychotic episodes due to hypnosis. At first, some were a bit fearful but a careful explanation, and the observation of others in the group under hypnosis, quickly led to all the members being hypnotized.

Forer (1961) notes that, "schizophrenics fight against the identifications which they require to function as human beings . . ." (p.193). We feel that the above method is of great help in assisting the patient to make these fundamental identifications. The process leads to more meaningful relationships as indicated in the following statement by one patient who dreamt all the group were horses and the therapist was herding them into a corral, "We were going willingly. You had a kind look on your face."

The present orientations and techniques further the therapy of experiencing which Gendlin[4] stresses, and hence, the experiencing is

[4]Gendlin, E. Client-centered developments in psychotherapy with schizophrenics. Unpublished report.

more meaningful. For example, one patient remarked, "So that's why I feel so phony?" He was experiencing a deeply felt emotion, furthered by insight, and shared with the group. The patient was referring to his feelings when he made efforts at being good—it was phony, because basically he wasn't any good (as his mother reiterated) and his efforts were therefore a farce.

This patient recalled that his mother constantly remarked, "There isn't anything I wouldn't do for you." At the age of 10, his father was sent to prison and, "My mother started to shack up with a guy. I knew what was going on. I felt like a pimp." Hypnosis was used to go back beyond this period of time, to contact his healthy self. A common practice was to give the suggestion to the group, while under hypnosis, to say "I like me." This has proved to be an effective method, since several of the patients have not only reported the therapeutic effects, but demonstrated this while in the group.

The point is, that these patients originally felt so bad, hated themselves so much, that their efforts at self love were phony. The hypnotic techniques employed have served a most useful method in breaking through.

For the past three years, group therapy for schizophrenic alcoholics has been conducted at a state-operated clinic. Specific theoretical orientations and therapeutic modalities have been utilized to assist these patients in their pathological problems. It must be stressed that this study represents a novel approach which is potentially useful. No claim is made that it represents an established method. Rather, the data seem to indicate that it is worthwhile for other therapists to explore.

REFERENCES

ABRAMS, S. The use of hypnotic techniques with psychotics. *Amer. J. Psychother.*, 1964, *18*, 79-97.

BOWERS, MARGARETTA K. Theoretical considerations in the use of hypnosis in the treatment of schizophrenia. *Int. J. clin. exp. Hypnosis*, 1961, *9*, 39-46.

FORER, B. Group psychotherapy with outpatient schizophrenics. *Int. J. Gr. Psychother.*, 1961, *11*, 188-95.

FRANK, J.D. Group psychotherapy with chronic hospitalized schizophrenics. In E.B. Brody and F.C. Redlich (Eds.) *Psychotherapy with schizophrenics.* New York: International Universities Press, 1952. Pp. 216-30.

FROMM-REICHMANN, FRIEDA. *Principles of intensive psychotherapy.* Chicago: Univer. Chicago Press, 1950.

HILL, L.B. *Psychotherapeutic intervention in schizophrenia.* Chicago: Univer. Chicago Press, 1955.

PARKER, J.B., Jr., MEILLER, R.M., & ANDREWS, G.W. Major psychiatric disorders masquerading as alcoholism. *Sth. med. J.*, 1960, *53*, 560-64.

SCOTT, E.M. A special type of group therapy and its application to alcoholics. *Quart. J. Stud. Alcohol*, 1956, *17*, 288-90.

31
Group Hypnotherapy Techniques with Drug Addicts*

Arnold M. Ludwig, William H. Lyle, Jr., and Jerome S. Miller

There is surprisingly little written on the use of group hypnosis as a treatment method. Much of the previous work in group hypnosis *per se* has been limited to the field of obstetrics (Kroger, 1953; Kroger & Schneider, 1959) and its main use in psychiatry and psychology has been as a screening procedure to gauge the susceptibility of subjects for individual hypnotic treatment or experimentation. More recently, this procedure has been employed in the treatment of alcoholism (Friend, 1957; Paley, 1952; Wallerstein, 1958), selected psychoneurotic patients (Peberdy, 1960), and chronic schizophrenics (Ilovsky, 1962).

As to the specific group hypnotic techniques employed, most reports give a sketchy, general description, and it is difficult to evaluate the therapeutic efficacy of any particular technique. Wolberg (1948), for example, mentions the importance of such general principles as guidance, reassurance, desensitization, and persuasion. Paley (1952), working with alcoholics, emphasizes the use of suggestions for (a) heightened group transference, (b) the relief of tension and to facilitate sleep, (c) pleasant fantasies associated with sobriety, (d) constructive fantasies associated with the mature acceptance of responsibilities, and (e) nega-

*Reprinted with permission from the authors and the publisher. Originally published in *The International Journal of Clinical and Experimental Hypnosis* (1964), Vol. 12, No. 2, pp. 53-65.

tive affect or anxiety associated with the idea of drinking. The use of hypnotic suggestion to enhance "therapeutic ventilation," reassurance, a greater objectivity concerning fearful experiences, and the necessity for understanding others, has likewise been mentioned (Friend, 1957; Illovsky, 1962; Peberdy, 1960).

Since there are no systematic descriptions of group hypnotherapy techniques, it is the purpose of our study to explore a number of possible techniques which might be employed in treating persons with character disorders or, more specifically, drug addict patients. Moreover, we hope to make some comments on the philosophy underlying the choice of this technique as a treatment approach.

Our impressions were gathered from three experimental hypnotherapy groups on whom various hypnotic procedures were tried. All groups had the same therapist and met once a week for one and one-half to two-hour sessions. Either one or two of the investigators served as observers for these sessions, and detailed notes and recordings were taken—the main emphasis being on the response of the group to the particular techniques employed. Group I met for six sessions, while Groups II and III met for twelve sessions each.

Two procedural questions governed the organization of these three groups: (a) Should group members be individually or collectively hypnotized? (b) Should such treatment efforts mainly be confined to patients who volunteer for group hypnotherapy?

Accordingly, we attempted to investigate these questions by organizing the groups as follows:

Group I   Six volunteer patients, each individually trained in hypnosis béforehand.

Group II   Six volunteer patients, trained in hypnosis collectively.

Group III Ten nonvolunteer patients, trained in hypnosis collectively.

In short, we soon learned that the method of hypnotic training, whether individually or as a group, had little distinguishing effect on subsequent group performance. In Group III, moreover, although the members had not volunteered for hypnotic treatment and did not do quite as well as those in the other groups, we were surprised to find as much cooperation as we did. Seven members of this group were able to achieve various depths of hypnosis, while the remaining three members, although they attended all sessions, took the treatment program lightly and were later found to be obviously faking during several of the hypnotic sessions.

All patients, regardless of their group, were encouraged to discuss and ventilate their fears or conceptions of hypnosis during the initial session and before the group induction procedure began. A short educational and supportive talk was given by the therapist on the phenomenon of hypnosis, and any of the patients' conscious misconceptions concerning hypnosis were dealt with.

During the first two sessions with Groups II and III, we attempted to train them in hypnosis by employing the method of high eye fixation while making continual suggestions for tiredness, relaxation, drowsiness, and sleep.

It was our impression that the time necessary for trance induction was shortened during the group induction procedure, compared to individual induction, and that the presence of the group enhanced suggestibility for various challenges—at least in the lighter stages of hypnosis. As a part of the induction procedure, and in an effort to deepen the level of trance, we employed various standard hypnotic challenges. Challenges of eye catalepsy, arm rigidity, jaw immobility, arm levitation, arm heaviness, leg immobility, hand rotation, and memory loss for a specific number were given during the first several sessions, and these various challenges were repeated periodically throughout the course of therapy. We refrained from employing the more difficult challenges since there seemed little practical necessity for using them. Even so, the trance level achieved by individuals varied considerably, and although a few individuals entered a profound trance state, most individuals remained in what might be clinically described as a light-medium to medium trance.

We made a special point of conducting most of the challenges and other hypnotherapeutic techniuqes while subjects kept their eyes closed in the trance state. This technique had several practical advantages. While the subjects' eyes remained shut, they were unable to tell who might have failed a particular challenge. Thus, the hypnotist became their main source for monitoring and testing reality. If the hypnotist told any number of persons that "only one of you has not yet achieved the task," (even if the whole group had failed on the particular challenge), each unsuccessful person interpreted the remark as applying solely to him and soon was under great group pressure to comply with the specific suggestion or challenge. This technique was used frequently and with great success to enhance or facilitate the responses to certain suggestions of any refractory or slowly-acting patients.

Another advantage of having the patients' eyes closed throughout most of the sessions pertained to a frequently encountered difficulty which arises in early sessions of regular group therapy. With their eyes closed, a certain amount of anonymity could be maintained, thereby relieving somewhat the patients' fear that the confidentiality of their personal emotional problems would be violated. As long as their eyes remained closed, patients were told that they would have difficulty identifying the source of the voice and that whatever another person said would be generalized and have specific meaning to each and every one of them. When responses to specific challenges or therapeutic questions were required, instead of calling the person by name, the hypnotist would designate who was to speak next by touching the person's hand.

SPECIFIC TECHNIQUES

Educational Talks

While patients were in trance, the therapist gave a number of short homilies or talks on the practical problems of drug addiction, such as how drugs fouled up their lives and those of their families and loved ones. It was explained that drug addiction mainly represented a symptom of underlying emotional problems and that taking drugs enabled them to escape from mature responsibility, boredom, tension, and depression. Inspirational talks and positive suggestions were given to enhance their sense of self-confidence, to encourage the resumption of adult responsibilities, to evaluate themselves frankly, to live up to their potentialities, to derive self-satisfaction by resisting the craving for drugs, and to discontinue their self-destructive behavior and attitudes.

Most patients were relatively unsophisticated about the virtues of self-understanding and had little tendency for introspection or for being "psychological-minded." Therefore, additional talks emphasized the importance of early, traumatic childhood experiences on later character development and problems. They were told that they all possessed a tendency to project their blame on society and other persons for their particular problems and that they shirked the task of evaluating how they themselves were responsible for their difficulties. The ultimate responsibility for their future lives, they were told, rested on their own shoulders, and if they wanted to keep off drugs and stay out of jail, the decision was theirs. They were told not to become too easily discouraged by rejection or the lack of job opportunities and to avoid the tendency to make excuses for returning to drugs. The therapist clearly pointed out the "evils" of taking that "first shot" of drugs and emphasized the need for an absolute drug-free existence.

Moreover, suggestions to increase group cohesiveness and to facilitate positive feelings toward the therapist were given. Patients were told that the common purpose of the group was to overcome the craving for drugs, to increase self-understanding, and to help each member lead a more constructive and happier life. The therapist, along with each member in the group, would be working toward these avowed ends.

Specific Anamnestic Questions

All patients were given an equal opportunity to think about and answer a number of questions designed to elicit "meaningful" material. Such questions as "What are the real reasons for your taking drugs?" "What early childhood experiences may have contributed to your present problems?" and "What major events in your life may have altered its course?" were asked. Generally, for these groups of patients, this technique seemed poor, since most patients tended to answer these questions in a detached, superficial, and unemotional manner. For example, in response to the question concerning the "real" reason for drug use, glib answers, such as "I was a victim of circumstances," were commonly encountered.

Specific Reality-Oriented Questions

Slightly better success was attained on questions designed to deal with practical problems. Subjects were required to answer such questions as, "Why I should not use drugs again," "What other alternatives besides drugs are available?" and "What must I change about myself?" These questions were asked in the hope of getting patients to do some practical thinking about themselves, and although they invested some emotion in responding to these questions, their answers proved shallow and platitudinous. For example, responses to the question concerning changing themselves included wishes for "more drive," "to resist temptation," "ambition to do something," "to find a love greater than drugs," "to change my environment," and "to help my people."

Fantasy Situations

Suggestions were given to have the patients mentally return to a time in their lives when they were leading a happy, drug-free existence. The virtues and advantages of this type of life were stressed and patients were encouraged to share their fantasies with the group. This technique, however, met with only limited success since a number of patients mentioned that they could not remember ever really being happy off drugs.

In another fantasy-type situation, patients were instructed to mentally watch a TV show in which the hero, played by them, was a drug addict who was trying to overcome his addiction. They were to see a situation in which the hero was tempted to take drugs after some type of rejection. Instead, he would overcome this craving, and this TV program would show how he achieved this. In the one group (Group II) in which this technique was tried, the results proved discouraging since the majority of patients reported that the hero of the program tried to resist but eventually succumbed to his temptation. In the instances where the hero was able to resist, this was accomplished mainly by escaping from the enticing situation.

Branding Iron

Two approaches with an imaginary branding iron were employed. In the first approach patients were told that they were tightly holding a branding iron over the fire, that they could feel the heat of the fire being transmitted up the handle, that the iron was becoming red hot and that, depending on their desire to give up drugs, they would soon be branding their brains with the words, "I must never take that first shot of drugs," which were on the branding iron. After a suitable suggestive groundwork had been laid they were told to take the iron, apply it to their forehead, feel the heat of these words being seared on their brains, and that these words would be indelibly stamped on their brains forever. If ever they should experience a craving for drugs again, these words would blaze in their brains and enhance their will power to resist drugs.

In another approach, with essentially the same technique, patients were encouraged to put their own words on the branding iron and then to brand their brains. Patients tended to choose such phrases as "I will never take that first shot," "self-love," "avoid getting depressed so that I won't take that first shot," "stay away from the old environment," "drugs and jail are married together, there's no divorce," "prove to myself that I can do what I want," "understanding," "achieve the goals I'm striving for," and "get rid of weaknesses."

The branding iron technique was used in a number of sessions and seemed to have a great deal of appeal to patients. The magical aspects of this technique seemed appropriate to their conceptions of therapy, and almost all patients, when questioned after the completion of their therapy sessions, believed that this hypnotic branding afforded them more will power to resist drugs in the future. Some patients went so far as to say that whenever the craving for drugs arose while in the hospital, the branding words would come to mind and alleviate the craving.

To reinforce the use of this technique, we had patients in the group regress to a time when their craving for drugs was at a peak, at which point they were to overcome this craving with the heightened will power which their hypnotic branding gave them.

Training in Autohypnosis for Relaxation and Sleep

Patients were trained during several sessions in how to relax or how to put themselves to sleep. Many patients, prior to the beginning of therapy, complained of tension, difficulty in relaxation, and insomnia, and this technique was highly successful in overcoming these problems. Almost all patients learned to use these autohypnotic techniques effectively and frequently.

Posthypnotic Suggestions with Positive Hallucinations

After attempting to deepen the trance level of the group, the therapist gave suggestions to the patients that they would soon be awakened, that on awakening their craving for drugs would become unbearable, that a complete "kit," along with some bags of heroin or other narcotic drugs of their choice, would be on a designated empty chair, that on seeing the drugs each person would arise from his chair, take one step forward and reach for the drugs. Just as they found themselves reaching for the drugs, they were to overcome their craving through their will power, force themselves to relax, and put themselves back to sleep through the autohypnotic techniques they had learned.

We had employed this technique with the rationale of "desensitizing" patients to the craving for the drug by training them to overcome the craving through relaxation. This technique proved effective with one or two persons in each group who displayed a great deal of conflict and anxiety in resisting the hallucinated drugs, but as an overall group technique, it was probably not too useful. The majority of patients realized that the situation was highly artificial and felt somewhat foolish as they responded to the group pressure to arise from their chairs and reach for a drug which they actually could not see. Despite the "contagion" of suggestion due to group pressures, a couple of the patients were able to completely resist arising from their chairs and reaching for the drug.

Memory Loss Training

After training patients in achieving a memory loss for a specific number (patients were to indicate success by raising their hand), the therapist progressively taught them to erase letters, nonsense syllables, and non-affect laden words from "the blackboards of their minds." When most of the members in the group were able to achieve this, they were told to erase the words "narcotic drugs," along with the associated craving, from their minds. Just as they were able to develop a specific amnesia for the numbers or words, suggestions were given that with the erasure of the words "narcotic drugs" they would develop a permanent amnesia for the craving.

Patients were also encouraged to put their own words, which were to represent their major problem, on their mental blackboards, and then to visualize themselves erasing these words and the affect associated with them from their minds forever. Commonly-selected patient words were "hate," "drugs," "incarceration," and most patients reported success in employing this technique—at least, during the time lapse of the therapy session.

The patients were also told that this particular technique could also be used by them, autohypnotically, to erase from their minds, at least once a day, all the small tensions and resentments which accumulated during the course of the day. To employ this technique effectively, patients were instructed to try to describe the cause or source of their tensions in a few words, to write these words in chalk on their mental blackboards, and then to erase these words and tensions from their minds.

It was our impression that although this technique seemed novel, simple, and practical, it was not employed by patients, perhaps with the exception of one or two persons, outside of the treatment sessions and proved to have only limited usefulness.

Interpersonal Coping Situation

In Group III, patients were instructed to mentally relive a situation with some important person in their past lives with whom they had always had difficulty coping and then to fantasy new, more constructive ways for dealing with this person. Although patients tended to picture themselves with one or the other parent, a sibling, or teacher, the most characteristic way in which they now handled the situation "constructively" was to avoid these persons. Despite the previous "educational" hypnotic talks by the therapist, the vast majority of patients could not seem to grasp the concept that interpersonal problems could be handled by sitting down and talking over differences with another person. A solution to interpersonal problems for them was simple—escape!

Homework

During one of the sessions, patients were given the posthypnotic suggestion to write a detailed account of an important incident in their lives which affected them profoundly and to hand their accounts in at the beginning of the next session. Although this technique was tried with only one group, all patients conformed to the suggestions and seemed to handle the task seriously. Several of the patients felt that this hypnotic homework assignment was valuable for them since it forced them to sit down and organize their thinking about themselves—a task in which they had little practice.

Hypnodrama

With group II we tried several techniques which met with great success. First, a particular patient was chosen and told that he had just been released from the hospital and was back home on the "streets." The other five members of the group were to be dope peddlers and former friends who were instructed to try, by whatever means possible, to get the designated person back on drugs. The peddlers were told that they could "hit below the belt," and to use all their cunning, intelligence, and knowledge of this particular person's weaknesses to convince or persuade him to take a shot of drugs.

Each member of the group was given the opportunity of changing roles after approximately 15 minutes in a particular role. The sessions soon became exceedingly lively, highly realistic, and produced a good deal of heated, meaningful interpersonal interaction. Although the selected individual tried to resist the enticements and arguments of the group of dope peddlers, their arguments at times and insights into the weaknesses of their prey were so powerful that the designated individual almost weakened and capitulated to their cajoling.

In another hypnodrama setting, individuals were selected to appear before a personnel board, consisting of the remaining members in the group, and to apply for a job. Not only was group participation enthusiastic, but the affect and insights presented were appropriate to the situation. The personnel board interviewed and reviewed the qualifications of the applicant with a penetrating thoroughness. When they suspected lying, they soon broke down the story, and when the applicant admitted his history of drug addiction, they were skeptical as to his ability to stay off drugs. Of interest was the fact (although no suggestions for the personnel board's behavior were given) that the members of the board refused to hire any "dope fiends" since they considered all addicts liars and unreliable.

In a third setting, posthypnotic suggestions were given to have a particular person, who had just come home from the hospital, be in the presence of his immediate family. The chosen person was to designate which role the other members of the group were to play, and after this was done, each person was to throw himself into the particular role and react to his "relative" accordingly. Although this setting did not prove as lively as the previous ones, the members of the family soon began leveling realistic complaints against the chosen person, mentioning all the money he had stolen from them, the number of times in the past he had disappointed them, and their doubts about his presently giving up drugs, despite his protests to the contrary.

It was our general impression that this technique seemed highly appropriate as a treatment method and that hypnosis facilitated the role-playing considerably. Our impressions seemed confirmed by the patients themselves who not only enjoyed participating in these role-playing sessions but found it very enlightening to switch roles and see themselves through the eyes of another person. Moreover, the role-playing seemed to give them a greater awareness of the great realistic pressures and problems they would face once they went back to the street or their old environment.

When the hypnodrama technique was employed on Group III it met with somewhat less success. We felt that the large size of this group, as well as the uncooperativeness of four members, were distracting influences and made realistic interaction more difficult.

Regular Nonhypnotic Discussion Sessions

In several sessions posthypnotic suggestions were given to stimulate conscious discussion of some of the material dealt with during hypnosis. These sessions proved relatively unproductive since patients not only displayed an increased tendency to direct all their remarks specifically to the hypnotist (this tendency was probably heightened by the authoritative relationship between the hypnotist and patients) but also were much more passive and uncommunicative than patients seem to be in ordinary group therapy sessions. Despite our innate therapeutic bias that patients should deal with meaningful material consciously, or at least have the opportunity for doing so, we found no advantage (nor did most patients) in combining regular group discussion sessions with group hypnotherapy. It seemed probable that the very structure of our group hypnosis sessions somehow exerted an antagonistic effect on free, conscious discussion and interaction, which represent ideal goals for any ordinary group therapy situation.

Summarizing Talks

In the last session, many of the previous autohypnotic techniques were practiced and approximately a half-hour talk, summarizing some of the material elicited in previous sessions, was given. The content of the talk emphasized the need to avoid the first shot, to learn how to handle rejection, to learn how to get "kicks" out of being a "square," to lead a productive life, and to assume adult responsibilities. Following this last group session, all subjects were interviewed individually about their impressions of the particular techniques employed and were carefully questioned on the possible therapeutic benefits.

RESULTS

Since many of the patients selected for group hypnotherapy were long-term prisoners, and the real test of possible therapeutic benefit would take place after release from the hospital, it was impossible to adequately evaluate the real benefits of this treatment approach. Furthermore, because of the geographic location of the hospital, it was extremely difficult to follow-up the progress of the few patients who had been released from the hospital. Therefore, although long-term follow-up studies are essential for any valid evaluation of the therapeutic efficacy of group hypnosis, and any other treatment method for that matter, we can presently offer only our clinical impressions, based on interviews with each patient, on the possible benefits of these procedures.

There is another difficulty which confronted us in evaluating our results. Depending on the particular goals of therapy, especially within the context of a short-term treatment program, varying results were obtained. For example, if we consider the acquisition of the ability to relax and go to sleep by means of autohypnotic techniques a worthwhile goal (which, in fact, we do), then group hypnosis proved highly successful in achieving this goal. Moreover, when patients claim that they are more at peace with themselves as a result of having gained a better understanding of themselves and others through the various hypnotic techniques, this also seems a worthwhile goal, regardless of "proving" these claims through actual follow-up studies.

As to the matter of "curing" drug addiction, or enabling the patient to lead a productive, drug-free existence after release from the hospital, we are forced to present our results as impressionistic. In listing our results (see Table I), we have attempted to group patients according to their degree of "conviction" concerning their ability to give up drugs and lead a better life after discharge. In our individual interviews we tried to test the strength of this conviction and attitude change, and in a number of instances, although patients protested marked change, our own clinical impressions did not conform to their claims. When a discrepancy arose between our impressions and the patient's claims, we erred on the side of placing them in a category which indicated less therapeutic benefit than the claims warranted.

When we look at the total results of our treatment effort, we find the familiar ratio of 1/3:1/3:1/3 of marked, moderate, and no improvement often reported in the treatment of psychiatric patients with most treatment methods. These results, therefore, would cause us to speculate whether the beneficial over-all effects of group hypnotherapy might be nonspecific and related more to the enthusiasm of our efforts than to the specific techniques employed. At present, we are uncertain of the "direct" efficacy of our treatment program.

TABLE I

Clinical Evaluations of Patients' Degree of Conviction to Give Up Drugs

	Marked	Moderate	Slight or None
Group I	3	2	1
Group II	1	3	2
Group III	3	2	5
Total	7	7	8

DISCUSSION

There were a number of technical difficulties in employing group hypnotherapeutic techniques which should be mentioned. Although trance depth seemed adequate for the execution of the particular techniques used, patients in Group I indicated that they could not achieve as deep a trance in a group setting as when they were hypnotized individually. In addition, one or two members in each group claimed that the group setting inhibited their frank responses to specific questions and felt that they would have derived more benefit from additional individual hypnotic sessions. This complaint concerning the inhibitory influence of the group, however, did not seem specific to group hypnosis since this same complaint is often made by drug addict patients who are receiving regular group therapy.

As mentioned previously, the sense of nominal anonymity which our approach engendered, along with the dependent relationship with the hypnotist, tended to diminish group interaction when the patients were not in hypnosis. They related passively to the therapist and seemed to have little regard for the opinions of their peers. The lack of group cohesiveness was marked, and even following the completion of each session, the usual behavior of patients pairing off and chatting with each other was not seen.

It was also our general impression that hypnotic techniques, especially with these particular patients, designed to uncover early traumatic material or to facilitate insight into emotional problems did not seem appropriate or particularly useful. The patients tended to respond to specific probing or anamnestic questions with rather bland, automatic, and superficial answers and did not seem to derive any apparent benefit from their answers.

For those drug addict patients with the diagnosis of sociopathy, passive-aggressive personality disorder, or inadequate personality, "insight-oriented" treatment seems to hold little meaning. Rather, they are more concerned with answers to such practical questions as how to increase their will power, how to stay on a job and assume responsibilities, how to increase their motivation to stay off drugs, how to relax, and how to overcome boredom. Introspection is not one of their virtues, and they view therapy as "getting something" from the doctor. This magical expectation for receiving some outside, authoritative direction seems to become more pronounced in a group hypnosis setting. Therefore, it appeared that the hypnotherapeutic techniques which seemed most successful in eliciting positive responses from the patients were those which seemed more "magical," more "authoritative," and oriented more toward dealing with current, practical, reality problems.

We are not prepared to compare the efficacy of these techniques to those employed in ordinary group therapy sessions with addicts (Osberg & Berliner, 1956; Thorpe & Smith, 1953), yet we believe that group hypnotherapy offers a number of advantages, especially for short-term treatment programs. Certainly, it undermines most of the destructive "griping" which seems characteristic of many group meetings with addicts and also allows members of the group to participate equally in all aspects of the treatment program. Since the direction and form of each session are under the control of the therapist, it enables the therapist to structure the sessions so that an enormous amount of material, covering a wide range of topics, can be presented and at least briefly dealt with in a relatively limited number of sessions. The nature of group hypnotherapy allows the therapist to offer a relatively standardized therapy program to groups of patients, should this be his inclination.

The group hypnotherapy structure seems to have an additional advantage in that it relieves the individual of the burden of being considered a "square" or "brown-nosing" if he participates too actively in the treatment meeting. Because of the many conscious and unconscious biases which patients have about the nature of the hypnotic relationship, the initiative for participating is taken from them since they believe that they must conform to the suggestions of the hypnotist and that this somehow relieves them of the responsibility for their actions and verbalizations.

The hypnotic group setting also seems conducive for extending the duration of the therapeutic session beyond its ordinary limits through posthypnotic suggestions, such as by giving various writing assignments or issuing instructions for practicing certain autohypnotic techniques.

There is no doubt that group hypnosis has severe limitations as a conventional type of psychotherapeutic procedure. It did not prove useful as a method for dealing with deep, insightful material, nor did it seem to encourage much meaningful introspection. However, despite the apparently superficial techniques employed, it was of interest that no patients, even those who claimed no benefit from treatment, criticized the superficial, practial orientation or expressed the need for a more probing, uncovering type of therapy. It may well be that group hypnotherapy may be a choice treatment for patients who are very dependent, alloplastic in their attitudes, possess little psychological-mindedness or tendency for productive introspection, and have an authoritative orientation toward interpersonal relationships.

Some brief comment should be made on the therapist's feelings in conducting group hypnotherapy. Usually, after a long hypnotherapy session there is often a feeling of being emotionally drained, similar to the feelings that many psychotherapists report after spending a treatment session with a very dependent, clinging or masochistically depressed person. The therapist is required to be much more active than in ordinary group therapy sessions and is also deprived of the emotional feedback and more spontaneous interaction which add an element of challenge and stimulation to most individual and group treatment sessions. After the first blush of novelty with this treatment approach wears off, the therapist must be prepared to *work* and postpone most of his therapeutic gratification until the course of treatment is complete and patients can be interviewed on the efficacy of their therapy.

In conclusion, we believe the structure of the group hypnotherapy setting to be plastic and flexible since it is capable of being molded to fit the needs of the particular patients in treatment. The sessions can be lengthened or shortened or combined with individual or ordinary group therapy, depending upon the therapeutic rationale of the therapist. The specific hypnotic techniques we have employed are far from exhaustive, and new, perhaps more effective, techniques can be designed. Although group hypnotherapy will never replace ordinary group therapy, it certainly deserves to be considered and investigated as another useful therapeutic tool in the treatment of psychiatric patients.

REFERENCES

FRIEND, M.B. Group hypnotherapy treatment. In R.S. Wallerstein (Ed.), *Hospital treatment of alcoholism.* New York: Basic Books, 1957. Pp. 77-120.

ILLOVSKY, J. Experiences with group hypnosis on schizophrenics. *J. ment. Sci.*, 1962, 108, 685-93.

KROGER, W.S. Hypnosis in obstetrics and gynecology. In J.M. Schneck (Ed.), *Hypnosis in modern medicine.* Springfield, Ill.: Charles C Thomas, 1953. Pp. 116-142.

KROGER, W.S., & SCHNEIDER, S.A. An electronic aid for hypnotic induction: A preliminary report. *Int. J. Clin. exp. Hypnosis*, 1959, 7, 93–98.

OSBERG, J.W., & BERLINER, A.K. The developmental stages in group psychotherapy with hospitalized narcotic addicts. *Int. J. group Psychother.*, 1956, 6, 436-46.

PALEY, A. Hypnotherapy in the treatment of alcoholism. *Bull. Menninger Clin.*, 1952, 16, 14-19.

PEBERDY, G.R. Hypnotic methods in group psychotherapy. *J. ment. Sci.*, 1960, 106, 1016-20.

THORPE, J.J., & SMITH, B. Phases in group development in the treatment of drug addicts. *Int. J. group Psychother.*, 1953, 3, 66-78.

WALLERSTEIN, R. Psychological factors in chronic alcoholism. *Ann. intern. Med.*, 1958, 48, 114-22.

WOLBERG, L.R. *Medical hypnosis.* Vol. I. *The principles of hypnotherapy.* New York: Grune & Stratton, 1948.

32
A Behavioral Analysis of a
Group Hypnosis Treatment Method*

Susan DeVoge

Hypnotherapeutic literature contains a number of references to the use of hypnosis in conjunction with the application of learning principles (Sachs, 1971; Dengrove, 1973; Woody, 1973). However, as Weitzenhoffer (1972) points out, most psychotherapists who use hypnotic techniques extensively in their therapy are not aware of this literature. He feels that not only do most hypnotherapists fail to integrate learning principles into their therapy in a planned systematic way, but in addition they show only an elementary knowledge of the principles and in some cases are even unaware of using them. Spanos, DeMoor, and Barber (1973) have recently presented a conceptual analysis of some of the parallels between hypnosis and behavior therapy, specifically focusing on those situations that make subjects' imaginings the pivot of therapeutic change. In their estimation, more precise delineations of these parallels are needed.

The purpose of this paper is to describe a group hypnosis treatment

*Reprinted by permission of the author, who presented this chapter as a paper at the annual convention of the American Psychological Association on August 30, 1975, in Chicago. At the time it had been accepted for publication by *The American Journal of Clinical Hypnosis* and was published in the October, 1975, issue Vol. 18, No. 2, pp. 127-131. Copyright 1975 by the American Society of Clinical Hypnosis. Reprinted with permission of *The American Journal of Clinical Hypnosis*.

method which will be illustrated by a report of its application in a clinical setting, and then to provide a behavioral analysis of the hypnotherapeutic techniques employed. The issue of hypnosis as a "state" will not be discussed in this paper. Rather, the aim is to provide a behavioral analysis of a hypnotherapy treatment method, with the hope of generating a greater awareness of, and a more systematic use of learning principles in hypnotherapy. It is not suggested that the concepts discussed here outline a system of group hypnotherapy; rather, it is believed that they constitute techniques which may be adapted to various therapeutic settings. The following description is a clinical report of the therapy procedure.

At the time this group was conducted, the author was a postdoctoral fellow at the University of North Carolina School of Medicine and a participant in the group. The therapist, Shirley Sanders, Ph.D., was primarily responsible for the development of the techniques. The behavioral analysis is entirely the responsibility of the author.

Description of the Group Hypnosis Treatment Method

Subjects involved in the therapy group were four female psychologists at the University of North Carolina School of Medicine who were interested in the clinical uses of hypnosis. The therapist was a clinical psychologist who was trained in the use of hypnotherapy. The therapy was described as a personal adjustment or growth oriented group. Weekly meetings of one hour were held for a period of six months.

The therapist began by discussing conceptions and misconceptions about hypnosis. Second, she described the treatment process itself. She explained that the group would be able to talk and to interact while under hypnosis. In addition, each person would be asked to focus on a problem area in her life while under hypnosis and to verbalize the situation to the group. Next, the therapist stated that she herself would be functioning as a group member involved in the hypnotic process. In addition, she explained that the leadership of the group, more specifically responsibility for the trance induction, would rotate as members felt comfortable taking this role. Finally, training in the use of auto-hypnosis was described as an integral part of the therapy procedure. All of the above explanations regarding the therapy process preceded the hypnotic induction.

In the initial discussion of hypnosis, as well as during the later sessions, a permissive rather than an authoritarian approach was followed, and the contribution of all members was encouraged. Barber (1964) discusses a study by Secter which suggests that this permissive approach is more effective in achieving a deep hypnotic state than one which depends more on the control of the therapist. This approach also had the additional advantage of minimizing the dependence of subjects on the therapist.

The first stage of therapy began with the therapist initiating a standard induction technique, beginning with the eyes closed and with instructions to withdraw attention from the outside world. The subjects were asked to focus on their muscles and to progressively relax them from feet to head. In addition, the clients were instructed to focus on their breathing, with the suggestion that they were breathing out tension and breathing in relaxation. These relaxation induction methods (Cheek and LeCron, 1968) were followed by deepening techniques involving counting a descent of stairs and instructions for the subjects to imagine themselves in a place where they felt safe and relaxed. Each session was conducted entirely under hypnosis with the subjects' eyes closed at all times.

Following the induction, attention was turned to the subjects' specific problem areas. Each subject was asked to focus on a situation which was a source of anxiety for her. The therapist suggested that it would be easy to vividly imagine all details of the situation as if it were actually happening. In turn, each client was asked to verbalize to the group the situation she was imagining. She was instructed to describe all details of the situation, in particular, her thoughts, fears, and responses while in the situation.

After each client's description of her visualization of the anxiety situation, the therapist remained silent for a brief period of time. Based on the description, she then began to provide contrary imagery. The therapist suggested that she was able to visualize the client interacting in a different manner. The following example illustrates the process: One client described herself as feeling very intimidated and inadequate about speaking in front of a large staff group, yet it was frequently necessary for her to do so. The contrary imagery provided by the therapist was as follows: Imagine yourself standing in front of that large group. You are feeling confident and sure of yourself because you are in control of the situation. A question arises where you don't know the answer, but you simply state that you do not know. You are not upset by this, because it is not necessary to have all the answers. You remain calm and confident, experiencing this as a challenge.

At this stage in the therapy, the client was asked to continue the fantasy and to verbalize the manner in which she imagined herself dealing with additional anxiety-producing events in the same situation. The group members were encouraged also to contribute to the fantasy by describing the subject confidently handling other threatening events. In this manner, the subject visually rehearsed more appropriate behavior in the kinds of situations she found threatening, switched off her usual negative affective response, and substituted a positive one for it. Walker and Rippingale (1973) have described a similar therapeutic procedure based on physiological evidence that affective responses can be changed readily by the appropriate instructions in hypnosis.

As the final step in the therapy process, the therapist asked the client to focus on or to create one visual image that symbolized the feelings she was having as she experienced herself as confident and in control of the problem situation. In the case of the client just discussed, the image was a red balloon which symbolized vibrancy, confidence, and extroversion for her. The therapist suggested to the subject that when she was placed in anxious situations she would be able to breathe deeply, exhale, release tension, and visualize the red balloon and further, that as she visualized it, she would experience the same feelings of confidence and control that she now felt. Other clients in the group were encouraged to add to her image in positive ways: For example, one client visualized the balloon made of heavy rubber, indicating its strength.

In every session, each client in turn presented a situation that was a problem for her and the same procedures as described above with group involvement were repeated. At the end of the first session, simple techniques of auto-hypnosis were presented (LeCron, 1964) and the therapist suggested that the clients would find it easy to recall their own specific visual cue.

During the sessions, it appeared that the use of visual imagery was easier for some clients than for others, but as the group progressed, those who originally found imagining to be difficult reported improvement after listening to descriptions of other clients' visual images. As therapy continued, the group members assumed increasing responsibility for the initial induction of the group and became progressively more involved in visualizing one anothers' problems and in building each others' visual imagery cues.

A BEHAVIORAL ANALYSIS

In the following discussion, the case will be made that the hypno-therapeutic techniques which I have just described are explicable in terms of learning principles. I am not proposing that all of the hypnotic phenomena can be directly translated into standard learning theory terms; it shall be noted, however, that unrecognized forms of learning exist. This concept is supported in a review and discussion of learning categories by Melton (1964).

The behavioral analysis of the previously described hypnotherapy method will be structured around the role of the therapist. The therapist's first task was to discuss expectancies about hypnosis and the therapy process. Part of these expectancies (that imagery would be vivid, that relaxation would be easy) were integrated into the formal induction itself. Spanos, DeMoor, and Barber (1973) have described the entire induction process simply as one of developing task motivational instructions and creating heightened responsiveness to test suggestions. There is evidence to show that behavior therapists such as Cautela (1970, 1971) are able to encourage clients to perform maximally well with similar motivational instructions: "Try to imagine everything as vividly as possible, as if you were really there [Cautela, 1970]." In other words, there is a notable similarity between task motivational instructions and the induction procedures used in the therapy group described above. The therapist's second task was the formal induction method used in the group, more specifically the focus on breathing and muscle relaxation. This induction procedure was almost identical to the behavioral relaxation instructions of Lazarus (1971).

The third task of the therapist was to elicit from the client under hypnosis a description of the problem situation and the client's thoughts and fears concerning it. This process is similar to a behavioral analysis of a problem area in learning terms (Cautela, 1968). In both cases, the therapist can assess the antecedent cognitive variables eliciting the anxiety. After the client's verbalization of her fears and maladaptive responses in the visualized situation, the therapist was silent—a response which served as an extinction procedure.

The fourth task of the therapist was to provide contrary imagery or new stimuli in behavioral terms. As the therapist described the client interacting in more adaptive ways, a positive reconditioning process (Wolpe, 1969) began which formed a more adaptive model to fill the gap of the extinguished response.

Next, the therapist asked the client to continue the fantasy and to verbalize the imagery of herself coping adequately with the situation. This "involved imagining" is very closely related to behavioral role-playing or role-rehearsal (Sarbin, 1970; Klinger, 1971; Skinner, 1953). In fact, Spanos (1971) has reported that the more subjects are involved in the process of imagining, the more they fail to indicate to themselves that the imaginings are not actual, external occurrences. At this point, the therapist commented positively on the subject's more adaptive imagery rehearsal and in this way served as a strong social reinforcer. The contribution of the group members' additional imagery of the client coping adequately with the situation enhanced the power of the social reinforcement.

The final task of the therapist was to instruct the client to focus on one visual image which symbolized the positive emotional state which had been constructed. It was suggested that focusing on this image later would recreate the same emotional feelings. In this manner, classical conditioning principles were used to pair a visual image with an emotional set. The posthypnotic suggestion in a learning framework involved the use of the visual image as a discriminative stimulus. Weitzenhoffer (1972) has noted that posthypnotic suggestions given in the course of hypnotherapy establish responses to cues which resemble learning. Posthypnotic suggestions themselves may be interpreted as techniques used for the generalization of learning from therapy to actual situations.

Two advantages of this group hypnotherapy method are easily explicable in a learning framework. First, it was observed that some clients began with better abilities to use visual imagery than others, but that over time, subjects who originally found it difficult reported an improvement in their own use of imagery. Sachs (1971) has demonstrated that hypnotic susceptibility can be increased by modeling. Sheehan (1972) has proposed that imagination and hypnotizability bear a strong, positive relation to one another. It is proposed that modeling of the use of visual imagery by the therapist and by some subjects improved the use of imagery for other group members. The second advantage of the treatment method was the rotation of leadership. In a learning framework, the sharing of leadership helped to extinguish dependence on the therapist and to reinforce assertive behavior.

Conclusions and Implications

Some common denominators between hypnosis and behavior therapy have been described by means of a behavioral analysis of a group hypnosis treatment procedure. The analysis of this treatment method has illustrated that a large number of hypnotherapeutic techniques are straightforwardly analyzable in behavioral terms. It is not proposed that hypnotic phenomena and behaviorial phenomena are identical; however, it is strongly suggested that a greater awareness of the use of learning principles by hypnotherapists would substantially increase the effectiveness of their therapy. By clarifying and specifying behavioral techniques that lead to effective change, therapists would be able to provide a more systematic use of hypnosis.

References

BARBER, T.X. Hypnotizability, suggestibility, and personality: V. A critical review of research findings. *Psychological Reports*, 1964, *4*, 299-320.

CAUTELA, J.R. Behavior therapy and the need for behavioral assessment. *Psychotherapy: Theory, Research, and Practice*, 1968, *5*, 175-79.

———— Covert reinforcement. *Behavior Therapy*, 1960, *1*, 33-50.

———— Covert extinction. *Behavior Therapy*, 1971, *2*, 192-200.

CHEEK, D., and LECRON, L. *Clinical hypnotherapy*. New York: Grune and Stratton, 1968.

DENGROVE, E. The uses of hypnosis in behavior therapy. *International Journal of Clinical and Experimental Hypnosis*, 1973, *21*, 13-17.

KLINGER, E. *Structure and functions of fantasy*. New York: Wiley, 1971.

LAZARUS, A. *Behavior therapy and beyond*. New York: McGraw Hill, 1971.

LECRON, L. *Self hypnotism*. New York: Signet, 1964.

MELTON, A.W. The taxonomy of human learning: Overview. In A.W. Melton (Ed.), *Categories of human learning*. New York: Academic Press, 1964.

SACHS, L. Construing hypnosis as modifiable behavior. In A. Jacobs & L. Sachs (Eds.), *The psychology of private events*. New York: Academic Press, 1971.

SARBIN, T.R. *Toward a theory of imagination*. Journal of Personality, 1970, *38*, 42-87.

SHEEHAN, P. Hypnosis and the manifestations of "imagination." In E. Fromm & R. Shor (Eds.), *Hypnosis*. Chicago: Aldine Atherton, 1972.

SKINNER, B.F. *Science and human behavior*. New York: Macmillan, 1953.

SPANOS, N.P. Goal-directed fantasy and the performance of hypnotic test suggestions. *Psychiatry*, 1971, *34*, 86-96.

SPANOS, N., DEMOOR, W., & BARBER, T. Hypnosis and behavior therapy: Common denominators. *American Journal of Clinical Hypnosis*, 1973, *16*, 45-64.

WALKER, W., & RIPPINGALE, C. The uses of hypnotically produced emotional responses in therapy. *Australian and New Zealand Journal of Psychiatry*, 1973, *7*, 27-31.

WOLPE, J. *The practice of behavior therapy*. New York: Pergamon Press, 1969.

WOODY, R. Clinical suggestion and systematic desensitization. *American Journal of Clinical Hypnosis*, 1973, *15*, 250-57.

33
Mutual Group Hypnosis for Creative Problem Solving*

Shirley Sanders

Creativity is indeed a multidimensional activity. In reviewing the literature, one can find any number of diverse definitions, each of which attempts to grasp the essentials of the creative act. Certainly the creative process is evident in paintings, in musical compositions, and in the choreography of a ballet. But is it not just as evident in the creation of a day dream, a fantasy, or a night dream? And certainly it is evident in the psychotherapy hour, as a patient arrives at a new level of personal understanding. To integrate all these diverse definitions I shall borrow Carl Rogers' (1959) understanding of the creative process, *i.e.*, "The mainspring of creativity appears to be man's tendency to actualize himself, to become his potentialities, whether it be to solve problems in life, in therapy, or to produce symbolic works of art." In this view, everyone has creative potential which can be elicited under the proper conditions.

Most theories of creative thinking agree on the importance of the following conditions which seem to foster creative activity:

1. Clear definition of a problem: By clearly defining the problem and investigating it from all possible vantage points it is possible to more easily find a creative solution. Indeed, clarity of definition more easily triggers clarity of solution. Wallas (1926) and Bartlett (1958) among others emphasize the importance of clarity.

2. *Setting aside Blocks and Interferences:* For creative thinking to occur, many theorists agree that a particular context is essential, *i.e.*, a situation that is non-judgmental and non-evaluative (Gordon, 1956, Rogers, 1959).

Certainly we know from everyday experience as well as from the clinical situation, that evaluation can present a threat which may cause some aspect of experience to be blocked. In the non-evaluative situation, the subject is liberated, more open to new possibilities. According to Wallach (1957) freedom that permits the "generation of possibilities is the beginning of the creative product".

3. *Brain-storming:* Brain-storming is the production of a large number of ideas or possible solutions. According to Osborn (1953), quantity leads to quality so that the more ideas produced, the more likely a novel solution will be produced. This technique permits the combining of diverse ideas.

4. *Utilizing Imagery:* Imagery is the protype for all thinking. Language itself becomes a vehicle of thought only with maturation. Thinking first occurs on a visual, kinesthetic, olfactory, tactile, auditory, and gustatory level. Thinking in pictures as an adult, then, can be considered regressive since it reflects the basic primitive unconscious ideas which are indifferent to logic, contradiction and the obvious. Nevertheless, regression can be in the service of constructive goals.

At the same time, imagery is liberating. It fosters fluidity of thinking which permits easy recombining and integration of ideas. Einstein, for example, was admittedly a poor verbal thinker; rather he described himself as a visual thinker and attributed his discoveries to thinking in images. The emergence of imagery in creative thinking is well documented (Koestler, 1964).

5. *Spontaneous Dreams:* Dreams and dream-like states permit escape from the usual ways of thinking. Dreams have their own logic which defy our usual waking logic. Dream logic permits recombination of ideas by virtue of their irrationality, particularly by the use of hidden analogies, concreteness, and reversal of causal sequences. By such unconventional combination, problems may be solved in the unlikely contradictions seen. Many artists and scientists have described solving a problem in their dreams.

6. *Utilizing imagery and metaphor to role play or try out solutions:* There is considerable literature describing the utility of role play in solving problems (Moreno, 1964, Greenberg, 1974). By combining the use of imagery and metaphor as the vehicle to carry out role play, it is

possible to more freely experiment without fear of failure. It makes possible the juggling of concepts and ideas and can amplify motivation for success, increased self-confidence, and more accurate prediction of outcome in real life situations.

7. *Validation:* Validation in real life occurs when the subject feels confident enough to put his new learning to the actual test of life.

BLOCKS AND INTERFERENCES TO CREATIVE THINKING

For convenience, I shall categorize these blocks as Emotional, Cultural, Cognitive.

Emotional blocks consist in large part of fears such as making mistakes or failure. Also fears of the new and different or fears of criticism and rejection by others are interferences.

Cultural blocks include, for example, the push for conformity that society demands. Also included is the social imperative to compete and out-do others. The conflicting dictum to be cooperative or to be like everyone else is a cultural block as is the excessive faith in reason, logic and verbal communication. Cultural expectation educates us away from creativity.

Cognitive blocks consist in large measure of rigid thinking and preconceived mind sets. One-sided thinking for example is a failure to use all the senses in observing in preference for one way of looking. Certainly these lists are not exhaustive, but they include some of the more obvious interferences of problem solving.

HYPNOSIS AS AN ENVIRONMENT
TO FACILITATE CONDITIONS
FOR CREATIVE THINKING

The hypnotic trance appears to provide an ideal atmosphere to minimize blocks and to maximize the operation of creative thinking. Bowers, 1957, described the facilitating effects of hypnosis on creativity. First, in a trance state, the subject is more able to clearly define the problem by actively focusing on it. Secondly, there is considerable clinical evidence to demonstrate that hypnosis can aid in putting aside interfering thoughts or concerns about criticism. Also in trance, the subject is able to think of a number of possible solutions at a symbolic level.

Third, hypnosis has been demonstrated to foster imagery of all types: visual, auditory, kinesthetic, olfactory, and tactile. Sheehan, 1972, had described the hypnotic enhancement of imagery. Fourth, hypnosis has frequently been used in both psychotherapy and research situations to facilitate dreams which are spontaneous in the sense that the subject himself provides the theme of dreams, or dreams which can be facilitated that are directly related to a given theme. Moss, 1967, reviews many studies.

Fifth, hypnosis through relaxation and concentration allows the subject to be less self-critical or self-conscious. Sixth, hypnosis can intensify role playing or acting out solutions in fantasy so that emotions are mobilized and the subject acts and feels as though it is actually happening (vivification of feeling). Thus, a successful experience at problem solving during hypnotic role playing can provide the necessary self-confidence and motivation for the subject to try out the newly found solution in real life.

APPLICATION

These techniques were applied in a hypnotic group aimed at fostering creative problem solving in life. I shall briefly report on two such group experiences.

The development of a method.

A growth-oriented group using the principles of hypnosis was initiated at the University of North Carolina School of Medicine. The group members were four female psychologists who were interested in the clinical use of hypnosis. Sessions were held weekly for an hour or more per week over a six month period.

The techniques included, (1) Clarification: asking each member to focus on a problem while in hypnosis and then to describe the problem to the group, using imagery, affect and metaphor to aid in the description. (2) Group brain-storming: each person in the group was asked to share her problem and to offer a possible solution so that everyone including the member with the problem offered a solution. (3) Mutual group hypnosis: everyone, including the group leader, participated in all aspects of the group while in hypnosis. After one month, leadership of the group was rotated so that each member participated as a group leader. Suggestions given by one hypnotized group member to another group member during trance is a modification of mutual hypnosis, described by Tart, 1969. Mutual hypnosis appears to have particular utility in providing social support and feedback to the member. (4) Dream: suggestions were given to have a dream about the solution after which the member rehearsed the solution in fantasy. Each member created an image which served as a cue or symbol of confidence or success in dealing with a particular problem. For example, the image of a "stop sign" signified control of anger for one group member. (5) Rehearsal of solution: the group leader initiated imagery suggestions in which the member was described as finding a solution to the problem or as coping with the problem in a successful way. Each group member contributed similar imagery descriptions of the member handling the problem. The member then was asked to describe herself in a situation whereby she was handling the problem. For example, one member felt unable to speak in front of a large group and described considerable anxiety. Each group member described an image of the member speaking calmly, fluently and clearly in front of a large group. The member then was able to visualize herself speaking comfortably in front of a group. (6) Finally, each member was encouraged to practice self hypnosis every day utilizing the techniques described above: (1) visualizing her problem, (2) experiencing imagery and dreams reflecting mastery, (3) rehearsal of solution by imagery (4) and daily practice of hypnosis. The group members looked forward to meeting and felt that the techniques fostered solutions of problems such as preparing an article for publication; completing a thesis; becoming more assertive. Because the emphasis in this group was on the development of techniques, no formal evaluation was made.

Pilot Study:

Eleven subjects from the University of North Carolina volunteered to participate in mutual group hypnosis aimed at problem solving. Since this was a preliminary pilot study the subjects comprised a variable group consisting of four men and seven women with a mean age of 31 (range 19-42); five subjects were nurses, three medical technicians and three were undergraduates. They were divided into three matched groups. Before group training was initiated all subjects were given the Welsh Figure Preference Test (1959). This instrument reflects basic personality factors correlated with creative thinking, such as openness, independence, fluidity, symbolic expression and high achievement (Welsh, 1975). After the test was administered, the subjects were asked to select a current life problem they wanted to solve but had not been able to resolve in the previous four weeks. Examples of life problems included (1) writing the data chapter of a thesis; (2) setting realistic limits on work assumed; (3) blocking on words while speaking in public. See Table 1 for complete listing.

The techniques described earlier were practiced in mutual group hypnosis for four consecutive weeks, one hour per week. Following the test session, the Welsh Figure Preference Test was readministered. Since all three groups performed in a similar manner, the scores of the three groups were pooled yielding an N of 11. The results of the Figure Preference Test demonstrated that one subject had decreased slightly in

Table 1

Life Problems Selected

1. Setting limits on work assumed.
2. Blocking on words when speaking in public.
3. Writing data chapter in thesis.
4. Confront someone more directly when angry.
5. Becoming a more consistent leader.
6. Finding direction and goals in school.
7. Finding something to be interested in.
8. Wasting time.
9. Fear of putting face in the water.
10. Irritation with co-worker.
11. Talking to professor.

the creativity measure, while 10 of 11 subjects showed an increase (See Table 2). This finding is significant according to the Sign Test, a non-parametric analysis useful in studies were there is a small N and a diverse population. In addition all subjects solved the defined problem within the four week training period.

These results suggest that creative problem solving techniques used in combination with mutual group hypnosis appear effective in helping subjects to arrive at solutions to problems they felt unable or unmotivated to resolve earlier. At the same time their performance improves on an independent measure of creativity.

The specific goals of creative problem solving are to teach the subject to "generate new possibilities in the face of a problem" and to reduce anxiety over expressing action that may not match cultural expectation. One subject learned that she could speak calmly, fluently and clearly in front of a group. Another subject learned that she could control her anger symbolically by visualizing a stop sign.

In this creative problem solving approach, within the context of mutual group hypnosis, fantasy becomes a positive, curative force providing clarification, hope, and possible solutions to heretofore unresolved problems. Frequently, fantasies have been described as unconscious often forbidden wishes (Freud, 1908) or habits (Sternbach, 1966). In the current view, fantasies can also be viewed as creative productions which the subject can use to solve problems.

Because all subjects defined their own problem and had voluntarily joined a problem-solving group, they were committed to "solving" their problems. This demand constitutes a double bind situation. Erickson

Table 2.
**Scores for the
Welsh Figure Preference Test**

Subjects	Pre	Post	Sign
1	46	58	+
2	58	64	+
3	56	59	+
4	40	64	+
5	77	78	+
6	109	116	+
7	40	44	+
8	76	79	+
9	49	80	+
10	79	86	+
11	72	71	-

Significant by the Sign Test, $P < .01$

and Rossi (1975) discussed the utility of such positive double binds in fostering change.

Needless to say, more controlled studies need to be made to determine the duration of changes over time and of the applicability of these techniques to people who have problems of a more serious nature.

REFERENCES

BARTLETT, F.C. *Thinking: An Experimental and Social Study.* New York: Basic Books, 1958.

BOWERS, K.S. and BOWERS, P.G. Hypnosis and Creativity. In E. Fromm and R. Shorr (Eds.), *Hypnosis: Research Developments and Perspectives*. Chicago: Aldine Press, 1972.

ERICKSON, M.H. and ROSSI, E.L. Varieties of the Double Bind. *American Journal of Clinical Hypnosis*, 1975, *17*, 143-157.

FREUD, S. Creative Writers and Day-dreaming. In J. Strachey (Ed.), *Standard Edition of the Complete Works of Sigmund Freud* (Vol.9). New York: Hogarth Press, 1959.

GORDON, W.T. An Operational Approach to Creativity. *Harvard Business Review*, 1955, *34*, 41-51.

GREENBERG, I.A. (Ed.), *Psychodrama: Theory and Therapy*. New York: Behavioral Publications, 1974.

KAGEN, J. Personality and the Learning Process. In J. Kagen (Ed.), *Creativity and Learning*. New York: Beacon Press, 1968.

KOESTLER, A. *The Act of Creation*. New York: Dell Publishing Company, 1964.

MORENO, J.L. *Psychodrama, Vol. I*. Beacon, N.Y.: Beacon House, Inc., 1964.

OSBORN, A.F. *Applied Imagination*. New York: Scribner, 1953.

ROGERS, C. Toward a Theory of Creativity. In H. H. Anderson (Ed.), *Creativity and its Cultivation*. New York: Harper Press, 1959, pp. 69-82.

SHEEHAN, P. Hypnosis and the Manifestations of the Imagination. In E. Fromm and R. Shorr (Eds.), *Hypnosis: Research Developments and Perspectives*. Chicago: Aldine Press, 1972.

STERNBACH, R.A. Psychosomatic Diseases. In Shean, G.D. (Ed.) *Studies in Abnormal Behavior*. Chicago: Rand McNally & Co., 1971.

TART, C. Altered States of Consciousness. New York: John Wiley and Son, 1969.

WALLACH, M.A. Creativity and the Expression of Possibilities. In J. Kagen (Ed.), *Creativity and Learning*. New York: Beacon Press, 1968.

WALLAS, G. *The Art of Thought*. New York: Harcourt, Brace & Co., 1926.

WELSH, G.S. *Preliminary Manual: The Welsh Figure Preference Test* (Research edition). Palo Alto, California: Consulting Psychologists Press, 1959.

WELSH, G.S. *Creativity and Intelligence: A Personality Approach*. University of North Carolina at Chapel Hill: Institute for Research in Social Science, 1975.

Part VII

CONCLUSION:
Appraisals and Predictions

34
Group Hypnosis:
Present Imperfect,
Future Indicative

Ira A. Greenberg

THE PRESENT

The current state of group hypnotherapy and hypnodrama, together with some of the by-products—group hypnosis for management consulting, academic achievement, and organizational analysis—is less than perfect, Yet there is much that one can be pleased with. As represented in the first six sections of this volume and among the thirty-three chapters they contain, the state of the art is such that it may be offered with confidence as a method of treatment for overeating and for such addictions as those of alcohol, narcotics, and nicotine, even though much research remains to be done to facilitate the better understanding and treatment of these problems.

Group hypnotherapy and hypnodrama have been used with some effect in the treatment of schizophrenics and even more so in the treating of neuroses that are manifested by such syndromes as depression, anxiety, hysteria, and phobia. However, these therapeutic modalities have not been used often enough to meet the clinical needs of patients who come for treatment or the continued educational needs of the medical or psychological practitioners who learn from the reported successes and failures of their colleagues in the field and from the laboratory findings of their academic colleagues. The principal problem of the present, so far as this writer sees it, is that far too little is being done in the area of hypnosis with groups while the presumed need for this among people seeking help continues to grow.

TOWARD THE FUTURE

Although the present exists in its own right, it is also the springboard to the future, and as such it contains much that may be of benefit in the years ahead. For example, this writer, who began doing group hypnosis workshops and group hypnotherapy in 1969, has in individual hypnotherapy sessions devised a way to help two men in their fifties who were suffering from high blood pressure, two women in their twenties suffering flying phobia, and several people of varied ages suffering psychosomatic or hysterical pain reactions. The method was simple. It called for the individuals while in hypnosis to use a zero-to-ten scale, with zero representing a state of perfect comfort and ten representing a state of maximum discomfort and then to learn through desensitization techniques to control the blood pressure or anxiety or discomfort and to decrease it at will while in self-hypnosis or in the waking state.

These techniques could easily be employed and taught in large groups. One researcher already has reported some success in one of these areas. He is psychologist Albert G. Forgione, Ph.D., of Tufts University, Department of Social Dentistry. Dr. Forgione informed me in 1974 that he has devised his own technique, which he was in the process of testing, of working with large groups of people suffering flying phobia, with the means of treatment being group hypnosis. In another area, O. Carl Simonton, M.D., the Fort Worth, Texas, physician who employs guided fantasy techniques to help terminal cancer patients fight and *vanquish* their once-fatal disease, has told this writer in 1975 of having used hypnosis to teach an elderly person to lower his blood pressure, also using a method of his own devising.

An additional use of group hypnosis is found in bust-development or breast-enlargment procedures, as investigated and reported on by James E. Williams, M.S. (Stimulation of Breast Growth by Hypnosis, *The Journal of Sex Research*, Vol. 10, No. 4, Nov. 1974, pp. 316–26). Williams, a counselor at the Gregg-Harrison Mental Health and Mental Retardation Center, in Longview, Texas, employed group hypnosis in his pilot project (Experimental N=3) and individual hypnosis in the formal study (Experimental N=13), with significant size increases achieved over the twelve-week period in which suggestions for breast enlargment were combined with hypnosis. Williams is continuing his work in this area for his doctoral research and is considering further use of group hypnosis. Another doctoral student, Harvey Hodge, M.A., enrolled at the California School of Professional Psychology, Los Angeles campus, also is considering employment of group hypnosis procedures for his dissertation research in the area of suggestions for female breast development in a formal training situation. Hodge, who is a staff associate of the Group Hypnosis Center for Los Angeles, founded by this writer in 1976, is to direct a program of training for breast enlargement for the Center, which also has scheduled group hypnosis programs concerned with weight control, study habits, sexual dysfunctions, and cigarette addiction, among others.

Without question, there probably is much work being done today in individual hypnotherapy and guided fantasy sessions that might effectively be employed in large group sessions. What is needed is the opportunity for these individuals doing the important work to master group hypnotherapy techniques, which actually are quite simple to do and easy to learn, so that these practitioners may spread and enlarge their therapeutic effect. Another approach is for energetic group hypnotherapists to learn the treatment approaches of the innovative physicians and psychologists and bring these methods from individual hypnotherapy sessions to the group sessions so that larger numbers of people may receive the treatment.

It is also highly likely that a review of the literature of clinical and experimental hypnosis, as published in the journals of the American Society of Clinical Hypnosis and the Society of Clinical and Experimental Hypnosis, as well as the journals of their corresponding societies abroad, would uncover treasures of treatment techniques which have been developed and employed in individual hypnotherapy sessions that might be as well employed in group hypnotherapy sessions. Such is what the present may hold in store for the future.

THE FUTURE

If the future is seen as a progression from where we are to something better, then the tools of group hypnotherapy and hypnodrama and the techniques they contain can be expected to blossom forth to bear bountiful fruits for mankind. To begin with, self-hypnosis is a method that enables individuals to help themselves in many ways, but at present only a very small number of people can avail themselves of this tool. With group hypnotherapy conducted in large numbers and on occasion on a large scale, self-hypnosis could be taught to many people easily as a by-product of the therapy. At the same time, just as there are many distinguished university professors in the nation who make available to large groups of people their learning and their unique qualities as teachers by means of educational television programs, so there are distinguished hypnotherapists—for example, psychiatrist Milton H. Erickson, M.D., of Phoenix, Arizona—who could bring their particular genius for treatment to large groups of people.

However, because of the obvious need for safeguards, the great hypnotherapists could present their offerings on closed-circuit television channels with the showings being attended by groups of patients guided by highly qualified local hypnotherapists who are present to facilitate the work of the great or nationally acclaimed therapists and to be available to help individuals deal with emerging traumatic material or other effects of this type of therapy. Naturally, and in accord with existing Federal Communications Commission regulations, hypnotic inductions would not be presented over public television but only in a limited way where the effect of a great hypnotherapist may be spread over large areas to the benefit of many groups that would experience this form of therapy with their own group hypnotherapists in attendance and closely involved.

An offshoot of group hypnotherapy is the employment of group hypnosis for the facilitation of creative problem solving, and in the future this could be done in many places by many trained group leaders. Another utilization of group hypnotherapy techniques, among the many that might be thought of or which already are in existence, is in the exploration of C. G. Jung's concept of the *collective unconscious*—or what J. L. Moreno calls the *co-unconscious*—as a means of learning more about human personality and also as a means of helping individuals in groups who are seeking treatment. This writer has made some preliminary explorations by means of the Cheek-LeCron Ideomotor Response technique and has found that a few patients and subjects have while in the hypnotic state been able to make certain diagnostic and prognostic responses in behalf of others in the group with some small degree of validity and consistency. This of course requires further study, and it may happen that other explanations for this phenomenon will emerge as a result of rigorous laboratory experimentation. But at the moment the possibilities seem interesting and additional study might prove beneficial in the examination of the concepts involved and in the possible development of a new group hypnotherapeutic treatment modality. The ideomotor response approach to studying the collective unconscious may turn out to be an extreme and unfeasible idea, but through group hypnotherapy innovations many more mundane and possibly more valid forms of treatment might be formulated, studied, and, where warranted, developed.

Group hypnotherapy may hold interesting treatment and other possibilities for the future, but this can only be determined if an increasing number of skilled group psychotherapists and skilled individual hypnotherapists learn to employ this modality and then make their findings known to others.

AUTHOR INDEX

SUBJECT INDEX

Abreaction, 75, 167, 171
Aesculapius, 3
Affect bridge, 63-64
Alcoholics Anonymous (AA), 436
Alcoholism, 18, 20, 24, 30-31,
    43-44, 84, 335-45, 381
Allen, Doris Twitchell, 249
American Journal of Clinical
    Hypnosis, 19, 29, 47, 117, 137,
    363, 371
American Medical Association, 19
American Psychological
    Association, 265, 363
American Society of Clinical
    Hypnosis, xiii, 10, 19, 131,
    313, 371, 382-83
American Society of Group
    Psychotherapy and
    Psychodrama, 290 ff.
Anaesthesia, 39
Anderson, Maurica, 248, 251
Anderson, Walt, 248-52, 271-72
Anger, temper, 18
Anima, 279

Anxiety, 49, 128-30, 213
Archetypes, 279
Assagioli, R., 285, 343
Assertive training, 120-21
Association for Humanistic
    Psychology,´8-9, 250-51, 264
    ff., 267, 292, 294
Audience, 234, 241
Audience sharing, 239, 259
Auxiliary ego, 171-72, 175, 209,
    234, 238-39
Axiodrama, 278

Barber, Theodore Xenophon, 23
Beacon Hill Sanitarium, 176
Behavior Science Education Center
    (BSEC), 8, 108, 111-12, 114
Behavioral Studies Institute (BSI),
    8, 108-9, 295
Bernheim, H., 39
Braid, James, 39
Brainstorming, 107, 372, 374
Breast enlargement, 382
Breuer, J., 39, 166

About the Editor

Ira A. Greenberg is a clinical psychologist practicing hypnotherapy in West Los Angeles and a management consultant using group hypnosis for creative problem solving. He is founder and executive director of the Psychodrama Center for Los Angeles, Inc., and co-founder of the Group Hypnosis Center for Los Angeles, a clinic for treating weight and other disorders. Dr. Greenberg heads Behavioral Studies Institute, which employs role training and psychodramatic techniques for executive and organizational development and uses group hypnosis and guided fantasy as steps beyond brainstorming to help corporations overcome obstacles, whether in product development and manufacturing or in financing and marketing. A staff and supervising psychologist at Camarillo State Hospital for six years and a part-time staff member since 1973, he continues to direct weekly televised psychodrama sessions there and has conducted twice-a-week group hypnotherapy sessions since 1969. He is on the faculty of the California School of Professional Psychology and has been elected a fellow of the American Society of Clinical Hypnosis. He received his Ph.D. from Claremont Graduate School in 1967 and a year later his book, *Psychodrama and Audience Attitude Change,* was published, followed in 1974 by *Psychodrama: Theory and Therapy.* Currently he is at work on the book, *Action Methods for Management Consulting.*

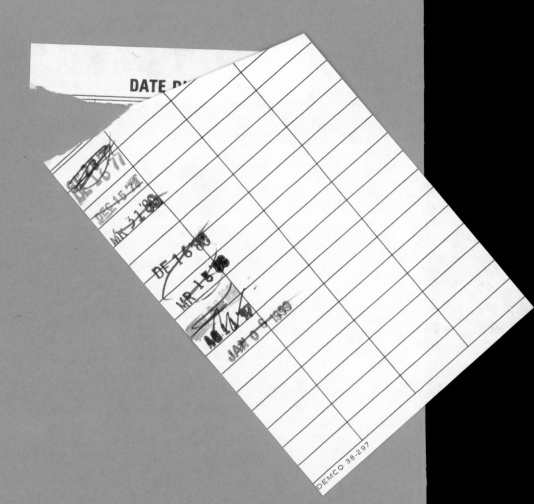

DATE DI

DEMCO 38-297